HOMEOSTASIS, NEPHROTOXICITY, AND RENAL ANOMALIES IN THE NEWBORN

DEVELOPMENTS IN NEPHROLOGY

Cheigh, J.S., Stenzel, K.H., Rubin, A.L., eds.: Manual of Clinical Nephrology of the Rogosin Kidney Center. 1981. ISBN 90-247-2397-3.

Nolph, K.D., ed.: Peritoneal Dialysis. 1981. ISBN 90-247-2477-5.

Gruskin, A.B. and Norman, M.E., eds.: Pediatric Nephrology. 1981. ISBN 90-247-2514-3.

Schück, O., ed.: Examination of the Kidney Function. 1981. ISBN 0-89838-565-2.

Strauss, J., ed.: Hypertension, Fluid-Electrolytes and Tubulopathies in Pediatric Nephrology. 1981. ISBN 90-247-2633-6.

Strauss, J., ed.: Neonatal Kidney and Fluid-Electrolytes. 1983. ISBN 0-89838-575-X.

Strauss, J., ed.: Acute Renal Disorders and Renal Emergencies. 1984. ISBN 0-89838-663-2.

Didio, L.J.A. and Motta, P.M., eds.: Basic, Clinical and Surgical Nephrology. 1985. ISBN 0-89838-698-5.

Friedman, E.A. and Peterson, C.M., eds.: Diabetic Nephropathy: Strategy for Therapy. 1985. ISBN 0-89838-735-3.

Dzurik, R., Lichardus, B. and Guder, W., eds.: Kidney Metabolism and Function. 1985. ISBN 0-89838-749-3.

Homeostasis, Nephrotoxicity, and Renal Anomalies in the Newborn

Proceedings of Pediatric Nephrology Seminar XI
held at Bal Harbour, Florida
January 29-February 2, 1984

edited by

José Strauss, MD
Division of Pediatric Nephrology
University of Miami
School of Medicine
Miami, Florida, USA

with the assistance of

Louise Strauss, MS, MA

Martinus Nijhoff Publishing
a member of the Kluwer Academic Publishers Group
Boston / Dordrecht / Lancaster

Distributors for North America:
Kluwer Academic Publishers
190 Old Derby Street
Hingham, Massachusetts 02043, USA

Distributors for the UK and Ireland:
Kluwer Academic Publishers
MTP Press Limited
Falcon House, Queen Square
Lancaster LA1 1RN, UNITED KINGDOM

Distributors for all other countries:
Kluwer Academic Publishers Group
Distribution Centre
Post Office Box 322
3300 AH Dordrecht, THE NETHERLANDS

Library of Congress Cataloging-in-Publication Data
Pediatric Nephrology Seminar (11th : 1984 :
Bal Harbour, Fla.)
Homeostasis, nephrotoxicity, and renal anomalies in the newborn.

(Developments in nephrology)
Includes indexes.
1. Pediatric nephrology—Congresses. 2. Infants (Newborn)—Diseases—Congresses. 3. Kidneys—Abnormalities—Congresses. 4. Kidneys—Diseases—Congresses. 5. Homeostasis—Congresses. I. Strauss, José. II. Strauss, Louise. III. Title. IV. Series.
[DNLM: 1. Homeostasis—in infancy & childhood—congresses. 2. Infant, Newborn, Diseases—congresses. 3. Kidney Diseases—in infancy & childhood—congresses.
W1 DE998EB / WS 320 P373 1984h]
RJ476.K5P435 1984 618.92'61 85-24576

ISBN-13: 978-1-4612-9647-8 e-ISBN-13: 978-1-4613-2637-3
DOI: 10.1007/978-1-4613-2637-3

LUCILE GOODSON MASSEY

who is who she is quietly

***

in her 80th year

of

gracing the earth

and

possibilities

***

for all

AN EXAMPLE

of

"I can" and "I will"

KNOWING THE WAY INTUITIVELY

CONTENTS

FOREWORD xi

ACKNOWLEDGEMENTS xiii

I CONTROL OF BLOOD PRESSURE AND SODIUM HOMEOSTASIS

Development of Adrenergic and Dopamine Receptors in the Kidney 3
Robin A. Felder and Pedro A. Jose

Prostaglandin-Angiotensin Interactions for Blood Pressure Regulation 11
Billy S. Arant, Jr.

Renal Handling of Sodium During Development 17
Pedro A. Jose, Robin A. Felder, Robert D. Fildes, Gilbert M. Eisner and Philip L. Calcagno

Clinical Overview of Neonatal Hypertension 23
Raymond D. Adelman

Panel Discussion 33
Jose Strauss, Moderator

II INTOXICATIONS - NEPHROTIC AGENTS

Risk Factors in Nephrotoxicity 49
Carlos A. Vaamonde

Aminoglycoside Nephrotoxicity - Clinical and Experimental Observations 87
Raymond D. Adelman

Management of Acute Renal Failure Due to Nephrotoxic Agents. Sorbent Hemoperfusion 97
Charles L. Stewart, James F. Winchester and Pedro A. Jose

Acute Dialysis and Ultrafiltration in the Newborn 107
Carolyn Abitbol, Michael Freundlich, Gaston Zilleruelo and Jose Strauss

Panel Discussion 115
Jose Strauss, Moderator

III CONGENITAL DISORDERS

Syndromes with Renal Malformations....................135
P. J. Benke, A. Feuer, R. Fojaco, J. Misiewicz and M. E. Carlin

Natural History of Congenital Anomalies of the Kidney and Urinary Tract....................147
Gaston Zilleruelo, Michael Freundlich, Carolyn Abitbol, Nuria Dominguez, Brenda Montane and Jose Strauss

Renal Tubular Acidosis....................157
James C. H. Chan and Uri Alon

New Diagnostic Imaging Procedures in Neonatal Renal Disease....................165
G. N. Sfakianakis

Panel Discussion....................169
Jose Strauss, Moderator

IV MINERAL METABOLISM

Early Neonatal Hypocalcemia....................183
Billy S. Arant, Jr.

Late Neonatal Hypocalcemia....................189
Michael Freundlich, Gaston Zilleruelo, Carolyn Abitbol and Jose Strauss

Pharmacologic Agents to Reverse Hypercalcemic and Hypocalcemic States....................199
Robert J. Geller and James C. M. Chan

Renal Hypophosphatemic Rickets....................223
James C. M. Chan and Uri Alon

Continuous Peritoneal Dialysis in Infancy with Particular Emphasis on the Neonatal Period....................235
Michael Freundlich, Carolyn Abitbol, Gaston Zilleruelo and Jose Strauss

Insufficiency and Resistance to Parathyroid Hormone....................241
Uri Alon and James C. M. Chan

Panel Discussion....................259
Jose Strauss, Moderator

V SPECIAL LECTURES

Functional Immaturity of the Newborn Kidney--Paradox or Prostaglandin? 271
Billy S. Arant, Jr.

Continuous Ambulatory Peritoneal Dialysis in Infants and Children 279
Edward C. Kohaut and Diane Appell

VI WORKSHOP

Case Presentations and Discussion 297
Jose Strauss, Moderator

PARTICIPANTS 323

AUTHOR INDEX 327

SUBJECT INDEX 329

FOREWORD

This is the 11th of the Pediatric Nephrology series created to help us be in touch with developments which are relevant to the problems we face daily in clinical practice and the questions we ask and try to answer in clinical and experimental research. Like volume IX, this one focuses on one of the subgroups to which we are committed--the neonates' special fluid and electrolyte requirements. This volume has more on blood pressure and renal function and looks at the hormonal regulators. There is greater depth about intoxications and nephrotic agents, congenital disorders and mineral metabolism. The exchanges were stimulating and the controversies were brought out without need of much of my usual prodding.

At Julie Ingelfinger's suggestion, at the end of each panel discussion I have added a comment to highlight the main points as I see them. Otherwise, the format remains as in past editions: the papers given related to the four major topic areas, each followed by panel and registrant discussion. Although the transcription is almost verbatim, you will not find the names of the discussants, purposely omitted to ease my editorial work and to encourage everyone to speak candidly. Some of the questions and answers are those submitted to the panelists after the sessions, incorporated here by request. Also, frequent references are made to others' work but their names have been omitted. Those of you who know the faculty will be able to distinguish the comments of one from the other by the content. Those of you who do not will find that knowing exactly who said what is irrelevant; the point is to grasp the ideas expressed and judge them yourself as stimuli to your own thoughts. However, if you would like to know statement sources or further details, this information is available upon request.

The guest faculty was comprised of Ray Adelman, Diane Appell, Billy Arant, James Chan, Pedro Jose, and Edward Kohaut; the local faculty was a representative cross-section of those interested in the newborn and his renal-GU disorders. It is interesting to experience the uniqueness of each year's special combination of people—faculty and registrants. As you read the papers and the resulting discussion this year, you will share in what proved to be an unusually dynamic, balanced exchange marked by insights and challenges stimulating to everyone. Many questions were asked; some were answered. Those that were not, hopefully remain as seeds in the minds of those who can help clarify the questions, find the answers, and ask new questions. If, indeed, this has been accomplished, Seminar XI and this book will have fulfilled our goals.

José Strauss

ACKNOWLEDGEMENTS

A key person for the success of Seminar XI in its planning stages and actualization was Pearl Seidler who endured even though she carried the burden of her husband Wally Seidler's tragic illness during the year and his untimely death during the seminar. Her devotion to her duties and ability to work with and through others has been an example for us to follow. Like her, all other staff members of the Division of Pediatric Nephrology cooperated to fructify this annual effort. Besides participating in the seminar, Drs. Gaston Zilleruelo, Michael Freundlich and Carolyn Abitbol took care of all administrative and clinical requirements during the seminar and the Pediatric Dialysis nurses functioned well with less than the usual resources available to them (in the sense that normally, decisions are made <u>with</u> them, not for or by them). Bonnie Ladich, as always, carried with distinction more than her share both in the office and at the seminar. Linda Lane, beautiful to see blossoming in confidence and skills, used her computer abilities to prepare much of the photo-ready copy for the book.

Also outstanding was the contribution of each faculty member who prepared camera-ready manuscripts for this volume and assumes complete responsibility for the content of his paper(s). Neither the seminar nor the book would have been possible without their keen interest and cooperation.

These are the companies whose commitment to medical education was expressed in financial support to help cover this year's seminar expenses:

Abbott Laboratories
American McGaw
Beach Pharmaceuticals
Burroughs Wellcome Company
Ciba Pharmaceutical Company
Cordis Dow Corporation
Erika
Hoechst-Roussel Pharmaceuticals, Inc.
Mead Johnson Nutrition Division
Merck, Sharp & Dohme
Ross Laboratories
Schering Corporation
Smith, Kline & French Laboratories
E. R. Squibb & Sons, Inc.
Travenol Laboratories, Inc.
Upjohn Company
William R. Rorer, Inc.
Wyeth Laboratories

Translation equipment was loaned by Ed Onorati and Dick Iacano of the Mailman Center. Translators were Dr. Zilleruelo, Dr. Freundlich and Dr. Lydia Masud. Only those who have attempted this feat can appreciate what being a translator requires.

Finally, we would like to acknowledge the role played by Children's Medical Services of the State of Florida's Department of Health and Rehabilitative Services and its director, Dr. William Ausbon. All year long they provide funds for the care of many of our patients whose problems, in turn, stimulate our educational efforts--including this seminar and book series.

Standing as a foundation for all, giving moral support and encouragement, are Dr. Bernard Fogel, Dean of the University of Miami School of Medicine and Vice President for Medical Affairs, and Dr. William Cleveland, Chairman of the Department of Pediatrics.

As the one who is doing the detail work for these volumes for the eleventh year, and without the editor's knowledge, I would like to acknowledge the role he plays as one who thinks like a man of action but acts like a man of thought* in relation to this series of seminars and books. What you see in a seminar in process and a published book is only a glimpse of what is there. In this case, seething underneath are his basic attitude of excitement over certain ideas, his vision of how these ideas might come together, his confidence in his ability to create a significant whole out of loose parts, his deep-down optimism about possibilities and willingness to creatively shift with reality, his genuine respect for others and genuine appreciation of the efforts of others. This is the Jose Strauss I know and admire--the fount from which these seminars and books evolve year after year.

*an anonymous quote from the Page a Day Wall Calendar, Workman Publishing, New York.

I

CONTROL OF BLOOD PRESSURE AND SODIUM HOMEOSTASIS

DEVELOPMENT OF ADRENERGIC AND DOPAMINE RECEPTORS IN THE KIDNEY

Robin A. Felder and Pedro A. Jose

The mechanism for the age related effects of adrenergic neurotransmitters, including dopamine, on the maturing kidney has not been fully evaluated. Since maturational changes in renal hemodynamics and sodium excretion cannot be entirely correlated with levels of renal or circulating catecholamines, changes at the receptor or postreceptor levels have to be considered.

ADRENERGIC RECEPTORS

Catecholamines can occupy specific receptors at the pre and postsynaptic sites. Presynaptic adrenergic and dopamine receptors may regulate the release of norepinephrine at the noradrenergic-neuroeffector junction (1). Occupation of presynaptic alpha adrenergic or dopamine receptors inhibits norepinephrine release while occupation of presynaptic beta adrenergic receptors enhance norepinephrine release (1, 2). Occupation of vascular postsynaptic alpha 1 and alpha 2 adrenoceptors induces vasoconstriction while postsynaptic beta 2 adrenoceptors induce vasodilatation (3). Presynaptic beta adrenoceptors are associated with vasoconstriction because of enhanced norepinephrine release while the opposite effect is associated with presynaptic alpha 2 adrenoceptors. Both postsynaptic alpha 1 and beta 1 adrenoceptors increase renin release while alpha 2 adrenoceptors decrease renin release (4). Postsynaptic dopamine 1 and presynaptic dopamine 2 receptors are both associated with arterial vasodilatation (5). Occupation of adrenal dopamine receptors by dopamine results in a decrease in aldosterone secretion (6).

Postsynaptic receptors may influence each other. Hormones such as estrogen and thyroxine, and ions such as sodium and magnesium can regulate adrenoceptor number and/or affinity (2, 7). The signal that results from the occupation of specific receptors by neurotransmitters may be amplified by certain intracellular messengers (3). Alpha 1 adrenoceptors release calcium from storage sites and are without effect on cAMP levels. Alpha 2 adrenoceptors open up calcium channels and decrease cAMP levels. Beta 1 and Beta 2 adrenoceptors as well as dopamine 1 receptors increase cAMP levels while the opposite effect may be observed following occupation of dopamine 2 receptors (4, 7, 9).

RENAL HEMODYNAMICS DURING DEVELOPMENT

Previous studies from our laboratory have indicated that

the adrenergic control of renal hemodynamics is different in the young and the adult (10-13). We have suggested that the low renal blood flow and high renal vascular resistance in the newborn are in part due to increased sensitivity of the neonatal renal vasculature to alpha adrenergic effects (1, 13). Similar conclusions have been made by Gootman et al. using the piglet model (14). In our studies, the intrarenal administration of the alpha adrenergic antagonist, phentolamine, increased renal blood flow in puppies in a dose related manner, starting at 0.5 ug/kg/min in younger puppies and 1.0 ug/kg/min in older puppies. In adult dogs no effect of phentolamine on renal blood flow was noted (13). The renal vasoconstrictor effect of epinephrine was also greater in puppies than in adult dogs (10). In addition, intrarenal epinephrine induced a redistribution of renal blood flow to the inner cortex in puppies but not in adult dogs. Norepinephrine also produced a greater vasoconstrictor effect in younger than older piglets (14). Gootman et al. also reported that renal nerve stimulation was associated with a greater reduction in renal blood flow in younger than older piglets (14). The renal vasodilatory effects of dopamine and isoproterenol, a beta adrenergic agonist, also increase with age (15, 16). Thus, the high renal vascular resistance in the newborn may be related to increased alpha adrenergic influence, and decreased dopamine and beta adrenergic influence. Studies on renal vascular adrenergic receptors during development are not yet available using radioligand binding studies.

ADRENERGIC RECEPTORS AND RENAL SODIUM TRANSPORT

Recent studies have confirmed a role of the adrenergic nervous system on renal sodium transport (17, 18). Innervation of proximal tubule, loop of Henle and distal tubule have been shown (19). Occupation of postsynaptic alpha adrenergic receptors by agonists increase sodium reabsorption while occupation of dopamine receptors by agonists decrease renal sodium transport (17, 20-22). Occupation of beta adrenergic receptors by agonists in rabbit and rat nephron increase sodium reabsorption, while they seem to mediate the opposite effect in dogs (21, 24, 25).

The alpha 1 adrenoceptor subtype has been identified as the mediator of increased renal sodium transport (26). In the kidney, however, alpha 2 adrenoceptors are more numerous than alpha 1 adrenoceptors (27). Although Osborn et al. have reported that the antinatriuresis during 1 Hz renal nerve stimulation did not seem to be mediated by alpha 2 adrenoceptors, there is evidence that these receptors may mediate renal sodium reabsorption in other experimental conditions (13, 26, 28). Fildes and coworkers recently showed that the alpha 2 adrenergic antagonist, yohimbine, given directly into the renal artery of hydropenic dogs increased sodium excretion without altering renal blood flow or glomerular filtration rate (13). The addition of the alpha 1 adrenergic blocker prazosin to yohimbine further increased sodium excretion indicating that both alpha 1 and alpha 2 adrenoceptors modulate sodium reabsorption by the kidney. Alpha adrenoceptors appear to mediate sodium transport in proximal convoluted tubule and ascending limb of Henle.

The effects of beta adrenergic agonists on sodium transport has not been consistent from species to species (21, 23, 25). In the proximal tubule of the rabbit and rat, ascending limb of Henle in the mouse and the cortical collecting tubule of the rabbit (21, 23, 24) beta adrenergic agonists mediate and increase in sodium or chloride transport. In the dog, however, beta adrenergic agonists decrease sodium reabsorption (25). It is likely that the beta 1 adrenoceptor subtype mediates the change in sodium reabsorption associated with beta adrenergic agonists, since this is the predominant beta adrenoceptor found in the kidney in radioligand binding studies (29, 30).

Stimulation of dopamine receptors has been shown to invoke a natriuresis. We have demonstrated that cis-flupenthixol, but not its stereoisomer, trans-flupenthixol, attenuated the natriuresis associated with an acute sodium load. It appears that dopamine exerts its natriuretic effect by occupation of specific renal tubular dopamine receptors (20, 31). Micropuncture studies showed that the effect of dopamine was beyond the superficial proximal convoluted tubule. Bello-Reuss et al. have also reported that dopamine decreases fluid transport in the rabbit pars recta (22). However, Felder et al. have reported dopamine 1 receptors in proximal convoluted tubule of the rabbit (32). Dopamine 2 receptors have also been identified in glomeruli as well as renal tubular homogenates (31). Their role on renal sodium reabsorption remains to be determined. In the rabbit intestine, however, dopamine receptors (other than the dopamine 1 subtype) increase sodium reabsorption (33).

ONTOGENY OF ADRENERGIC REGULATION OF RENAL SODIUM TRANSPORT

The effects of various adrenergic agonists and antagonists on sodium transport in the developing kidney have been recently studied (10-13). The intrarenal administration of the alpha adrenergic blocker, phentolamine, induced a dose related increase in sodium excretion in puppies and adult dogs (13). The effect was greatest in adult dogs and least in younger puppies. In younger puppies, the combination of alpha and beta adrenergic blockade did not elicit any further change in fractional sodium excretion. However, in mature puppies, the imposition of beta adrenergic blockade attenuated the natriuresis seen after alpha adrenergic blockade alone. These studies suggest that the natriuretic consequence of the occupation of beta adrenergic receptors was seen in mature but not young puppies. The natriuretic effect of dopamine has also been demonstrated in our laboratory to increase with age (16).

These changes in sodium excretion induced by adrenergic agents were related to the number of specific renal neurotransmitter receptors in the developing puppy (12, 24, 35). These receptors were characterized by radioligand binding studies. In renal cortical membranes, alpha adrenoceptors decrease while beta adrenoceptors increase with age. Renal cortical dopamine receptors did not change with age (35).

According to the receptor studies, the newborn kidney is under greatest alpha adrenergic influence. Therefore alpha adrenergic blockade per se should result in a greater natriuresis in younger puppies than adult dogs. However, the opposite was seen. It is possible that increased distal tubular avidity for sodium in the newborn obscures proximal tubular events. Another possibility, however, should be considered. Alpha adrenergic receptors may induce natriuresis not only by blocking alpha adrenoceptors but also by allowing the expression of the natriuretic consequences of uncovering endogenous beta adrenergic and dopamine effects. The newborn kidney has not yet developed the beta adrenergic and dopamine coupled natriuretic activity seen in the adult dog. Therefore, blockade of alpha adrenoceptors, while eliminating an antinatriuretic effect, is not accompanied by the natriuresis associated with beta adrenergic and dopamine receptors. In contrast, in the adult dog with minimal alpha adrenoceptors and full complement of beta adrenergic and dopamine receptors, alpha adrenergic blockade allows full expression of the natriuretic consequences of stimulation of beta adrenergic and dopamine receptors. Thus blockade of a specific adrenoceptor may have the additional effect of uncovering the effects of other adrenoceptors. Change in renal nerve activity may also influence endogenous neurotransmitter levels (36). Thus we suggest that the changes in alpha and beta adrenoceptors with age correlate well with the alpha and beta adrenergic effects on sodium excretion during development. In contrast, the increasing natriuretic effect of dopamine is not related to changes in dopamine receptor number and presumably relates to post receptor events.

Although the variations in responses to catecholamines may explain the differences in salt handling between the young and the adult animal, other factors have been postulated for the increased avidity of the neonatal distal tubule to sodium. These factors need not be exclusive of each other. Increased sodium avidity may be due to increased sodium retaining hormones (e.g. aldosterone)(37). It may also be due to a limited ability of the newborn to elaborate a natriuretic factor(s) or a failure of this factor(s) to effect a natriuretic response. An interaction among natriuretic and antinatriuretic factors is known, including dopamine, kinins and aldosterone. For example, in the adult, dopamine inhibits aldosterone secretion (38). A relationship may exist among the adrenergic nervous system, substance P and kinins (38, 39). We have reported that the ability of the newborn to excrete a sodium load is enhanced by substance P. The increased sodium excretion in these puppies correlated well with urinary kallikrein levels (40).

The sympathetic nervous system regulates substance P levels (38). If this situation occurs in the kidney, it is anticipated that the increased alpha adrenergic activity in the newborn would decrease substance P levels, and therefore renal kallikreins and limits the ability of the puppy to excrete a salt load.

We conclude that a changing pattern of adrenergic and dopaminergic control occurs with maturation. It is possible that the decreased ability of the newborn to excrete a salt load might be related to (1) increased alpha and decreased beta adrenoceptors (2) decreased dopamine effects (post receptor site), (3) decreased substance P effect and subsequently renal kallikrein activity (possibly by alpha adrenergic inhibition), (4) increased mineralocorticoids (in part due to decreased inhibitory effects of dopamine?).

This paper was supported in part by grants from the National Institutes of Health HL-07213 and HL 23081, American Heart Association, Nation's Capital Affiliate and National Kidney Foundation of the National Capital Area, Inc.

REFERENCES

1. Langer, S.Z., Covero, I., and Massingham, R.: Recent developments in noradrenergic neurotransmission and its relevance to the mechanism of action of certain antihypertensive agents. Hypertension 2: 372, 1980.

2. Hoffman, B.B., and Lefkowitz, R.J.: Radioligand binding studies of adrenergic receptors: New insights into molecular and physiological regulation. Annu. Rev. Pharmacol. Toxicol. 20: 581, 1980.

3. Minneman, K.P., Pittman, R.N., and Molinoff, P.B.: B-adrenergic receptor subtypes: Properties, distribution, and regulation. Annu. Rev. Nleurosci. 4: 419, 1981.

4. Olson, R.D., Nies, A.S., and Gerber, J.G.: Catecholamine induced renin release in the anesthetized mongrel dog is due to both alpha and beta adrenoceptor stimulation. Evidence that only the alpha adrenoceptor component is prostaglandin mediated. J. Pharmacol. Exp. Thera. 224: 483, 1983.

5. Goldberg, L.I., and Kohli, J.D.: Differentiation of dopamine receptors in the periphery. In Kaiser, C., and Kebabian, J.W. (eds.): Dopamine Receptors. Washington, D.C.: American Chemical Society, 1983, p. 101.

6. Carey, R.M., Thorner, M.O., and Ortt, E.M.: Dopaminergic inhibition of metoclopramide-induced aldosterone secretion in man. Dissociation of responses to dopamine and bromocryptine. J. Clin. Invest. 66: 10, 1980.

7. Creese, I., Sibley, D.R., Hamblin, M.W., and Leff, S.E. The classification of dopamine receptors: Relationship to radioligand binding. Annu. Rev. Neurosci. 6: 43, 1983.

8. Rasmussen, H. Calcium and cAMP as Synarchic Messengers: New York, John Wiley and Sons, 1981.

9. Kebabian, J.W., and Calne, D.B.: Multiple dopamine receptors. Nature 277: 93, 1979.

10. Jose, P., Slotkoff, L., Lilienfield, L., Calcagno, P., and Eisner, G.: Sensitivity of the neonatal renal vasculature to epinephrine. Am. J. Physiol. 226: 796, 1974.

11. Jose, P.A., Slotkoff, L.M., Montgomery, S., Calcagno, P.L., and Eisner, G.M.: Autoregulation of renal blood flow in the puppy. Am. J. Physiol. 229: 796, 1975.

12. Felder, R.A., Pelayo, J.C., Calcagno, P.L., Eisner, G.M., and Jose, P.A.: Alpha adrenoceptors in the developing kidney. Pediatr. Res. 17: 177, 1983.

13. Fildes, R.D., Eisner, G.M., Calcagno, P.L., and Jose, P.A.: Renal alpha adrenoceptors and sodium excretion in the dog. Accepted for publication, Am. J. Physiol.

14. Gootman, P.M., Buckley, N.M., and Gootman, N.: Postnatal maturation of neural control of the circulation. In Scarpelli, E.M., and Cosmi, E.V. (eds): Review of Perinatal Medicine. New York: Raven Press, p. 1.

15. Buckley, N.M., Brazeau, P., and Frasier, I.D.: Cardiovascular effects of dopamine in developing swine. Biol. Neonate 43: 50, 1983.

16. Pelayo, J.C., and Jose, P.A.: The influence of age on renal dopamine effects. Pediatr. Res. 16: 310A, 1982.

17. DiBona, G.F.: The functions of the renal nerves. Rev. Physiol. Biochem. Pharmacol. 94: 75, 1982.

18. Moss, N.G.: Renal function and renal afferent nerve activity. Am. J. Physiol. 243 (Renal Fluid Electrolyte Physiol. 12) F425, 1982.

19. Barajas, L., Wang, P., Powers, K., and Nisho, S.: Identification of renal neuroeffector junctions by electron microscopy of reembedded light microscopic autoradiograms of semi-thin sections. J. Ultrastruc. Res. 77: 379, 1981.

20. Pelayo, J.C., Fildes, R.D., Eisner, G.M., and Jose, P.A.: The effects of dopamine blockade on renal sodium excretion. Am. J. Physiol. (Renal Fluid Electrolyte Physiol. 14) F247, 1983.

21. Bello-Reuss, W. Effect of catecholamines on fluid reabsorption by the isolated proximal convoluted tubule. Am. J. Physiol. (Renal Fluid Electrolyte Physiol. 1) F357, 1980.

22. Bello-Reuss, E., Higashi, Y., and Kaneda, Y.: Dopamine decreases fluid reabsorption in straight portions of rabbit proximal tubule. Am. J. Physiol. 242 (Renal

Fluid Electrolyte Physiol. 11) F634, 1982.

23. Chan, Y.L.: The role of norepinephrine in the regulation of fluid reabsorption in the rat proximal tubule J. Pharmacol. Exp. Thera. 215: 65, 1980.

24. Iino, Y., Troy, Y.L., and Brenner, B.M.: Effects of catecholamines on electrolyte transport in cortical collecting tubule. J. Membr. Biol. 61: 67, 1981.

25. Gill, J.R, Jr., and Casper, A.G.T.: Depression of proximal tubular sodium reabsorption in the dog in response to renal beta-adrenergic stimulation by isoproterenol. J. Clin. Invest. 50: 112, 1971.

26. Osborn, J.L., Holdaas, H., Thames, M.D., and DiBona, G.F.: Renal adrenoceptor mediation of antinatriuretic and renin secretion responses to low frequency nerve stimulation in the dog. Circ. Res. 53: 298, 1983.

27. Graham, R.M., Pettinger, W.A., Sagalowsky, A., Brabson, B.D., and Gandler, T.: Renal alpha-adrenergic receptor abnormality in the spontaneously hypertensive rat. Hypertension 4: 331, 1982.

28. Smyth, D., Umemura, S., and Pettinger, W.A.: Alpha$_2$-adrenoceptors and sodium reabsorption in the isolated perfused rat kidney. Proc. Am. Soc. Nephrol. 16th Annu. Meet., Washington, D.C.: 1983, p. 179A.

29. Snavely, M.D., Motulsky, H.J., Moustafa, E., Mahan, C., and Insel, P.A.: B-adrenergic receptor subtypes in the rat renal cortex. Selective regulation of B$_1$-adrenoceptors by pheochromocytoma. Circ. Res. 51: 504, 1982.

30. Montgomery, S., Jose, P., Spiro, P., Slotkoff, L., and Eisner, G.: Regional differences in the binding affinities of beta adrenergic receptors in the canine kidney cortex. Proc. Soc. Exp. Biol. Med. 162: 250, 1979.

31. Felder, R.A., Blecher, M., Eisner, G.M., and Jose, P.A.: Cortical tubular and glomerular dopamine receptors in the rat kidney. in press. Am. J. Physiol.

32. Felder, R.A., Blecher, M., Calcagno, P.L., and Jose, P.A.: Dopamine receptors in the proximal tubule of the rabbit. Submitted to the Am. J. Physiol.

33. Donowitz, M., Cusolito, S., Battisti, L., Fogel, R., and Sharp, G.W.C.: Dopamine stimulation of active sodium absorption in rabbit ileum. J. Clin. Invest. 69: 1008, 1982.

34. Felder, R.A., Schoelkopf, L., Sporn, D.P., Connell, M., Eisner, G.M., Calcagno, P.L., and Jose, P.A.: Renal beta adrenergic receptors in the maturing canine. Pediatr. Res. 16: 321A, 1982.

35. Felder, R.A., Blecher, M., Schoelkopf, L., Calcagno, P.L., and Jose, P.A.: Renal dopamine receptors during maturation. Pediatr. Res. 17: 148A, 1983.

36. Morgonuv, N., and Baines, A.D.: Effects of salt intake and renal denervation on catecholamine catabolism and excretion. Kidney Int. 21: 316, 1982.

37. Spitzer, A.: The role of the kidney in sodium homeostasis during maturation. Kidney Int. 21: 539, 1982.

38. Kessler, J.A., Adler, J.E., Bohn, M.C., and Black, I.B.: Substance P in principal sympathetic nerves: regulation by impulse activity. Science 214: 335, 1981.

39. Mills, I.H., McFarlane, N.A., and Ward, P.E.: Increase in kallikrein excretion during the natriuresis produced by arterial infusion of substance P. Nature 257: 108, 1974.

40. Fildes, R.D., Solhaug, M., Tavani, N., Jr., Eisner, G.M., Calcagno, P.L., and Jose, P.A.: Enhancement of sodium excretion by substance P during saline loading in the canine puppy. Pediatr. Res. 17: 737, 1983.

PROSTAGLANDIN-ANGIOTENSIN INTERACTIONS FOR BLOOD PRESSURE REGULATION

Billy S. Arant, Jr., M.D.

Blood pressure (BP) measured on the first day of life varies directly with the gestational age of the infant (1). Arterial BP is the product of blood flow through a vessel, which varies directly with cardiac output, and the resistance to flow, which varies inversely with the cross-sectional diameter^4 of the vessel. Cardiac output can be altered by changes in blood volume (BV), heart rate or stroke volume, but BP in the neonate is predominantly low when BV, cardiac output, heart rate and stroke volume are high relative to the adult (Table). Mean arterial BP divided by cardiac output is the calculated arbitrary value which reflects total peripheral resistance (TPR). In the newborn, TPR is lower than in the adult. In order for the newborn to maintain BP at 40 mmHg if cardiac output were reduced to that of the adult (100 ml/min/kg), TPR must increase from 0.3 to 0.4 units. On the other hand, if BP in the newborn were reduced to 20 mmHg but cardiac output remained unchanged (300ml/min/kg), TPR must decrease to 0.07 units.

Table. Comparison of hemodynamic determinants of blood pressure in the human.

	MAP mmHg	CO ml/min/kg	TPR units	HR min^{-1}	SV ml/kg	BV ml/kg
Neonate	40	300	0.13	120	2.50	100
Adult	100	100	1.00	80	1.25	75

MAP=mean arterial pressure, CO=cardiac output, TPR=total peripheral resistance, HR=heart rate, SV=stroke volume, BV=blood volume

Of the vasoactive factors in the circulation which may influence TPR in the newborn, plasma epinephrine and norepinephrine concentrations are higher than adult values at delivery and decrease during the first 48 hours of life when BP is increasing (2). Vasopressin is increased in infants at birth and decreases over the first three days of life to adults values (3). Plasma renin activity is 20-50 times greater in the newborn than the adult (4), and angiotensin II concentrations are also higher at birth than in older infants or adults (5). Since circulating vasopressor substances are increased in the neonate compared to the adult, a deficit in their production cannot explain the lower TPR and BP of newborn infants. On the other hand, certain prostaglandins, especially prostacyclin, which is a potent vasodepressor substance, have been shown to be increased in both the plasma (6) and urine (7) of newborn infants compared to adults. TPR in either the newborn or the adult, therefore, may not be determined by the amount of any single circulating vasopressor or vasodepressor substances, but may rather be the net effect of all vasoactive substances at any given time.

BV relative to body size is higher at birth when BP is lower than at any other time of life. In premature infants BV is about 100 ml/kg compared to 75 ml/kg (8) in the adult. Infants whose umbilical cord was clamped early had blood volumes following birth that were 20 to 30 ml/kg less than those whose cords were clamped only after pulsations had ceased. However, within two hours of life, BP was not different between the groups of infants. This observation suggested that either the capacity of the vascular space had increased following birth to accommodate the added BV or that plasma had been extravasated from the vascular space into the urine or the interstitial space. Evidence that BV decreases during after the first 24 hours of life in infants born at term includes rising hematocrits and declining plasma volumes (9). Morphologic evidence for differences in vascular resistance in fullterm infants deprived of placental transfusion includes electron microscopic studies of skin vasculature (10). Early-clamped infants exhibited narrow-lumened vessels, while the cross-sectional diameter of vessels from late clamped infants was markedly increased with thinning or compression of endothelial cells and with fenestrae in the capillary wall, which may facilitate plasma movement into the interstitial space.

When the BV of puppies at birth and during postnatal life were compared to the adult dog, an inverse relationship was observed between mean arterial BP and BV at every age (11). Even though BP increased with postnatal age, the same inverse relationship between BV and mean arterial pressure was observed at every age of study. In normal human adults, diastolic BP varied inversely with BV; however, patients with essential hypertension exhibited a direct relationship between diastolic BP and BV (12). In a study of sick premature infants (8), mean arterial BP did not increase when BV was expanded with 5% albumin solution, suggesting that TPR in the neonate is low even when BV is high. During intravenous 5% albumin/saline infusion, BP, central venous pressure and heart rate increased in adult dogs, and plasma renin activity decreased (11). However, the newborn puppy responded similarly to volume expansion by increases in central venous pressure and heart rate, but mean arterial BP actually decreased by 25%, and plasma renin activity increased. Moreover, arterial plasma concentrations of both PGE_2 and 6-keto$PGF_{1\alpha}$ (the stable metabolite of prostacyclin), both vasodilators and potent stimuli to renin release, were increased in both puppies and adult dogs after volume expansion, but their relatively greater increase in the puppy may account for the lowering TPR and BP as well as for the increase in plasma renin activity.

Arachidonic acid, released by the action of phospholipase on membrane phospholipid, is substrate for one of several enzymatic pathways. The cyclo-oxygenase pathway forms endoperoxide intermediates which are converted to the classical prostaglandins, PGE_2, $PGF_{2}\alpha$, PGD_2, prostacyclin (PGI_2), and thromboxane A_2. Prostaglandin synthesis can be reduced with nonsteroidal anti-inflammatory drugs such as indomethacin or aspirin which inhibit cyclo-oxygenase activity. Less familiar to some clinicians is the reduction in prostaglandin synthesis by glucocorticoids which inhibit phospholipase and reduce the availability of arachidonic acid for cyclo-oxygenase activity. It is this mechanism, perhaps, by which glucocorticoid therapy may benefit premature infants at risk of hyaline membrane disease since prostacyclin synthesis is increased this disorder (13). A relationship between the rate of fluid administration and patency of the ductus arteriosus in newborn infants was first reported in 1977 (14). When the rate of intravenous fluid administration was increased, a previously-closed ductus arteriosus opened, and when the rate was reduced, the ductus closed again. The decrease in BP following volume expansion in newborn puppies could have been due to increased left-to-right shunt through a patent ductus arteriosus. Angiographic studies found the ductus closed in 3-day-old puppies (15). Following the intravenous administration of 10 ml/kg of 5% albumin, however, BP decreased and the ductus arteriosus became patent. The ductus arteriosus in puppies pre-treated with meclofenemate, a cyclo-oxygenase inhibitor, remained closed. Ductal patency with volume expansion, therefore, appears to be prostaglandin-mediated. A similar decrease in BP after volume expansion in 60-day-old puppies, however, could not be explained by the same mechanism since the ductus arteriosus was anatomically closed at that age. The fall in BP following volume expansion of older puppies was accompanied by an increase in cardiac output, a decrease in TPR, and a rise in plasma 6-keto$PGF_{1}\alpha$ concentrations.

On the contrary, BP in newborn puppies did not change following an acute hemorrhage of 20 ml/kg body weight. In fact, systolic BP actually increased and was associated with increases in plasma renin activity and angiotensin II; however, PGE_2 and 6-keto$PGF_{1}\alpha$ concentrations decreased. Progressive hemorrhage in fetal lambs was associated with a gradual increase in plasma vasopressin and plasma renin activity (16). Therefore, changes in BV in the fetus and newborn can be associated with alterations in the circulating concentrations of vasoactive substances.

In conclusion, interpretation of data from previous or future cardiovascular studies in neonates must be done with the understanding that the hemodynamic changes which follow pharmacologic manipulation of a single vasoactive factor will not be an isolated response, but rather the net result of all vasoactive factors perturbed during the experiment.

REFERENCES

1. Kitterman, J.A., Phibbs, R.H. and Tooley, W.H.: Aortic blood pressure in normal newborn infants during the first 12 hours of life. Pediatrics 4: 959, 1969.

2. Eliot, R.J., Lam, R., Leake, R.D. et al.: Plasma catecholamine concentrations in infants at birth and during the first 48 hours of life. J. Pediatr. 96: 311, 1980.

3. Pohjavouri, M. and Fyhrquist F.: Hemodynamic significance of vasopressin the newborn infant. J. Pediatr. 97: 462, 1980.

4. Kotchen, T.A., Strickland, A.L., Rice, T.W. et al.: A study of the renin-angiotensin system in newborn infants. J. Pediatr. 80: 938, 1972.

5. Pipkin, F.B. and Smales, O.R.C.: A study of factors affecting blood pressure and angiotensin II in newborn infants. J. Pediatr. 91: 113, 1977.

6. Kaapa, P., Viinikka, L. and Ylikoohala, O.: Plasma prostacyclin from birth to adolescence. Arch. Dis. Child. 57: 459, 1982.

7. Seyberth, H.W., Muller, H., Ulmer, H.E. et al.: Urinary excretion rates of 6-keto-$PGF_{1\alpha}$ in preterm infants recovering from respiratory distress with and without patent ductus arteriosus. Pediatr. Res. 18: 520, 1984.

8. Barr, P.A., Bailey, P.E., Sumners, J. et al.: Relation between arterial blood pressure and blood volume and effects of infused albumin in sick preterm infants. Pediatrics 60: 282, 1977.

9. Gairdner, D., Marks, J., Roscoe, J.D. et al.: The fluid shift from the vascular compartment immediately after birth. Arch. Dis. Child. 33: 489, 1958.

10. Pietra, G.G., D'Amodio, M.D., Leventhal, M.M. et al.: Electron microscopy of cutaneous capillaries of newborn infants: effects of placental transfusion. Pediatrics 42: 678, 1969.

11. Arant, B.S., Jr.: The relationship between blood volume, prostaglandin synthesis and arterial blood pressure in neonatal puppies. <u>In</u> Spitzer, A. (ed.):

The Kidney During Development. Morphology and Function. New York: Masson, 1981, p. 167.

12. London, G.M., Safar, M.E., Weiss, Y.A. et al.: Volume-dependent parameters in essential hypertension. Kidney Int. 11: 204, 1977.

13. Engle, W.D., Arant, B.S., Jr., Wiriyathian, S. et al.: Diuresis and respiratory distress syndrome: physiologic mechanisms and therapeutic implications. J. Pediatr. 102: 912, 1983.

14. Stephenson, J.G.: Fluid administration in the association of patent ductus arteriosus complicating respiratory distress syndrome. J. Pediatr. 90: 257, 1977.

15. Arant, B.S., Jr.: Unpublished observations.

16. Robillard, J.E., Weitzman, R.E., Fisher, D.A. et al.: The dynamics of vasopressin release and blood volume regulation during fetal hemorrhage in the lamb fetus. Pediatr. Res. 13: 606, 1979.

RENAL HANDLING OF SODIUM DURING DEVELOPMENT

Pedro A. Jose, Robin A. Felder, Robert D. Fildes, Gilbert M. Eisner, and Philip L. Calcagno

Normally growing term infants remain in positive sodium balance while on widely varying salt intakes (1). However, in healthy preterm infants below 35 weeks gestational age a negative sodium balance resulting in hyponatremia has been observed in the first 1-3 weeks of life (2,3). The negative sodium balance in preterm infants is mainly due to renal sodium wasting exacerbated by inefficient intestinal sodium reabsorption (4). It has been estimated that infants less than 33 weeks gestational age require a minimum of 4-5 mEq sodium/kg/day to offset these losses in the first weeks of life. Al-Dahhan et al reported that supplementations of 4-5 mEq/kg/day in premature babies prevented hyponatremia, maintained a positive sodium balance, improved early growth, and allowed earlier discharge from the hospital. No adverse effects were seen and supplementation was not needed after the second post-natal week (4). In contrast, Lorenz et al showed that very low birth weight infants taking as little as 1.6 mEq/kg/day were able to maintain a normal serum sodium concentration. They suggested that the estimation of sodium requirement in the first week of life must take into account not only actual urinary sodium excretion which is influenced by gestational age but also the anticipated change in water balance (5).

The mechanism for the high fractional sodium excretion in preterm infants was studied by Rodriguez-Soriano et al using clearance techniques (6). They reported lower reabsorptive rates of sodium in more proximal segments of the nephron resulting in a marked increase in distal tubular load. The mechanism for the lower reabsorptive rates in the proximal nephron was not assessed in their report but some insight may be gained from the studies in developing rats (7). Solomon showed that the adult plasma to proximal tubule sodium gradient was only achieved when the proximal tubular length was greater than 1500 um, the length seen in adult rats. It is possible that the very short proximal tubules in very premature infants behave in a similar fashion with decreased proximal tubular reabsorption and increased distal tubule delivery. Since the increased delivery of fluid to the distal tubule in very premature infants is not compensated by increased distal reabsorption, an increased sodium excretion results. This occurs in spite of much higher circulating aldosterone levels in very premature infants. It has been suggested that the relatively lower distal tubular sodium reabsorption in very premature infants may be due to (a) decreased ability of the distal tubule to respond to aldosterone per se, or (b) that the distal tubule is already under maximal aldosterone stimulation and thus no additional effect would be noted with higher aldosterone levels. Whatever the mechanism involved, positive sodium balance in these very low birth weight infants is attained quickly so that after 20 days of postnatal age, a positive sodium balance is expected (8).

Both preterm and term infants have a limited ability to excrete a salt load when compared to the adult. This limitation can not be entirely explained by differences in glomerular filtration rate (9). However, the difference, if any, in the changes in glomerular filtration rate after a saline load between term and preterm infants are not known. Previous studies have also shown that differences in renal blood flow or filtration distribution do not fully explain these age related differences in sodium handling. The major mechanism seems to be related to differences in renal tubular response to an acute salt load (9, 10).

In the adult proximal tubule two-thirds of sodium reabsorption is by active mechanisms while the other third is by passive mechanisms (11). The mechanism for solute solvent coupling in this nephron segment is best explained by the coexistence of luminal hypotonicity and lateral intercellular hypertonicity (11). Osmotic water permeability of the proximal tubule markedly influences passive sodium and water transport. Horster and Larsson have shown that the hydraulic hydrostatic conductance is high in the neonatal proximal tubule (12). Two to six day old rabbit proximal tubules had the highest decrease in hydraulic conductivity. There was a marked decrease in hydraulic conductivity at 10-14 days and reached mature values by 30-38 days. The importance of hydraulic conductivity during differentiation was further studied by these investigators (3). The imposition of hyperoncotic serum in the medium bathing the isolated proximal tubule resulted in a greater increase in fluid reabsorption in 2-6 day old than more mature animals (3). These studies indicate that the hydraulic conductivity of the proximal tubule is a very important modulator of net volume flow during differentiation. These studies suggest that there should be enhanced proximal tubular reabsorption in the young. This tendency however is counterbalanced by decreased active transport at this site. For example, the area available for active transport, the basolateral membrane and the activity of Na-K-ATPase in this membrane are low compared to the mature animal (13, 4). Aperia et al have shown that Na-K-ATPase activity in the proximal tubule of young rats can be induced by mineralocorticoids. This is accompanied by an increase in proximal tubular transport. This effect is not seen in older rats.

The relative permeabilities of the proximal tubule for sodium and chloride also changes with development. The ratio of sodium to chloride permeabilities was 0.55 in superficial proximal tubule and 1.11 in juxtamedullary proximal tubule (15). The value in superficial tubule resembled that for ions at free solution boundaries whereas the value for the juxtamedullary nephron was close to that in final adult proximal convoluted tubule. Whereas the tubular fluid to plasma sodium ratio does not change with age, the ratio for chloride increases with age. Surprisingly, given these differences in sodium transport in the proximal tubule between the newborn and the adult, the fraction of glomerular filtrate reabsorbed in this segment is similar; that is, two thirds of the glomerular filtrate is reabsorbed by the proximal tubule (11). In very premature infants, however, the proximal tubular reabsorption is probably less. After saline loading, the depression in proximal tubular reabsorption is similar in newborn and adults (1). Thus the limited ability of the newborn to excrete a salt load is not due to inherent differences in proximal tubular solute transport.

The thick ascending limb of Henle transport chloride and sodium without accompanying water reabsorption. This low hydraulic conductivity is also present during development (15). However, the ability of this segment to transport sodium and chloride is much less in the newborn compared to the adult (16, 17). The decreased ability of the newborn thick ascending limb of Henle to reabsorb sodium results in a relatively greater sodium delivery to the distal tubule than in the adult. In the preterm infant distal sodium delivery is enhanced even more.

The changes in distal solute delivery were studied by Aperia and Elinder in rats (18). They showed increased distal tubular delivery in 20 day and 40 day old rats. However, at the late distal tubule, the fraction of filtrate remaining was similar in both groups of rats, indicating greater reabsorptive rates in this segment in 20 day old rats. This increased avidity of the distal tubule for sodium is considered to be the major reason for the limited ability of the newborn to excrete a salt load (19). Using clearance methods, a similar phenomenon has been reported in both term and preterm human infants (19). The mechanism for the increased avidity of the distal tubule for sodium is under intensive investigation. This may be due to increased mineralocorticoid effect (1). Indeed, there is an increased activity of the renin-angiotensin-aldosterone system in the newborn (20). The role of aldosterone in the newborn was studied by Elinder and Aperia in rats by observing the effects of aldosterone blockade on distal sodium reabsorption (21). After aldosterone blockade, the fraction of filtered sodium reabsorbed between the early and late distal tubule was not different between younger and older rats. Thus, the increased distal tubular avidity for sodium in the young could not be explained by increased aldosterone effects.

Following a salt load, the newborn may be unable to elaborate natriuretic factors including natriuretic hormone, oxytocin and renal kallikrein to the same extent as in adults (22-24). Renal prostaglandins have not been shown to be a factor. We have recently shown that the ability of the newborn to excrete a salt load was enhanced by substance P (24). Substance P is an undecapeptide with neurotransmitter and natriuretic properties. The addition of substance P during saline loading in puppies significantly increased sodium excretion. This was associated with an increase in urinary kallikrein. Urinary kallikreins are low in the newborn (25, 26). Renal kallikreins may be natriuretic (27). We propose that an interaction of several hormones on the distal tubule may explain the differences in sodium handling after an acute salt load between newborns and adults.

This paper was supported in part by grants from the National Institutes of Health HL 07213 and HL 23081, American Heart Association, Nation's Capital Affiliate, and National Kidney Foundation of the National Capital Area, Inc.

REFERENCES

1. Spitzer, A.: The role of the kidney in sodium homeostasis during maturation. Kidney Int. 21: 539, 1982.

2. Sulyok, A.: The relationship between electrolyte and acid-base balance in the premature infant during early postnatal life. Biol. Neonate 17: 227, 1971.

3. Roy, R.N., Chance, G.W., Radde, I.C. et al.: Late hyponatremia in very low birth weight infants (<1.3 kgs). Pediatr. Res. 10: 526, 1978.

4. Al-Dahan, J., Haycock, G.B., Nichol, B. et al.: Renal and gastrointestinal salt handling in the newborn: The effects of salt supplementation. Int. J. Pediatr. Nephrol. (In Press).

5. Lorenz, J.M., Kleinman, L.I., Kotagal, U.R., and Reller, M.D. Water balance in very low birth weight infants: Relationship to water and sodium intake and effect on outcome. J. Pediatr. 101: 423, 1982.

6. Rodriguez-Soriano, J., Vallo, A., Oliveros, R., and Castillo, G.: Renal handling of sodium in premature and full-term neonates: a study using clearance methods during water diuresis. Pediatr. Res. 17: 1013, 1983.

7. Solomon, S.: Maximal gradients of sodium and potassium across proximal tubules of kidneys in immature rats. Biol. Neonate 25: 327, 1974.

8. Ross, B., Cowett, R., and Oh, W.: Renal functions of low birth weight infants during the first two months of life. Pediatr. Res. 11: 162, 1977.

9. Goldsmith, D.I., Drukker, A., Blaufox, M.D., Edelmann, C.M., Jr., and Spitzer, A. Hemodynamic and excretory responses of the neonatal canine kidney to acute volume expansion. Am. J. Physiol. 237 (Renal Fluid Electrolyte Physiol. 6): F387, 1979.

10. Jose, P., Pelayo, J., Felder, R. et al.: Maturation of single nephron filtration rate in the canine puppy; the effect of saline loading. In Spitzer, A. (ed.) The Kidney During Development. Morphology and Function. New York:

Masson Publishing USA Inc., 1982, p. 139.

11. Berry, C.A.: Water permeability and pathways in the proximal tubule. Am. J. Physiol. 245 (Renal Fluid Electrolyte Physiol. 14): F279, 1983.

12. Horster, M., and Larsson, L.: Mechanisms of fluid reabsorption during proximal tubule development. Kidney Int. 10: 348, 1976.

13. Schwartz, G.J., and Evan, A.P.: Development of solute transport in rabbit proximal tubule. I. HCO_3^- and glucose absorption. Am. J. Physiol. 245 (Renal Fluid Electrolyte Physiol. 14): F382, 1983.

14. Aperia, A., Larsson, L., and Zetterstrom, R.: Hormonal induction of Na-K-ATPase in developing proximal tubular cells. Am. J. Physiol. 241 (Renal Fluid Electrolyte Physiol. 10): F356, 1981.

15. Horster, M.: Expression of ontogeny in individual nephron segments. Kidney Int. 22: 550, 1982.

16. Horster, M.: Loop of Henle functional differentiation. In vitro perfusion of the isolated thick ascending segment. Pflugers Archiv. 378: 15, 1978.

17. Lelievre-Pegorier, M., Merlet-Benichou, C., Roinel, N., and de Rouffignac, C.: Developmental pattern of water and electrolyte transport in rat superficial nephrons. Am. J. Physiol. 245 (Renal Fluid Electrolyte Physiol. 14): F15, 1983.

18. Aperia, A., and Elinder, G.: Distal tubular sodium reabsorption in the developing kidney. Am. J. Physiol. 240 (Renal Fluid Electrolyte Physiol. 9): F487, 1981.

19. Aperia, A., Broberger, O., Thodenius, K., and Zetterstrom, R.: Developmental study of the renal response to an oral salt load in preterm infants. Acta Paediatr. Scand. 63: 517, 1974.

20. Pelayo, J.C., Eisner, G.M., and Jose, P.A.: The ontogeny of the renin-angiotensin system. Clin. Perinat. 8:347, 1981.

21. Elinder, G., and Aperia, A.: Effect of aldosterone blocking on distal sodium reabsorption during development. Eur. J. Pediatr. 140: 166, 1983.

22. Kleinman, L.I., and Banks, R.O.: Natriuretic effect of oxytocin on saline-expanded neonatal dogs. Am. J. Physiol. 239 (Renal Fluid Electrolyte Physiol. 8): F589, 1981.

23. Solomon, S., Hathaway, S. and Curb, D.: Evidence that the renal response to volume expansion involves a blood-borne factor. Biol. Neonate 35: 113, 1979.

24. Fildes, R.D., Solhaug, M., Tavani, N., Jr., et al.: Enhancement of sodium excretion by substance P during saline loading in the canine puppy. Pediatr. Res. 17: 738, 1983.

25. Godard, C., Valloton, M.B., and Favre, L. Urinary prostaglandins, vasopressin, and kallikrein excretion in healthy children from birth to adolescence. J. Pediatr. 100: 898, 1982.

26. Robillard, J.E., Lawton, W.J., Weisman, D.N., and Sessions, C.: Developmental aspects of the renal kallikrein-like activity in fetal and newborn lambs. Kidney Int. 22: 594, 1982.

27. Mills, I.H., McFarlane, N.A., and Ward, P.E.: Increase in kallikrein excretion during the natriuresis produced by arterial infusion of substance P. Nature 257: 108, 1974.

CLINICAL OVERVIEW OF NEONATAL HYPERTENSION

Raymond D. Adelman, M.D.

Hypertension in the newborn is being more frequently recognized by pediatricians (1,2,3,4). There is increased physician awareness of the existence of elevated blood pressures in this population; accurate, simple methods of measurement are now available, and the monitoring of systemic blood pressure in neonatal care units has become fairly routine. Although most neonatal hypertension reported in the pediatric literature has been due to renal artery thrombosis, as a consequence of indwelling umbilical artery catheters, an increasing number of infants are being detected with hypertension either from another cause or an undetermined etiology. The true incidence of neonatal hypertension is not known. In our own intensive care nursery the incidence of hypertension is around 2.5% (4). A recent survey of premature infants discharged from a neonatal intensive care unit revealed that 8.9% had elevated blood pressures when seen on a followup visit (5).

Measurement of blood pressure

Systolic blood pressure in the neonate can be measured by palpation, auscultation, direct intra-arterial recording, Doppler ultrasound, or oscillometry. Auscultation is frequently difficult because heart sounds are faint. The Doppler and oscillometry methods are simple, noninvasive, and generally correlate well with the reference standard, direct intra-arterial measurement (6,7,8). Direct systolic recordings are usually the most accurate readings; however, they may register lower than actual values if the pressure wave is dampened due to impaired blood flow through the arterial line. This may be seen more often in the premature infant under 1500 grams in whom small 3.5 French umbilical catheters are used. Furthermore, when a peripheral artery is utilized, we have noticed significant differences in systolic pressure between Doppler and direct recordings with the latter as much as 20 mmHg higher. Such differences are less likely to occur with a more centrally placed arterial line.

Blood pressure values vary with cuff size and fit and with state of alertness (9), birth weight (10), presence or absence of agitation (11), and postnatal age (12). The blood pressure should always be taken with an appropriate size cuff on a quiet, resting infant. An inappropriately small cuff will give artifactually high blood pressure readings. The late onset of hypertension in a long-term nursery resident may only signify he/she has outgrown the original cuff! Blood pressure cuffs should be removed periodically or rotated to prevent development of peripheral nerve palsies.

Blood pressure in the full term infant rises with age (12); comparable data in the low birthweight infant on age related changes in blood pressure are unfortunately limited. Utilizing the best available published data and our own experience, we have defined systemic hypertension as the following: a systolic blood pressure >90 mmHg and a diastolic blood pressure >60 mmHg in the term newborn, and a systolic blood pressure >80 mmHg and a diastolic blood pressure >50 mmHg in the preterm newborn.

Causes of hypertension

Reports of a correlation between maternal and newborn blood pressures (13) suggest the possible identification and monitoring of infants at risk for later development of essential hypertension. Such correlations have not been demonstrated by others (12), and are so low as to preclude in a practical way identification of individual infants at risk. The incidence or existence of essential hypertension in the neonatal population is unknown.

Although hypertension of undetermined etiology is more frequently recognized, most published cases of hypertension have been of secondary causes: (Table 1) Vascular (renal artery thrombosis [Fig. 1], coarctation), renal parenchymal (renal insufficiency, obstruction) and miscellaneous (increased intracranial pressure, fluid and electrolyte overload, drugs [14], pulmonary disease [15]).

TABLE 1. Causes of Hypertension in the Neonate

Vascular:	Other:
Renal artery thrombosis	Increased intracranial pressure
Renal vein thrombosis	Fluid and electrolyte overload
Coarctation of the aorta	Neural crest tumor
Renal artery stenosis	Adrenogenital syndrome
Hypoplastic aorta	Cushing's disease
	Primary hyperaldosteronism
Renal:	Correction of omphalocele
Renal dysplasia	Pneumothorax
Renal hypoplasia	Hypercalcemia
Obstructive uropathy	Genitourinary tract surgery
Infantile polycystic disease	Thyrotoxicosis
Renal insufficiency	Drugs: Ocular phenylephrine, corticosteroids, theophylline, DOCA
Renal tumors	

Prior to the last 15 years renal artery thrombosis was uncommonly seen either clinically or in post mortem studies (16,17). The striking increase in the incidence of renal artery thrombosis over the last decade and a half is clearly associated with the use of thrombogenic indwelling umbilical artery catheters. Systemic hypertension secondary to renal

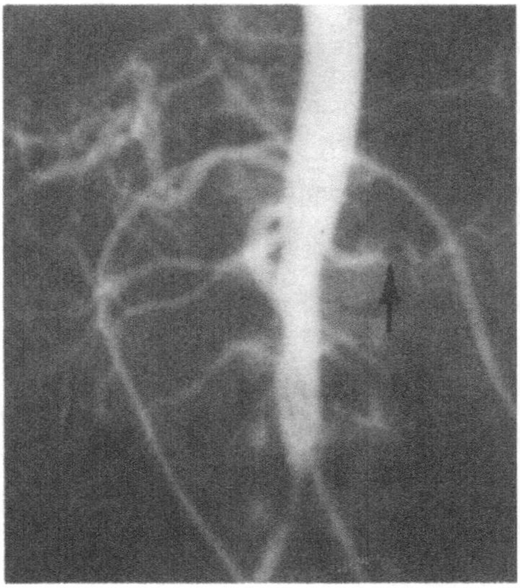

FIG. 1. Thrombotic occlusion of the left renal artery associated with a mural thrombus about an indwelling umbilical artery catheter.

artery thrombosis is clinically diagnosed in around 1 per thousand live born infants and in 3% of infants with indwelling umbilical artery catheters (3,4). Coarctation of the aorta, in contrast, is present in 0.2 infants per one thousand live births. Occult renal artery thrombosis may be even more common. Only a minority of infants with umbilical artery catheter related thromboses are clinically diagnosed (19), And only 25% of adults with renal artery thrombosis develop clinical hypertension (20). One can only conjecture as to the impact of silent renal artery thrombosis on renal growth and function and on a possible predisposition for subsequent renal related hypertension. Clearly, umbilical artery catheters should only be used when absolutely necessary. To reduce downstream renal embolization, catheter tips should be placed below the origin of the renal arteries.

We have also seen a number of neonates with chronic lung disease who developed hypertension. The hypertension is usually moderate and may relate to an increased systemic vascular resistance due to hypoxia and/or increased pulmonary vascular resistance.

Clinical features

Most newborns with systemic hypertension who were described in our earlier reports (3,4,21) were symptomatic and presented with cardiorespiratory problems such as tachypnea, cyanosis, or congestive failure and/or neurological symptoms such as lethargy, coma, tremors, apnea, seizures and hemiparesis. Hypertension in the very small premature was felt to be uncommon. Most hypertension had a renovascular origin. We have been impressed over the last few years, however, at the significant incidence of hypertension in the very low birthweight infant, the frequency with which hypertensive infants are asymptomatic, and the increasing number of infants in whom causes other than renal artery thrombosis are discovered or in whom no etiology is found.

Although many infants with hypertension are asymptomatic, a disturbing number of very low birthweight infants, approximately 40-50%, have clinical or ultrasound evidence of cerebral hemorrhage (22). Although many factors may contribute to these hemorrhages, modest changes in systemic blood pressure due to handling or acute volume expansion, may play a significant role. Such hemorrhages originate in the capillaries of the subependymal germinal matrix which are poorly supported by glial membranes and inadequately protected against changes in systemic arterial pressure because of impaired autoregulation of cerebral blood flow. Rapid increases in systemic arterial pressure following volume expansion are associated with intraventricular hemorrhage in the newborn beagle (23). In human newborns, Lou (22) has proposed a similar relationship between changes in systemic arterial pressure and cerebral hemorrhage.

Evaluation

Hematuria, proteinuria, azotemia, and elevated serum creatinine are commonly seen in hypertensive infants but are nonspecific findings. Peripheral plasma renin activity is often elevated. When hypertension occurs in an infant with an indwelling umbilical artery catheter and renal artery thrombosis is suspected, abdominal aortography by hand injection can be used to identify thrombosis of the renal arteries or other major vessels (21). A renal scan using 99^{m}Tc DPTA and/or I^{123} or I^{131} Iodohippurate is less invasive and also useful, especially in the infant no longer having a catheter. Computerized renal scans, allowing comparison of relative function and size in each kidney, increase the yield of the renal scan in diagnosing renovascular disease and are very helpful in the followup of renal function and growth (21).

In infants in whom renovascular hypertension is not suspected, urinary catecholamines, 17 hydroxysteroids, and 17 ketosteroids are obtained as well as an evaluation of the anatomy of the genitourinary tract either by intravenous pyelography or abdominal ultrasound. Ultrasound in the neonate is being employed more often because of ease of use, the potential toxicity of radiocontrast media, and the poor quality of pyelograms usually obtained in the neonate.

Medical management

The management of neonatal hypertension has been largely empiric based upon drug regimens successful in older children and adults (Table II). There is little data in the newborn concerning the levels of blood pressure requiring pharmacological therapy, the morbid consequences of nontreatment of mild to moderate hypertension, and the frequency and extent of adverse effects of currently used drugs.

Table II. Agents Used in the Management of Neonatal Hypertension

Agent	Range (mg/kg/24 hr)
Chlorothiazide	20-50 mg/kg p.o.
Furosemide	1-4 mg/kg i.v., p.o.
Hydralazine	1-9 mg/kg i.v., p.o.
Methyldopa	5-50 mg/kg i.v., p.o.
Diazoxide	2-5 mg/kg/dose i.v.
Propranolol	0.5-5.0 mg/kg p.o.
Captopril	0.05-0.4 mg/kg/dose P.O.
Nitroprusside	0.5-5.0 µg/kg/min i.v.

We generally treat neonates with persistent systolic and/or diastolic blood pressures above the 95th percentile for weight and age. Mild hypertension usually responds to diuretics and/or hydralazine which is increased in a stepwise fashion until blood pressure is controlled. High dosages are often needed. If blood pressure continues to be poorly controlled, methyldopa or propranolol is usually added. Captopril is quite effective in very low dosages. It is contraindicated with bilateral renal artery stenosis or unilateral stenosis involving a solitary kidney. Diazoxide and nitroprusside may be used with extreme hypertension. Precipitous drops in blood pressure have been associated with cerebral ischemia and cortical blindness and should be avoided by using graded dosages of diazoxide or a carefully monitored nitroprusside drip.

In our experience, most infants respond well to a single agent in combination with sodium restriction. One should be aware of hidden sources of sodium for the patient such as saline flushes and drugs. In some infants multiple antihypertensive medications are required. Medications can usually be tapered when blood pressure has remained normal for a period of one to two months. Most infants tolerate antihypertensive medications well, can be tapered off medications within the first four to eight months of life and remain normotensive. Hydralazine has been associated with diarrhea and emesis. One of our patients developed paroxysmal atrial tachycardia. Methyldopa can cause lethargy; propranolol can lead to bradycardia; and diuretics can produce hypokalemia, hyponatremia; and in the case of furosemide, significant hypercalciuria with nephrocalcinosis.

All hypertensive infants in our nursery have been successfully treated with medical management. Others have not had this experience (2,24). Nephrectomy may be needed for hypertensive neonates with unilateral renal involvement not responding to aggressive antihypertensive therapy or in whom there are unacceptable adverse drug side effects.

Although antihypertensive drugs are generally employed safely and efficaciously, additional information is needed on their pharmacokinetics in the newborn and on their impact on infant maturation, growth, and development. The neonate differs from the older child in the handling of many drugs, because of profound postnatal changes in organ development, maturation and function, the presence of coexisting pathological processes unique or exaggerated in the neonate, and properties of the individual drugs. We have studied in our laboratory the effect of chronic beta blockade with propranolol given for a period of six months to newborn beagle puppies. No changes in body or individual organ growth were noted but significant abnormalities in carbohydrate metabolism were detected (25). Animals treated with beta blockade showed a much more pronounced fall in blood glucose following insulin administration than control animals (Fig. 2). Differences between treated and control puppies were also noted in glucose disappearance rate.

Prognosis

Neonatal hypertension can be associated with significant morbidity and mortality. One third of earlier reported cases died from hypertension associated problems, presumably because of inadequate medical or surgical control of hypertension. In our experience hypertensive neonates respond well to medical management. Their long-term prognosis, however, is unclear. We have followed eleven infants over a 6½ year period. Two died from presumably unrelated causes but were normotensive prior to death. The remaining nine are normotensive and not receiving any antihypertensive medication. However, most have a significant reduction in size or an abnormality in function of the involved kidney. Whether these children will develop further deterioration in renal function over time is not known, nor is it known whether they will subsequently develop hypertension. Long-term followup is needed.

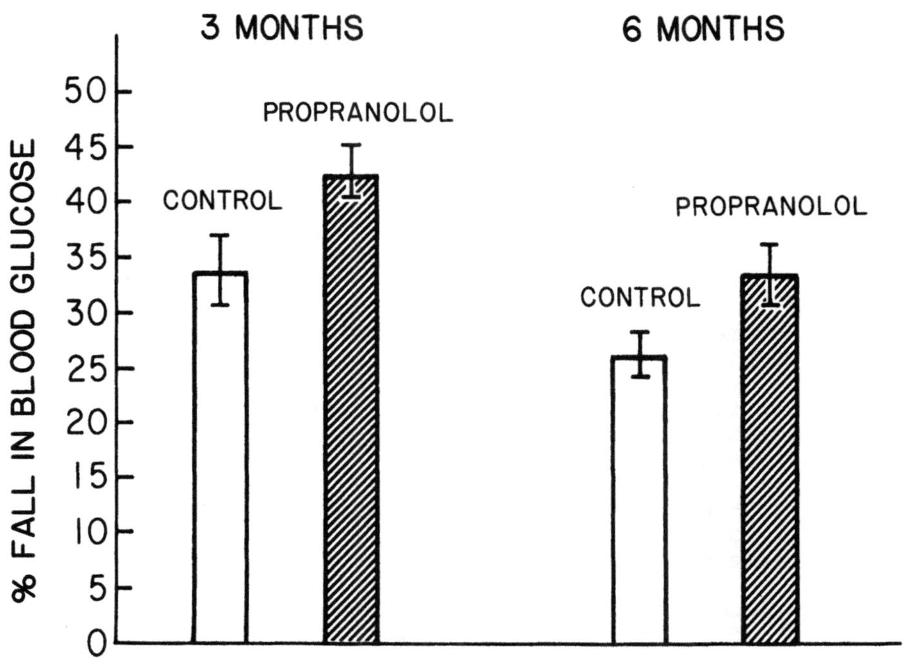

FIG. 2. % Fall in blood glucose levels following 0.1 U/kg insulin IV in puppies treated for 3 and 6 months with propranolol. (Adelman: Unpublished data)

SUMMARY

Reports of hypertension in the newborn have increased markedly, both as a complication of indwelling umbilical artery catheters and as a result of increased physician awareness. Antihypertensive medications are generally effective in controlling hypertension and usually need to be utilized for only a limited period of time. Additional data are needed on the handling of antihypertensive medications by newborns and on their potential acute and chronic adverse effects. The long-term prognosis of infants with renal artery thrombosis is not known.

REFERENCES

1. Bauer SB, Feldman SM, Gellis SS, et al: Neonatal hypertension: A complication of umbilical artery catheterization. New England Journal of Medicine, 293:1032, 1975.

2. Plummer LB, Kaplan GW, and Mendoza SA: Hypertension in infants--A complication of umbilical artery catheterization. Journal of Pediatrics 89:802, 1976.

3. Adelman RD, Merten D, Vogel J, Goetzman BW, and Wennberg RP: Nonsurgical management of renovascular hypertension in the neonate. Pediatrics 62:71, 1978.

4. Adelman RD: Neonatal hypertension. Pediatric Clinics of North America, 25:99-110, 1978.

5. Sheftel ON, Hustead V, and Friedman A: Hypertension screening in the followup of premature infants. Pediatrics 71:763, 1983.

6. Dweck HS, Reynolds DW, and Cassady G: Indirect blood pressure measurement in newborns. American Journal of Diseases in Children, 127:492, 1974.

7. Frieson RH and Lichtor JL: Indirect measurement of blood pressure in neonates and infants utilizing an automatic noninvasive oscillometric monitor. Anesthesia and Analgesics, 60:742, 1981.

8. Pellegrini-Caliumi G, Agostino R, Nodari S, Maffei G, Moretti C, Bucci G: Evaluation of an automatic oscillometric method and of various cuffs for the measurement of arterial pressure in the neonate. Acta Paediatric Scandinavia, Sep. 71(s):791, 1982.

9. Lee YH, Rosner B, Gould JB, Lowe EW, and Kass EH: Familial aggregation of blood pressures of newborn infants and their mothers. Pediatrics, 58:722-729, 1976.

10. Versmold HT, Kitterman JA, Phibbs RH, et al: Aortic blood pressure during the first twelve hours of life in infants with birth weight 610 to 4220 grams. Pediatrics 67:607, 1981.

11. Moss AJ, Duffie ER, and Emmanouilides G: Blood pressure and vasomotor reflexes in the newborn infant. Pediatrics, 32:175-179, 1963.

12. deSwiet M, Fayers P, and Shinebourne EA: Systolic blood pressure in a population of infants in the first year of life. The Brompton Study. Pediatrics 65:1033, 1980.

13. Ibsen KK and Gronback M: Familial aggregation of blood pressure in newly born infants and their mothers. Acta Paediatrics Scandinavia, 69:109, 1980.

14. DeStefano P, Bongo IG, Borgna-Pignatti C, et al: Factitious hypertension with mineralocorticoid excess in an infant. Helv. Paediat. Acta. 38:185-189, 1983.

15. Hill A, Perlman JM and Volpe JJ: Relationship of pneumothorax to occurrence of intraventricular hemorrhage in the premature newborn. Pediatrics 69:144, 1982.

16. Gross RE: Arterial embolism and thrombosis in infancy. American Journal of Disease in Children, 70:61, 1945.

17. Zeulzer WW, Kurnetz R, and Newton WA: Circulatory diseases of the kidneys in infancy and childhood. IV. Occlusions of the artery. American Journal of Diseases in Children, 81:21, 1951.

18. Fyler DC, Buckley LP, Hellenbrand MD, et al: Report of the New England Regional Infant Cardiac Program. Pediatrics, 65 (Sup.) 375, 1980.

19. Goetzman BW, Stadalnik RC, Bogren HG, et al: Thrombotic complications of umbilical artery catheters: A clinical and radiographic study. Pediatrics, 56:374, 1975.

20. Lessman RK, Johnson SF, Coburn JW, and Kaufman JJ: Renal artery embolism. Clinical features and long-term followup of 17 cases. Ann. Int. Med, 89:477, 1978.

21. Merten DF, Vogel JM, Adelman RD, Goetzman BW, and Bogren HG: Renovascular hypertension as a complication of umbilical arterial catheterization. Radiology, 126: 751, 1978.

22. Lou HC, Lassen NA, and Friis-Hansen B: Is arterial hypertension crucial for the development of cerebral hemorrhage in premature infants. Lancet, i:1215, 1979.

23. Goddard-Finegold J, Armstrong D, Zeller RS: Intraventricular hemorrhage following volume expansion after hypovolemic hypotension in the newborn beagle. J. Pediatr. 100(s):796, 1982.

24. Baldwin CE, Holder TM, Ashcraft KW, and Amoury RA: Neonatal renovascular hypertension - a complication of aortic monitoring catheters. Journal of Pediatric Surgery, 16:820, 1981.

25. Adelman RD and Wright JS: The effect of chronic propranolol on the growth and endocrine function of newborn puppies. Clinical Research 32:90A, 1984.

PANEL DISCUSSION

Jose Strauss, M.D., Moderator

MODERATOR: We have with us experts from Japan, Central and South America, and many parts of the United States. One of the doctors who worked with us last year and presented a paper about renal artery and vein thrombosis in the neonate is here today. Would you like to start the session by commenting about your work?

COMMENT: Last year I worked on a study about renal artery thrombosis in the newborn and we found that in those patients, the most important findings were hypernatremia and decrease in platelets. Of course, hematuria and proteinuria were found, too. We found that most of these patients had renal artery thrombosis. We concluded that all patients with umbilical catheters had to be evaluated for this complication.

COMMENT: I would agree that any infant who has an umbilical artery catheter should have his or her blood pressure monitored while catheterized, and even after the catheter is removed. They certainly are at risk for developing renal artery thrombosis.

COMMENT: We should mention the ultrasound evaluation in these patients.

COMMENT: If we suspect that the patient has a renal artery thrombosis and has a catheter in place, we tend to prefer angiography. If they don't have a catheter in place and we think they have renal artery thrombosis, we tend to use a renal scan, usually the I-123 Hippuran Scan with computerization of the data. If we don't suspect that it is renal artery thrombosis, then certainly we want to evaluate the anatomy of the kidneys. I think from that standpoint, the ultrasound is quite useful. Most of us find intravenous pyelograms in the newborn a mess to evaluate. Obviously, if the renal structure is normal and there is no evidence of obstruction, we look for other etiologies of the hypertension and determine ketosteroids, hydroxysteroids and catecholamines. There are some individuals who claim they can actually look at the renal artery with ultrasound and see whether there are abnormal pulsations. We are not quite that skillful from the standpoint of the neonate. We don't use renal ultrasound if we think there is a renal vascular problem.

MODERATOR: To continue with that general subject, you mentioned that your IVP's sometimes don't confirm the suggestion of some obstructive process that the scan suggested. What is the truth? Which method is telling us the actual situation? We did a study here. Dr. George Sfakianakis, our expert on renal scans and various modalities other than IVP, was the Principal Investigator. We found actually that the renal scan was giving us the best information. When renal function seemed to be decreased, whenever we had questions, we would go to the renal scan and have findings that the IVP often missed or even couldn't visualize the kidneys because the renal function was decreased. Would you care to comment about how you would do the assessment of a patient with suspected renal problems beginning with fetal life? Again, on the ultrasound we seem to be having more and more diagnoses made of renal anomalies in utero, some of which are not confirmed after the baby is born. Can you talk about the pitfalls of the various approaches? How would you go about working up a patient if you were called today for some suspected anomalies? It's a very complex subject. You need 30 minutes but you have about 30 seconds!

COMMENT-RESPONSE: With regard to infants who have renal artery thrombosis, I think the scan is much more helpful than the IVP. The IVP in the newborn is not very helpful when looking at renal vascular disease. If we are concerned about an obstructive uropathy as a cause of hypertension, the IVP can be helpful from that standpoint, but again the scan is often very revealing and the ultrasound is often very helpful. Part of this depends upon how skillful the various people in a given institution are to interpret these modalities and it depends on how sick the infant is. The ultrasound is easy to use because we can get that done in the unit whereas if we are going to do a nuclear scan the infant has to be taken out of the newborn intensive care unit. So, if we are evaluating an infant with hypertension, I think the renal scan is more helpful than the IVP; if we are ruling out obstructions as an etiology of hypertension, I would tend to go with ultrasound first and then maybe a renal scan. I would be less likely to use an IVP. The problem with ultrasound and the prenatal diagnosis of obstruction is that we all have experienced what you have experienced. That is, we get a lot of referrals of infants who usually have a unilateral obstruction detected during pregnancy, the mother is warned that there may be surgery ahead. The baby is delivered, we repeat the ultrasound and it is completely normal. There have been articles in the literature cautioning us about being overly aggressive and overly pessimistic based on the intrauterine ultrasound. Certainly, these infants need to have adequate evaluation postnatally.

QUESTION: Everybody talks about hypertension playing a role in failure to grow. In some of these children, hypertension has been incriminated as a contributing factor to renal failure. What is your experience in the follow-up of these patients? Is there a link between growth failure and hypertension?

RESPONSE: We have all seen failure to thrive in hypertensive children who do not have renal insufficiency. It is quite striking in some of these children whose hypertension is related to a vascular disease. When you correct their hypertension, they have a growth spurt or will enter puberty. I don't know if there are data available on the role of hypertension per se in the patient with chronic renal insufficiency and its impact upon growth.

QUESTION: I noticed that two out of ten of your patients, 20%, have growth failure. Do they have metabolic acidosis? As you remember, there is a report from Israel in the Journal of Pediatrics of two or three cases in which after unilateral renal vein thrombosis, there was acidosis. We also have a paper in the Journal of Pediatrics in which we reported four patients with unilateral renal vein thrombosis who developed metabolic acidosis. In fact, we were able to diagnose Type IV renal tubular acidosis and also growth failure until we began using sodium bicarbonate to correct the metabolic acidosis. The question is, was there hyperchloremic metabolic acidosis in the two patients out of ten of yours who had growth failure?

RESPONSE: I am aware of your studies. One child has had an evaluation that suggested that metabolic acidosis was not present. The other child is having those determinations done at this very moment. So, by tomorrow I should know.

QUESTION: I also would like to ask a question concerning arteriograms. You convinced us about how useful the renograms are. What are the indications for the arteriogram? I am asking because I have a case in point. I have now in my hospital a newborn who has hypertension without urinary abnormalities , without elevated plasma renin or aldosterone levels but the 17 ketosteroids were a little high. We did not see hematuria or proteinuria. We did an ultrasound; it looks normal. There was no deformity of any side of the kidneys. At what point should we do an arteriogram or should we do the renogram since you so convincingly showed us that it is so useful?

RESPONSE: In our experience, there has been a good correlation between the computerized renal scan and angiographic findings. If a patient has a catheter in place, I think the angiography still gives a more definitive answer. But if he doesn't have a catheter in place, I certainly would do a renal scan. If that were normal, I would be reluctant to do angiography unless the patient had a rather severe, sustained hypertension. In that case, it might be worth doing an angiography. We have done it on a few infants in whom we've done percutaneous femoral angiography. But generally, the computerized scans correlated very nicely. We haven't found that necessarily with the regular renal scan. If we just eye ball both kidneys often we don't see dissimilarities. If we look at the renogram per se we often don't. But we get quantitative data back on the computerized scan that compare effective renal plasma flow, tubular transit time and hippurate transfer comparing the right to the left kidney. We can often see subtle asymmetries that were not detected just by a visual inspection of the scan.

QUESTION: I would like to go back to the earlier discussion. I was interested in what seems to be the remarkable lack of effect of changes in blood volume on blood pressure for the various reasons and mechanisms that were explained. Am I right in believing that all these were physiologic studies done in either normovolemic or hypervolemic animals or babies? Also, what is the significance of these studies in relation to individuals or babies who may be hypovolemic? I think this is of interest from the clinical standpoint because of the widespread practice of supporting hypovolemic infants with dopamine, with fluids and the like. From the physiologic standpoint, I want to ask: what may happen to the various alpha mechanisms as was outlined in babies or animals who are experimentally made hypovolemic?

RESPONSE: The status of the animals and the babies was euvolemic for age. In other words, nothing was done to them prior to initiation of the study. The studies that have been done in human infants are taken at wherever they are and for whatever had been done but the early studies which were mainly those of comparing early and late cord clamping (to study the effect of placental transfusion) were normal babies and most of them were term, a few preterm. The other studies in the human infants from Alabama were mainly normal premature infants compared with those with respiratory distress syndrome, many of which at that time were given high fluid therapy and volume expansion. So, the studies were done in animals that were euvolemic for age but, compared to older and more mature infants or animals, they were relatively hypervolemic, which is the characteristic state of the fetal and neonatal animal. The apparent reason for the infants to seem to be hypovolemic or contracted, with low blood pressure or persistent fetal circulation, whatever else the rationale for giving a lot of fluid may have been originally, was just an observation because no one has measured lower blood volumes in those infants. It's not that the blood volume is low but that the capacity of the vascular system or resistance may be increased. Capillary fill may be decreased not because of vasoconstriction and poor peripheral perfusion, but actually decreased because of maximum vasodilatation and very sluggish blood flow through those vessels. As far as support for giving lots of fluids, if you look at it in reverse, when studies compared higher fluid intake versus "normal" fluid intake, respiratory distress, patent ductus arteriosus, congestive heart failure, necrotizing enterocolitis, and bronchopulmonary displasia were higher with the higher fluid intake. The more fluid an infant received, the greater the morbidity and mortality. Then, when you look at studies comparing the incidence of symptomatic patent ductus, depending upon what is the fluid practice in the nursery, you will see that in some nurseries the incidence is as high as 70% of infants under 1200 grams and they will have symptomatic patent ductus arteriosus. Those are infants who are receiving 150 to 200 cc of fluids per kg per day. Regardless of whether they are on radiant warmers or what the insensible losses are, it seems to be the volume of fluid that is actually administered, not the volume lost, that determines results. When you tabulate each Neonatal Unit's practice for fluid therapy, you see the decrease in the incidence of symptomatic ductus arteriosus when there is less fluid intake. Some years ago, the incidence at some good places was bout 40%; our own incidence is 16% and our practice is to start with 65 ml/kg on the first day to permit a weight loss. When the other groups stopped the babies' blood tranfusion or giving packed cells as a push, their incidence of patent ductus dropped from 40% to about 25% just with the cessation of that particular practice. Volume is important. I always say that you cannot say ahead of time how much fluid an infant should receive; it depends upon his needs. I think part of the explanation is due to the peculiar responses of the newborn that are quite different from what we would anticipate and would have predicted from what we know about, what we would like to know about from adult studies. They just don't seem to work. Part of the answer is the difference in receptor density and affinity and the post-synaptic transmission of message. Transmission is an area of fascination which I think will continue to confuse us for a little while.

RESPONSE: The problem with those animal studies, as you know, is that they are done in the anesthesized state which might not be applicable to the human being who is not anesthesized. Along these lines, there is an abstract submitted to the Society for Pediatric Research this year which presents results obtained with infusion of different adrenergic agents into the renal arteries of chronically catheterized sheep fetuses. Obviously, they are supposed to be in a state similar to the natural state. The results with infusion of dopamine indicate that the younger the fetus, the smaller the effect of dopamine was and that the adult lamb had a little bit better response than the fetus. So, these different responses were still seen in the chronically unanesthesized animal and presumably in an euvolemic state since nothing was done to them.

RESPONSE: In the animal studies that we have done, we first did them in anesthesized animals and then, too, we have done them in the chronic animal preparation, the unstressed situation as well, and we find the same directional responses. They are quantitatively a little bit different but the same type of responses are apparent.

COMMENT: I'd like to make two points. First of all, it's critically important that we know what "normal" is. As was mentioned earlier, a lot of the efforts for volemic expansion in newborns occurred because we were uncomfortable with blood pressures that were in fact normal for some of these low birth weight infants. They may run systolic blood pressures of 35 to 40 mmHg and that is perfectly normal for them. There have been some studies in acutely volume depleted beagle puppies. In those studies, the blood was acutely withdrawn from the puppies until they became hypotensive; then, the same volume was reinfused rapidly. What they found was that not only did the blood pressure return to normal; it actually exceeded normal. They found an increased incidence of periventricular and intraventricular hemorrhaging in those beagle puppies. That data and data from others would suggest that in the acutely volume expanded animal, who may in fact be hypotensive for a variety of reasons, rapid changes in blood pressure may contribute to the cerebral hemorrhages that are so common in the very low birth weight premature.

MODERATOR: In terms of the placental transfusion touched upon earlier today, I would like to ask a few questions related to that and to the question just asked in terms of volume. Stan James, Karlis Adamson, Sahla Daniel and myself at Babies' Hospital in New York, studied neonates during the first few minutes after delivery, comparing placental transfusion to cesarian section and to other vaginal deliveries without placental transfusion. Then, when the effect of the transfusion subsided, we assessed the effect of an infusion of 5% glucose. We obtained similar increases in urinary output, GFR, renal blood flow, etc. with the placental transfusion as with the infusion of 5% glucose. I was discussing this with a distinguished Swede who is comparing the role of volume with the role of osmolality in the effects on the kidney of the neonate. Since we are talking about sodium today and we are not going to go back in such an extensive manner during the rest of the Seminar, can you elaborate on the role of volume versus osmolality, composition, sodium, etc.? I know that some of you maintain that volume is the evil in these changes and we are going to talk about the role of those factors on renal function. But, do we change the role of volume by changing the composition of the fluid we administer?

RESPONSE: Let me digress from that just one moment to respond to the previous comment. I want to clarify that those characteristics apply only to the experimental animal; the dog particularly has a large spleen which contains an enormous amount of blood. So, you have to withdraw about 40 to 50 cc/kg of body weight of whole blood before you get any significant drop in blood pressure. In response to a slow bleed (as the terminology is loosely used in the nursery), this gradual hemorrhage results in a gradual volume contraction, stimulation of renin release, and constriction of blood vessels by catecholamines and angiotensin II. When this blood is reinfused, you have a greater circulating blood volume in a constricted vascular space which has a reduced capacity.

The other thing, depending upon how the blood is handled, renin and substrate are available in blood that is withdrawn; when you transfuse a patient, particularly a renal failure patient, he will become markedly hypertensive during transfusion. So, there you are--angiotensin I is present in transfused blood, and with converting enzyme present, as soon as it is reinfused into a vasoconstricted space, you have a tremendous increase in blood pressure which could blow out the vessels and produce disruption of cerebral circulation. So, I think that's a little bit different than volume expansion of all comers: euvolemic for age or whatever you want to call that. We are dealing with volume of the blood related to volume of the steady state vascular space. So, its hard to extrapolate from one study to the other unless you are dealing with splenectomized dogs. That is something that is important to the understanding of at least canine cardiovascular physiology.

As far as what happens with volume, we heard this morning that there is a decrease in proximal tubular reabsorption or rejection of sodium, and that fluid from the proximal tubule is delivered more distally for reabsorption. Although there is increased distal reabsorption or distal avidity for sodium to be isotonically reabsorbed, its capacity is limited. There will be a tremendous effect on the total amount of sodium that's rejected from the nephron when proximal reabsorption is reduced. If you begin with a term infant whose blood volume is decreased, blood pressure is higher, it depends upon not the volume that you give, either 10, 20 or 30 cc/kg or whether it's 5% albumin or whole blood or crystalloid or whatever else. It depends upon the baroreceptor response or some other response of the cardiovascular system that sends the message to the kidney as to whether or not the sodium is excreted or retained. So, without knowing exactly what the status of that particular baby is, it would be difficult to forecast exactly what the response will be. You can take a newborn animal, a day old puppy, and he may excrete a sodium load like an adult. All of them don't behave like we have characterized one day old puppies to behave. Occasionally you will get an adult who will not excrete 50 to 100 % of the sodium load, as you would have predicted from the mean values of various studies. So, there are ways of getting an adult or an older animal to respond like a premature, and there are ways of taking an immature animal and getting it to behave physiologically like an adult. One of those manipulations has to do with the responses that are produced by changes in blood volume.

COMMENT: A moment ago you mentioned an experiment you did with Stanley James with the infusion of glucose in water. I would like to raise a question concerning the possibility of producing acidosis when you do that. As we all know, the acid-base status of an infant usually has a mean CO_2 of about 22 mEq/Liter instead of the normal CO_2 content in adults of about 26 mEq/Liter. So, if one should infuse glucose in water, as you mentioned, would there be increased risk of further dilution and causing dilutional acidosis, aggravating the mildly lower CO_2? As we all know, acidosis can cause vasoconstriction, and perhaps changing baroreceptor responses. In your studies or in other studies, was acid-base examined?

MODERATOR: We looked at the acid-base status; Dr. Daniel may recall more specific details. As I recall, we could not identify any differences among the various groups by acid-base status; so, I would venture to say that the placentally transfused babies were not necessarily different from the babies who were infused with the solution, but I would not swear that that was the case. The urinary response, the GFR and renal blood flow responses were not different. To me, that suggests an area worth looking into. In terms of volume--I tend to agree with the previous commentator; that is what we said in the papers (Pediatrics, 1981). It makes sense to me that probably the kidney or the body is geared more to protect volume than composition or osmolality. I don't know that that has been actively studied and proven to be so.

COMMENT: You are right. I don't think that this has been studied in newborns, as far as I know. In adults, it has been shown that indeed volume takes precedence over osmolality. This was done a long time ago. In the studies that we did, pH, pCO_2 and pO_2 were monitored so that they were kept from straying too far from normal, including those animals who were unanesthesized. The two comments here would be that we talk about volume and composition, then the area that comes would be the maturational status or patterns of water loading versus sodium loading. We all know that the ability of the newborn to excrete a water load presumably matures faster than the ability to excrete a salt load. This is one difference. The other is with regards to acid base; some showed that the ability of a newborn to excrete sodium given as sodium chloride load was less than that given as a sodium bicarbonate load. At that point, I think that they were examining mainly the difference between bicarbonate ion and chloride ion. I don't recall them monitoring pH changes.

MODERATOR: By the way, Dr. McCance studied that many, many years ago. He probably was one of the first ones to call attention to the difference in the way the kidneys handle sodium chloride versus sodium bicarbonate.

COMMENT: He also was one of the first to show that volume took precedence over hypernatremia in those adults exposed to high temperatures. Even after the hypernatremia was corrected, they continued to drink water to maintain their blood volume.

MODERATOR: Fantastic! He has been the first in so many things! Sometimes a very few cases or an occasional observation but he put it together in such a creative way.

COMMENT: This strikes me as very interesting. Even much earlier on, in Homer Smith's book From Fish to Philosopher, he mentioned that phylogenetically we would always conserve. According to his philosophy of evolution, as we swim from the salt water to the fresh water estuary, the first thing we would conserve is, in fact, volume. And then, in the land, further on, acid-base as we begin climbing the trees.

MODERATOR: I know that you are a great admirer of Homer Smith. You wrote a review for one of the clinical series where you quoted Dr. Smith. It really reflects the importance of the kidneys (with a slight exaggeration)! Would you like to make a comment about those studies on the renal handling of sodium?

RESPONSE: In those studies about bicarbonate loading and sodium, we just compared chloride and bicarbonate; we didn't look at pH. I can't comment so much on that. What the commentator said was right.

COMMENT: Regarding the question a few minutes ago about change in acid-base status with volume. There are two things that I have observed (not studied but observed). One is from the studies on the effect of volume expansion in an effort to raise blood pressure. In those babies that were volume expanded, a trend toward respiratory acidosis was observed in infants that were volume expanded, suggesting that the alveolar-capillary distance or diffusion was impaired and therefore, there was retention of CO_2 and more difficulty in oxygenation of the blood. So, a respiratory acidosis or impaired gas exchange may result from an increased pulmonary interstitial fluid. That's one thing. The other thing regards volume expansion. We are looking at a lot of things to see how volume affects sodium handling in puppies. One of the things we observed was that from the beginning, when our animals were stable and we were monitoring acid-base just to report stability of the animal, we noticed that there was a mild respiratory acidosis and that also there was a change in the urinary pH and bicarbonate excretion, going from an acid urine with very little bicarbonate to an alkaline urine with a rather large amount of bicarbonate. All this was associated at the same time with a decreased blood bicarbonate. So, there was a dumping of bicarbonate following volume expansion in the puppies and there was also a decrease in alveolar capillary gas exchange. We had a combined respiratory and metabolic acidosis. Those were the preliminaries for our other studies on what volume can do to bulk reabsorption in the proximal tubule (as we understand it right now, although it may take place somewhere else). Increased blood volume can do a lot more than raise blood pressure; it can change acid-base status, sodium chloride and sodium bicarbonate handling by the tubule, it can affect renal blood flow and GFR, and many other things, depending on what else is done with the baby or the animal.

COMMENT: I would like to add that it can also increase parathyroid hormone secretion.

COMMENT: It is not surprising because even a small change in ionized calcium content (as small as 0.1 mg/dl) is a stimulus for parathyroid hormone secretion. It all seems to tie in together so well. The calcium or calcium entry probably has something to do with blood pressure, too.

MODERATOR: I want to go back to some of the comments made in a previous session. Since we are talking about the effect of "load", would you care to elaborate on that? You were describing the way in which the premature baby handles sodium (fractional excretion or in general terms), with a tendency toward hyponatremia; and then a discrepancy arises when you show us that the response to a sodium load is not so great. What makes that difference?

COMMENT-RESPONSE: Actually, that is a question I always think about. Why is it that a premature infant who under "basal state" is a salt waster, and then, when you give a saline load, actually he retains the saline load. Why is it that he can not respond to a saline load better than an adult, since he is always excreting a lots of salt? My theory is as follows: if one were to compare a very premature to a full-term infant, in their ability to excrete a salt load, I venture to guess that the one with lower gestational age would excrete that load a little bit better. The reason why these "salt wasting" infants can not excrete a salt load as well as the adult is because the major mechanism for excretion of a salt load is related to the distal tubule and beyond. Therefore, when one is given a sodium load, one would expect the distal tubule to decrease its reabsorption of salt and water. In the premature infant, the factors which decrease that sodium load do not occur as much; therefore, the decrease that you would expect in the adult, does not happen. The premature baby is starting at a different level, and that level is not decreased any further, while an adult will decrease it to a greater extent. The difference is really in the degree of the response.

QUESTION: I would like to know if there is any reason to use indium-tagged platelets in the diagnosis of thrombosis of the aorta in the newborn. Since the renal arteries are very small, probably it would be difficult to make the diagnosis of renal artery thrombosis with this method. My second question is when severe thrombosis of the aorta is diagnosed, should one use thrombolytic agents? Since all patients who had hypertension in the newborn period showed no hypertension later on, suggesting that there is not too much residual damage from the thrombosis which often accompanies the hypertension, do we need to treat them with agents which have dangerous side effects?

RESPONSE: We haven't used any indium labeled platelet studies or iodine labeled fibrinogen studies to detect the size or location of thrombi. We haven't used thrombolytic agents either. Some people have proposed the use of lacal streptokinase but we haven't done that. Another question which comes up is whether or not there is any role for surgery in these patients; we've been impressed with the ability of the vessels of the newborn to become patent over time. Whether that is because of fibrinolytic mechanisms, collateral circulation, or recanalization, we really don't know. There have been some reports in the surgical literature proposing thrombectomy especially in patients with bilateral renal artery thrombosis. Again, I don't know whether or not we have the answer to that. I have been asked about two infants somewhere else, who had bilateral renal artery thrombosis, were treated conservatively, and eventually opened up and did well. But, what to do in those cases is still an unanswered question.

COMMENT-QUESTION: I would like to make a comment about the last question and to raise another question. It would be interesting to see if the pro-urokinase works out--whether that might be a safe agent to use with the already high risk of intracranial bleed. My question is how does the panel feel about long term control of hypertension as far as progression of other renal diseases? If I might use a case to illustrate my own bias, I have a child that I followed from age three months and is now about a year of age who initially presented with bronchiolitis but was found to have a very large cardiac silhouette. During the work-up, she had just pericardial effusion, no other cardiac disease. The effusion was a transudate and the etiology was a nephrotic syndrome. We biopsied this baby because her renal function was a third normal for her age; she had diffuse mesangial sclerosis, an unusual and interesting congenital nephrotic syndrome. She had severe hypertension. It was embarrassingly found at cardiac catheterization; she ran mean arterial pressures of about 90 to 110, very high, which required multiple medications to control. Other measures instituted were diet modification, high biologic protein, some restriction of her total protein intake, salt restriction, phosphorus restriction with phosphate binders and, again, blood pressure medication. I've been amazed to find that her 1/serum creatinine line for renal function has remained stable for the last 9 months rather than declining rapidly as one would expect for diffuse mesangial sclerosis. A long-winded statement to point out that control of hypertension may be an important factor in altering progression of renal diseases. I would like to ask the panel members how they feel about that.

RESPONSE: I agree.

RESPONSE-QUESTION: I also. Which anti-hypertensives did you use? Diuretics alone or were you forced to use other substances including propranolol?

RESPONSE: The child is on multiple medications including maximal doses of furosemide, hydralazine, propranolol, captopril and quinidine.

COMMENT: You are using everything known to man!

COMMENT: She would not control with any of the agents alone, unfortunately. Withdrawal of any agent results in her blood pressure going back up. She does control though, really with few side effects from all those medications.

QUESTION: Before you started the anti-hypertensives, did you have a chance to determine the plasma renin and the aldosterone in this child? It was at three months. Granted, it's very hard to do at that age.

RESPONSE: No. Retrospectively, I certainly wish that we had.

COMMENT: You would have a reportable case if you had all these variables. I think that you have succeeded very well in treating a very difficult child. Starting at three months with nephrotic syndrome!

QUESTION: Which do you think is more important: reducing the phosphate load on the kidney, the hyperfiltration, or the sodium?

RESPONSE-QUESTION: I think they are all important and you have just done extremely well in controlling all these variables. We all know that hypertension is one of the reversible causes of kidney failure and you have histologic evidence of chronic renal insufficiency and for the cause of hypertension. So, by controlling the hypertension and the phosphate intake, I think you have helped the kidneys. Do you have any evidence of hyperparathyroidism or renal osteodystrophy?

RESPONSE: She has just very mild hyperparathyroidism and I'm having to keep her phosphorus a little bit lower than I feel comfortable doing and her ionized calcium a little bit higher than I ordinarily do.

COMMENT: A maneuver that you did not comment on was the reduction in protein intake. From our adult colleagues, now the popular concept or hypothesis for prevention of deterioration of renal function and glomerular diseases is protein restriction before you reach end-stage. Exactly how we are going to manage that in pediatrics I don't know because if we believe that protein is necessary for growth and if protein is bad for renal parenchymal disease, we may have a conflict! For sure, we've got the basis for doing some studies. That's another mechanism that may have been involved in your success.

MODERATOR: I would like to enter a rather strong word of caution in that regard. I think that that is still an unproven hypothesis. I was told that remarks have been made on the relative or absolute unimportance of growth provided you protect the kidneys (assuming that you did end up protecting the kidneys). I would like to think that what we should do is protect the whole patient rather than just protect the kidneys. Obviously, it makes sense in renal disease to reduce protein intake. Now, when it comes to the neonate, what applies to the older child may not apply here. Again, Sahla Daniel and Dr. Sonaka at Babies' Hospital, myself, and Dr. James sent an abstract to the SPR comparing babies that were taking about four grams of protein per kilogram versus babies that were taking about two grams and there were no differences in GFR that we could detect in a small group of babies. Now, these were normal babies that were being studied for other reasons but we interpreted the statements that protein restriction would protect the kidneys as applying to the neonate (in whom growth is so important), as meaning that the kidneys of the neonate would behave as kidneys of the diabetic or the patient that has overt renal disease.

COMMENT: I want to affirm what you all have said. The previous question, if my memory is right, is the 10 million dollar question. I think that's the amount NIH is putting for studies to look into protein intake and renal deterioration. Conveniently, they have omitted the pediatric population because of I'm not sure what--that some rule supreme or are too ticklish to modify protein intake and deal with growth factors as well. But clearly, there are a lot of animal data. There are some human data in the Italian literature that suggests that protein restriction will help to change the curve of 1/serum creatinine with time. There are animal data as well from Colorado with regard to phosphate restriction. There also certainly are lots of data in the pediatric literature and the adult literature about the adverse effects of severe hypertension on renal function. I would echo what has just been said; I think you are doing a wonderful job with the patient you described. We look forward to hearing about this patient in another five years.

MODERATOR: For the record, I want to ask a question about the captopril used in the neonate. The question has come up as to whether those drugs which have been extensively used in older children are experimental in the neonate. Particularly about captopril, the side effects--lowering GFR and so on, have been reported. Do you have any comments, any words of wisdom?

COMMENT-RESPONSE: Not really. Most of the drugs we use in the neonate probably have not been authorized by the FDA for use in the neonate. We clearly do have to follow these patients carefully and look at short and long term adverse side effects. The captopril that we have used has been first of all in very low doses. I think you want to avoid an overshoot. Second, we have not been forced to keep our patients on anti-hypertensive medication for a long period of time; we are fortunate from that standpoint.

MODERATOR: What is you operational approach? Do you ask for informed consent as an experimental drug or do you use those drugs even though they have not been approved by the FDA for use in the neonates? Do you prescribe them as for any other patient?

COMMENT-RESPONSE: I actually don't use that much captopril. I tend to use hydralazine and propranolol based upon a dictum that somebody told me years ago: "Use the poisons that you are familiar with." We have had a rather long history of using those drugs in neonates and we feel somewhat more comfortable about their safety. I don't think enough data have been gathered in regard to captopril.

COMMENT: I think you would notice that in the recommendations we heard that captopril is never the drug of choice as a first line drug. You use it when you have to use it, when something that you are most familiar with has failed.

MODERATOR: Thank you.

EDITOR'S COMMENTS

This Panel Discussion touched upon areas of current interest with questions on anatomical and on purely physiological-hormonal-chemical causes of hypertension. The very important aspect of volume of the extracellular fluid and its relationship to a changing capacity of its continent, was emphasized. This clearly suggested that no fixed amount of fluids can be prescribed for a neonate, especially when he is under conditions which have been identified as increasing insensible water losses. Finally, discussed in a rather philosophical and pragmatic manner was the dilemma faced by pediatricians in general and neonatologists in particular, of needing to prescribe medications which do not have specific Food and Drug Administration approval for that given age. This lack of approval usually exists not because of side effects or undesirable complications but because of poor incentive for most pharmaceutical companies who, faced with a relatively small market in the pediatric age group, opt for the "trickling down effect" of gradual non-approved application based on the experience gained in treating adult animals and patients.

II

INTOXICATIONS - NEPHROTIC AGENTS

RISK FACTORS IN NEPHROTOXICITY

C. A. Vaamonde, M.D.

The majority of drugs commonly used in clinical practice have a low incidence of renal toxicity. In assessing the frequency of nephrotoxicity, it is clear that most renal injury tends to cluster around certain patients and specific clinical situations. Because nephrotoxicity may limit the clinical usefulness of many diagnostic and therapeutic agents, recognition of factors associated with a greater risk for renal injury is important [1-3].

The exact frequency of nephrotoxicity is difficult to assess. Discrepancies between animal and clinical studies, availability (initially) of only isolated case reports of toxicity, clinical trials that are uncontrolled or poorly designed, lack of uniformity in defining the criteria for nephrotoxicity,are some of the important factors responsible for our uncertainty about how frequent a specific nephrotoxicity is.

Of great importance is the criteria used for defining renal injury. It is obvious that the criteria should be quantitative. It is well established that glomerular filtration rate (GFR) will be decreased by more than 50 percent of its normal value when serum creatinine concentration increases above the range of normal (see Fig 1 for relationship between GFR and serum creatinine concentration). Blood urea nitrogen (BUN) concentration is much less reliable as an index of renal function (GFR) because of the added influence that protein intake and catabolism, and the urea renal tubular reabsorption associated with the body's state of hydration have on its concentration. It is thus important, to define exactly the increase in serum creatinine that will be used clinically to signal nephrotoxicity (increase of 0.5, 1.0 mg/dl, or more, above baseline value). However, serum creatinine levels should only be used in the context of the relationship outlined in figure 1. The use of serum creatinine increases alone,rather than percent decreases in endogenous creatinine clearance (Ccr) may lead to relative overdosage and nephrotoxicity (aminoglycosides). Since the actual measurement of Ccr in hospitalized patients may be fraught with problems (inaccurate urine collections, uncooperative patients, need for indwelling catheters), and the availability of the results necessary to appropriately prescribe or modify dosage, is usually delayed (laboratory reports are available 12 (at best) or 24 to 36 hours after completion of the urine collection), other more practical methods should be used.

For a rapid approximation of the GFR the formula proposed by Cockcroft and Gault [4] can be used. This formula takes into consideration the age, body size (as

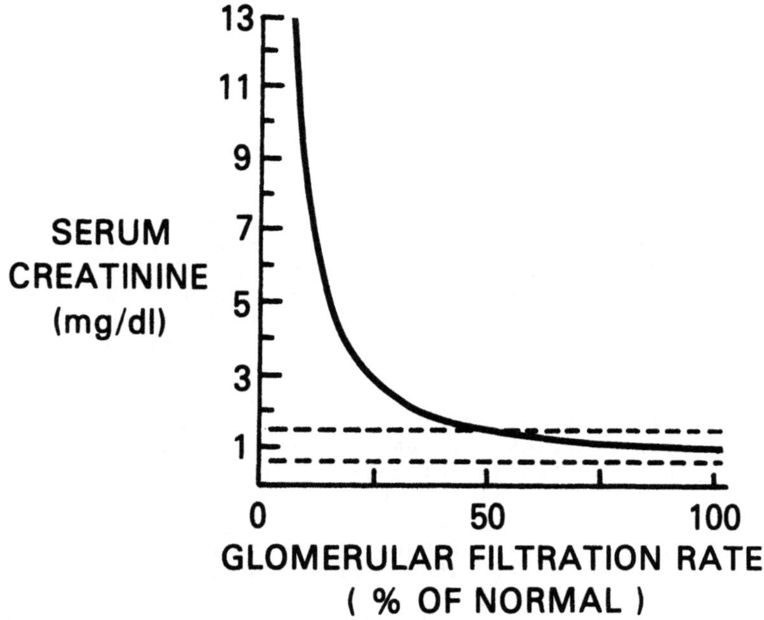

FIGURE 1. Relationship between glomerular filtration rate (GFR) and serum creatinine concentration. GFR is expressed as % of normal. Serum creatinine normal values are given as 0.5 to 1.5 mg/dl. (a) Note that serum creatinine levels will begin to increase when GFR decreases below 50 percent of normal. (b) Any factor (reversible or irreversible) affecting GFR at the normal end of this relationship needs to decrease GFR substantially before serum creatinine increases above the normal range. Factors of equal magnitude acting at the opposite (renal failure) end of this relationship produce rapid and sizable increases in serum creatinine, resulting in appearance of uremic symptoms. (c) Serum creatinine levels are influenced by the age, sex, and body built (lean body mass) of subjects.

assessed by body weight), and sex of the patient, in addition to the serum creatinine concentration (Table 1). Because renal function declines with age, and serum creatinine concentration depends on lean body mass (muscle), that varies with many circumstances (age, sex, body built,state of nutrition, disease), this formula provides an approximation of GFR. Because of over-estimation of GFR, however, the accuracy and practical value of this formula has been most recently questioned (Lerner, A., DeLos Angeles, A., Goldstein, S., Kramer, M., Raja, R.:

Correlation of predicted glomerular filtration rate (PGFR) with measured creatinine clearance and inulin clearance. Kidney Int., 27:145A, 1985). Until a rapid, reliable and practical method for the estimation of the GFR becomes available, great care should be exerted in clinically assessing GFR, when prescribing or modifying dosage of drugs which depend on GFR for excretion.

Table 1. Rapid Estimation of Creatinine Clearance (Ccr) by the formula of Cockcroft and Gault [4].

Men

$$\text{Estimated Ccr (ml/min)} = \frac{(140\text{-age})\ (\text{Body weight in Kg})}{72 \times \text{Serum creatinine in mg/dl}}$$

Women

$$\text{Estimated Ccr (ml/min)} = \frac{(140\text{-age})\ (\text{Body weight})}{72 \times \text{Serum creatinine}} \times 0.85$$

Serum creatinine concentration depends on lean body mass (muscle), a relationship which changes with age and body size. This formula [Cockcroft, D., Gault, M.H.: Prediction of creatinine clearance from serum creatinine. Nephron 16:31-41, 1976] permits an approximate correction of serum creatinine concentration for these factors. Since the formula was derived from observations on men only, the authors suggest to decrease the obtained value by 15% (multiply by 0.85), to correct for the different relationship between lean body mass and body weight in women.

As shown in Table 2, risk factors for renal injury may be patient-related, drug-related or the result of drug association or interactions. The later category is particularly important in seriously ill, complicated patients with multiple body systems failures, such as the patients usually treated in medical, surgical or pediatric intensive care units.

The question of the general susceptibility of the newborn or young infant to nephrotoxicity is far from resolved. Factors that a priori may be considered to increase this susceptibility are a lower plasma protein binding and prolonged half-life of drugs or toxins. The fractional plasma protein binding of many drugs is lower in infants than in adults (even after correction for the lower albumin levels of the former) [5,6]. It has been estimated that the half-life of any drug that is excreted only by GFR, such as inulin, would be prolonged in the young infant [7]. For any given dose, however, the expanded volume of distribution (due to the proportionally large extracellular fluid volume (ECFV) in infants) probably explains the prolonged t 1/2 of drugs or toxins at this age. As pointed out by Cafruny [8],the fact that the half-life of potential toxins is prolonged does not warrant the conclusion a priori that the

Table 2. Risks Factors in Nephrotoxicity

1. <u>Patient-related factors</u>
   Age, sex, race
   Prior renal insufficiency
   Specific diseases (diabetes mellitus, multiple myeloma, diseases with proteinuria, lupus)
   Sodium-retaining states (cirrhosis, heart failure, nephrosis)
   Dehydration and volume depletion
   Acidosis, potassium and magnesium depletion
   Hyperuricemia, hyperuricosuria
   Sepsis, shock
   Renal transplantation

2. <u>Drug-related factors</u>
   Inherent nephrotoxic potential
   Dose
   Duration, frequency, and form of administration
   Repeated exposure (i.e.,radiocontrast, anti-tumoral agents)

3. <u>Drug interactions</u>: Combined or closely associated use of diagnostic or therapeutic agents with added or synergistic nephrotoxic potential.
   - Aminoglycosides
   - Radiocontrast agents
   - Anti-tumoral agents (cisplatin, nitrosoureas)
   - Nonsteroidal anti-inflammatory agents
   - B-lactam antibiotics
   - Cyclosporin
   - Loop diuretics
   - Others (methoxyflurane, rifampin, amphotericin B).

risk of renal injury is increased. In fact, he advanced some justification for the concept that renal immaturity (or the particular level of morphological-functional development of the kidney) may constitute defense against renal injury [8]. A number of mechanisms may lead to a lesser exposure of renal cells to drugs or toxins in newborns and young infants. These are [8]: (a) the larger fractional ECFV resulting in larger volume of distribution and slower rate of renal excretion; (b) the reduced plasma protein binding resulting in more rapid delivery of drug to the kidney; (c) the lower GFR per glomerulus resulting in less drug in the nephron at any given time; (d) the limited proximal tubule active transport system for acids and bases, reducing the trapping in proximal tubular cells and decreasing the concentration of drug in the tubular fluid and urine; (e) a less efficient countercurrent multiplier system lowering the concentration of drugs in the renal medulla; (f) In addition, a delayed hepatic metabolism may slower renal excretion. Nevertheless, as attractive as this suggestion [8] may appear, further work is necessary to substantiate its implications.

The risk factors associated with the use of

radiocontrast media, aminoglycoside antibiotics, anti-cancer drugs and non steroidal anti-inflammatory agents will be considered in this review.

RISK FACTORS IN RADIOCONTRAST NEPHROTOXICITY

Acute renal failure is an uncommon but increasingly recognized complication of the use of iodinated radiographic contrast media. There is a growing awareness that its true incidence may be higher than previously thought (0 to 12 %), since only the more serious patients are seen by the nephrologists. This indeed has been our experience at the University of Miami Medical Center. A renewed attention has been given to this problem and numerous publications have appeared recently in major medical journals [9-13].

Renal dysfunction can occur following the administration of virtually any intravascular radiocontrast agent, and has been reported after urography, angiography, multiple dose cholecystography [14] and, most recently, computerized tomography with intravenous radiocontrast [13,15,16]. Of note, in a recent review seven of 23 patients who developed acute renal failure post-radiocontrast had been studied with computerized tomography [13].

In recent years a number of risk factors for the development of contrast media renal dysfunction have been identified (Table 3). Of those numerous risk factors, two are uniformly accepted as definite factors: pre-existing renal insufficiency and diabetes mellitus. Multiple myeloma, dehydration and prior contrast-induced acute renal failure are considered as probable risks. The remainder are controversial or less-likely to have a role. We will describe them in the order listed in Table 3.

Advanced age (60 years or older). Review of four recent series comprising 70 patients shows that 50 (71%) were 60 years of age or older [13]. It is not known if underlying vascular disease or progressive reduction in renal mass and renal blood flow associated with aging [17,18] are in part responsible. Since elderly patients are more likely to have other predisposing factors, such as diabetes and volume depletion, the contribution of advanced age alone to radiocontrast nephrotoxicity is unclear. It should be remembered, however, that serum creatinine in the elderly may not reflect the true level of GFR because of their smaller lean body mass (Fig.1., Table 1). Thus, a creatinine clearance should be obtained if possible, or GFR estimated by the Cockcroft and Gault formula (Table 1). It is possible that the higher susceptibility shown by elderly patients may be entirely related to a relative radiocontrast overdose due to an overestimation of their GFR.

Pre-existing renal insufficiency appears to be of great importance [19]. The majority of patients who develop radiocontrast nephrotoxicity have some degree of pre-existing renal insufficiency. In a recent study of the renal effects of angiography [20], patients with mild renal dysfunction (serum creatinine greater than 1.5 mg/dl) had a 6% incidence of radiocontrast-induced acute renal failure,

Table 3. Risk Factors in Radiocontrast Nephrotoxicity

Advanced age (60 years or older)
Pre-existing renal insufficiency *
Dehydration
Specific diseases Diabetes mellitus Multiple myeloma Vascular disease
Overdose (simple or multiple exposure)
Prior radiocontrast-induced acute renal failure
Epinephrine - assisted venography
Hyperuricemia, hyperuricosuria
Proteinuria

* Definite risk factor

whereas only 2% of those with normal renal function did. Similar results have been reported by others [9,11,13,21]. Of 129 patients with impaired baseline renal function summarized by Coggins and Fang [22] from eight studies from the current literature (1976-80), 72 percent developed nephrotoxicity after radiocontrast administration.

Dehydration, although not universally accepted as a risk [9,23], appears to contribute to renal impairment, particularly in susceptible patients [24-25]. Unfortunately, patients are usually kept hydropenic for many hours in preparation or during multiple x-ray studies. If follows, particularly in patients at risk, that a normal state of hydration should be assured in all patients prior to undertaken radiographic procedures.

The diabetic patient population has emerged as probably having the highest risk of developing contrast media renal dysfunction. This can occur whether the patients have normal renal function [26], pre-existing renal disease [11,13,15,16,23,27-29], were subjected to a major angiographic procedure or only computerized tomography with contrast [13,15]. A review of 88 reported patients with diabetes and radiocontrast-induced acute renal failure indicated that 89% had pre-existing renal insufficiency [13]. A more recent study [30], reveals that among 122 diabetic patients collected from the literature, 57% developed renal dysfunction after intravenous urography, and 91% of them had a serum creatinine level equal to or greater than 2 mg/dl prior to the radiographic procedure. Others, however, found that diabetes per se may not be a risk factor when patients were matched for pre-existent renal disease [20,21,30,31], and that diabetic patients without renal insufficiency appear not to have an exaggerated risk [21,30]. Experimentally, we have shown that the untreated diabetic rat with normal renal function did not exhibit enhanced sensitivity to the renal effects of radiocontrast media [32]. Others, have also found similar results [33].

Because a great proportion of diabetic patients are old, have renal disease, proteinuria, vascular disease, including hypertension, and may be dehydrated, it is mandatory in those patients to weigh very carefully the benefits to be derived from the radiographic studies against the definite risks. Whenever possible, alternate diagnostic procedures (ultrasound, computerized tomography without radiocontrast) should be prefered in the complicated diabetic patient.

Multiple myeloma is generally considered a risk factor; recent experience, however, casts some doubt about this [13,34]. Part of this controversy may originate in the multiplicity of causes potentially responsible for acute renal failure in patients with multiple myeloma. These include: hypercalcemia, hyperuricemia, dehydration, nephrotoxicity from other agents or the presence of prior renal disease (secondary to Bence Jones proteinuria, hypercalcemia, hyperuricemia, or amyloidosis). Although, the reported incidence of acute renal failure by retrospective evaluation is low, about 4 percent in more than 450 patients [22], great care should be exercised when performing radiocontrast studies in patients with multiple myeloma.

Other specific diseases, such as vascular disease, congestive heart failure and liver disease have been suggested as confering enhanced risk. There is no convincing evidence for the latter two. Peripheral vascular disease, nephrosclerosis and hypertension, however, are considered as possible risk factors by some [10,11,13,21], but they may only indicate the presence of other risk factors, such as pre-existing renal disease or diabetes.

The amount of radiocontrast media injected remains a controversial issue related to nephrotoxicity [10,13]. There are doubts if large doses of radiocontrast (greater than 2.5 ml/kg body weight or 0.9 g iodine per kg) in a single study may result in renal impairment in the absence of other risk factors. There is, however, general agreement that repeated radiographic studies performed in a short sequence (angiograms, IVP, renal venography, computerized tomography with contrast) may indeed, enhance the risk of nephrotoxicity. This has been our experience. Thus, it is very important to avoid large doses of radiocontrast (overzealous radiologists, second "passes" to obtain better X-rays, etc) or repeated studies without appropriate intervals (two or three days) between procedures.

It is not clear if patients with prior episodes of radiocontrast nephrotoxicity have an enhanced risk upon rechallenge with radiocontrast [9,13,27-29]. It is conceivable that those previous episodes may simply indicate the presence of other risk factors. A recent retrospective study [35] has suggested that epinephrine-assisted venography (EAV) is a more nephrotoxic procedure than renal angiography without EAV. EAV is a useful procedure for enhancing the visualization of the pheripheral renal veins in the diagnosis of renal cancer, inflammatory masses, pseudotumors, renal vein thrombosis, and other lesions.

Hyperuricemia and hyperuricosuria, although associated with radiocontrast nephrotoxicity may not be independent risk factors [13,36]. The current concensus is that proteinuria as a risk factor for radiocontrast nephrotoxicity is significant only as a marker of underlying renal disease (diabetes mellitus, multiple myeloma, nephrotic syndrome).

Radiocontrast-induced renal injury has been rarely reported in the newborn or infant [37,38].

Although, recent studies did not find an increased incidence of post-contrast media renal dysfunction [39-41], physicians should remain aware of this potential complication. Indeed, even in one if these studies [39], increased renal dysfunction was apparent in patients at risk. Furtermore, in another report [40],the lack of nephrotoxicity was attributed to careful, planned and aggressive hydration. Unfortunately, these authors did not follow their study beyond 24-hours post-angiography. Finally, in a recent prospective study [42], although no changes in GFR were detected in patients with or without prior renal insufficiency following renal arteriography, transient glomerular proteinuria and enzymuria were observed. The authors considered these findings as indicating tubular toxicity induced by radiocontrast [42].

In summary, the overwhelming risk factors related to radiocontrast nephrotoxicity are the presence of renal insufficiency and diabetes mellitus. Dehydration, because of its common occurrence, and age, because of usual underestimation of decreased renal function in the elderly are also important. Repeated exposure to radiocontrast in a short span should be avoided.

Figure 2 illustrates a typical case of radiocontrast-induced nephrotoxicity. The possible risk factors involved in this patient include: prior renal insufficiency, vascular disease and hypertension, congestive heart failure, age, dehydration (diuretics), and the concomitant use of other potential nephrotoxic agents: prostaglandin synthetase inhibitors (aspirin).

In general, contrast media-induced renal failure has a good prognosis. In some high risk patients, however, mortality may be as high as 5%-10% [13]. Some of these patients (diabetics with renal disease) may develop end-stage renal failure [23].

Prevention of this form of acute renal failure follows the same guidelines for nephrotoxins in general. Specific guidelines to prevent contrast media renal damage are outlined in Table 4. It has been suggested recently that prevention of renal failure may be achieved in diabetic patients at risk (older patients with pre-existing renal disease) by the administration of mannitol within one hour after intravenous pyelography [43-45].

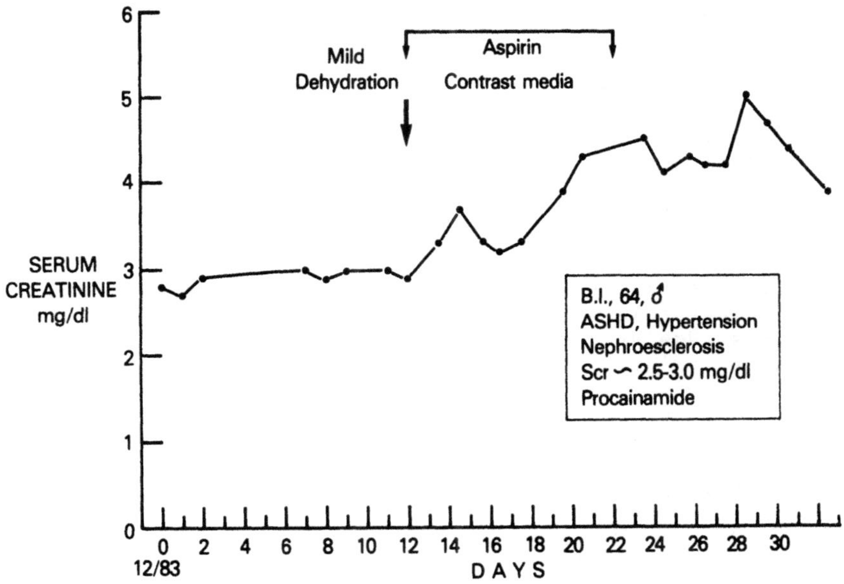

FIGURE 2. Risk factors in radiocontrast nephrotoxicity. A 64 year old patient with arteriosclerotic heart disease, mild hypertension and congestive heart failure, and renal insufficiency (serum creatinine concentration in the previous year ranged from 2.5 to 3.0 mg/dl) was admitted to the Miami VA Medical Center because of unstable angina. It was assumed that his chronic renal failure was secondary to hypertension and nephrosclerosis. In the 12 days preceeding the coronary angiographic study, his renal function remained stable, with a serum creatinine around 3 mg/dl. During this period he received thiazide diuretics and subsequently furosemide, and as judged by changes in body weight, it was possible that he was mildly dehydrated at time of angiography. Following the procedure (on day 12 with a standard dose of radiocontrast, and without procedural complications) there was an increase in serum creatinine within the first 24 hours. A decrease towards the pre-study level was observed by day 16, and a subsequent increase peaking at 5 mg/dl 10 days later. Subsequently, his serum creatinine decreased towards his baseline. It is not clear if aspirin (given from day 12 to 22) might have impaired renal function further by blocking renal vasodilator prostaglandins. The possible role of procainamide is unclear.

Table 4. Guidelines for the prevention of radiocontrast nephrotoxicity

1. Identification of patients at risk (renal insufficiency, diabetes, multiple myeloma)

2. Careful assessment of benefit of x-ray procedure against potential risk, particularly in high risk patients

3. Select other diagnostic procedures when possible (sonography, computerized tomography without contrast)

4. Avoid dehydration. This is mandatory in high risk patients: use vigorous hydration

5. Limit total dose of radiographic agent. Avoid multiple radiographic procedures within 24-hours or in subsequent days. Use epinephrine-assisted venography with great care

6. If hyperuricemia and hyperuricosuria use vigorous hydration and allopurinol

7. In high risk patients try mannitol

RISK FACTORS IN AMINOGLYCOSIDE NEPHROTOXICITY

Because nephrotoxicity may limit the clinical usefulness of aminoglycoside antibiotics recognition of factors associated with a greater risk for renal injury is important [1-3]. These risk factors are listed in Table 5.

Patient-related factors

Age. Advanced age often has been suggested as a risk factor for aminoglycoside toxicity in retrospective studies [46]. Not taking into consideration the patient's age and body size will result in a tendency to overdose older atients (Table 1, Fig 1). Indeed, two prospective studies using serum aminoglycoside levels as dosage guides have found no significant relationship between nephrotoxicity and age [47,48]. In addition, because older patients have a lower Ccr for each value of serum creatinine, they will be more likely to show an increase in serum creatinine after a renal injury than will younger patients. Therefore, Smith and Smith [3] have concluded that the false assumption that age itself is an independent risk factor for aminoglycosides is due to: (1) failure to use appropriate control groups, (2) overdosing of elderly patients based on serum creatinine levels, (3) failure to measure serum aminoglycoside levels, and (4) bias in ascribing nephrotoxicity caused by use of serum creatinine increases, rather than percent changes in Ccr, as the definition of toxicity. Nevertheless, these authors have recently reported that age correlated with gentamicin nephrotoxicity in a study of 214 patients

Table 5. Risk Factors in Aminoglycoside Nephrotoxicity *

<u>Patient-related factors</u>	
Age†	Potassium depletion
Prior renal insufficiency†	Magnesium depletion
Dehydration and volume depletion §	Liver disease
<u>Drug-related factors</u>	
Inherent nephrotoxic potential §	
Dose §	
Duration and frequency of administration §	
<u>Drug interactions</u> (drugs with a synergistic effect on aminoglycoside nephrotoxicity)	
Synergism strongly supported	
Cephalothin	
Cyclosporin A	
Probable association (unproven synergism)	
Cisplatin	Methoxyflurane
Other cephalosporins	Loop diuretics ‖
Nonsteroidal anti-inflammatory agents	Amino acids
<u>Unproven factors</u>	
Sex	Renal transplants
Metabolic acidosis	Shock
Prior aminoglycoside exposure	

* Modified from Vaamonde [1]
† Because of overestimation of GFR resulting in overdosing
§ Most important clinically
‖ Secondary to volume depletion

utilizing multivariate stepwise discriminant analyses [49].

Gentamicin renal damage is noted less often in <u>neonates and children</u> than in adults, althoug it may occur with prolonged therapy. Recent experiments in neonates [50] and puppies [51] have demonstrated that renal tubular damage (enzymuria, morphologic changes) may occur during gentamicin administration despite normal serum creatinine levels. It was suggested [51] that the normal redistribution of renal blood flow from deeper to superficial glomeruli that occurs after ten days of life in the dog,served to minimize gentamicin accumulation and damage to superficial nephrons and to preserve function. Younger rats accumulated less gentamicin in the kidney than adult animals receiving the same dosage of the aminoglycoside [52]. Furthermore, sexually immature rabbits treated with gentamicin did not develop acute tubular necrosis despite similar serum and renal tissue gentamicin levels in comparison to sexually mature animals (54% incidence) equally treated [53].

<u>Prior renal insufficiency</u>. The evidence supporting prior renal insufficiency as a risk factor is also flawed by methodologic problems [3]. Since excretion of gentamicin is very closely related to the GFR, the same considerations discussed above apply to patients with pre-existent renal

failure. Thus, unless aminoglycoside serum levels are used to adjust dosage, these patients are prone to overdosage. Although there are studies reporting a greater likelihood of increases in serum creatinine during aminoglycoside treatment in patients with pre-existent renal disease [46,47], three prospective studies could not find an increased risk with prior renal insufficiency [49,54,55].

Dehydration and volume contraction. Bennett et al [56] demonstrated that a low-sodium diet markedly increased gentamicin nephrotoxicity in the rat. This nephrotoxic potentiation was attributed to a higher renal cortical accumulation of gentamicin [56-58]. Other investigators have found increased renal dysfunction with intravascular volume depletion [59] or diuretic-induced natriuresis [58]; or, they suggested that chloride, rather than sodium depletion, is important [60]. High sodium intake [56], deoxycorticosterone acetate (DOCA)-saline or furosemide-induced sodium chloride diuresis [61], or sodium bicarbonate administration [62,63] failed to produce a functional or morphologic protective effect. The importance of volume depletion (usually diuretic-induced) was also demonstrated in a prospective clinical study [55]. A 46% incidence of aminoglycoside nephrotoxicity was found in patients with volume depletion, as compared with a 6% incidence in those without volume contraction ($P < 0.005$).

Potassium and magnesium depletion. Potassium and magnesium depletion have been suggested as risk factors for experimental aminoglycoside nephrotoxicity [64-66]. Since the clinical counterpart of these findings is not known, it seems prudent to maintain normal body stores of these cations in patients receiving aminoglycosides.

Liver disease. Two recent studies suggest increased susceptibility to aminoglycoside nephrotoxicity in patients with liver disease [49,67].

Drug-related factors

The type of aminoglycoside prescribed, the dose, duration of treatment, and frequency of administration are the most important determinants of aminoglycoside-induced nephrotoxicity.

Inherent nephrotoxic potential of aminoglycosides (Comparative nephrotoxicity. The factors determining the different nephrotoxic potential of aminoglycosides are incompletely understood, but they may relate to their intrinsic characteristics, degree of renal cortical accumulation, or other unknown factors. The former include: (a) the number, charge orientation, or position of the NH2+ groups [68],(b) an inherent propensity of the aminoglycoside molecule to cause toxic injury to intracellular organelles independent of the renal cortical levels [69,70], and (c) different transport rates for reabsorption and secretion in different nephron populations [71,72] or nephronal segments [73].

Comparative nephrotoxicity. Smith and Lietman [74] have summarized data from 24 prospective, controlled clinical trials reported in the British literature since 1969. The value of the majority of the studies is limited by failure to: (a) use a standard dosage and duration of therapy; (b) evaluate toxicity in an unbiased manner; (c) define nephrotoxicity uniformly; (d) frequently monitor renal function during and after therapy; (e) differentiate patients with other causes of acute renal failure from those with aminoglycoside-induced nephrotoxicity, and (f) enroll sufficient numbers of patients to draw meaningful conclusions.

Clinical comparisons have shown that tobramycin has the same or a lower toxicity than gentamicin [75-77]. Smith et al [77] reported that nephrotoxicity occurred in 26% of patients treated with gentamicin, but in only 13% of patients receiving similar dosages of tobramycin ($P < 0.025$). Sisomicin [74] and amikacin have no greater nephrotoxicity than gentamicin [78], whereas netilmicin appears to have toxicity similar to that of tobramycin [74,79].

A summary of the relative experimental aminoglycoside nephrotoxicities in rats derived from several studies [70,80-84] reveals the following rank order (from most to least):neomycin > gentamicin > sisomicin, kanamycin, and amikacin > tobramycin > netilmicin > streptomycin. The different results observed between some clinical and animal studies of comparative nephrotoxicity, such as those of tobramycin versus netilmicin, may be explained by the different species analyzed or by the rat strain used (the Fischer 344 rat being more sensitive to aminoglycosides).

It is apparent that (except for streptomycin) the degree of drug accumulation in the renal cortex does not correlate consistently with the differences in nephrotoxic potential of aminoglycosides. However, it is necessary to consider that in many studies, renal cortical aminoglycoside levels were measured a few or several days after commencing aminoglycoside administration; thus, cellular necrosis and regeneration may have interfered with the measurements. Furthermore, it is conceivable that the very initial cortical aminoglycoside concentration may be of crucial importance in determining cellular injury.

Dose. A strong correlation between the daily and total aminoglycoside dose and toxicity has been easily and consistently demonstrated in animal experiments [70,81,85,86]. Clinical studies using doses lower than 3 mg/kg/day for gentamicin or tobramycin demonstrated a clear relationship between dose and nephrotoxicity [1, 87]. Negative reports have corrected the aminoglycoside dosage according to increased blood levels [54,78]. At higher dosages (>4.5 mg/kg/day), such as those used to treat severe sepsis, the correlation has not been as good,perhaps, because the dose-response curve for toxicity is relatively flat in this dosage range or because of other confounding clinical events [3].

Duration and frequency of administration. Clinical studies have established that duration of therapy, usually beyond 10 days, is a risk factor for aminoglycoside nephrotoxicity [1,54]. Although a threshold duration of therapy has not been defined before which aminoglycoside nephrotoxicity does not occur, renal damage is unusual before 5 to 6 days of treatment. Animal studies have clearly established an increased toxicity with frequent administration of aminoglycoside [88,89]. However, the relationship between frequency of administration and nephrotoxicity has not yet been appropriately evaluated in patients [1]. It appears that aminoglycosides given to experimental animals in a continous infusion may be more nephrotoxic than similar daily doses administered intermittently [90]. For any given aminoglycoside, a relationship between dose, serum levels, and renal tissue concentrations has been suggested by Schentag et al [91] and others [87] as accounting for individual patient differences in susceptibility to nephrotoxicity. However, this attractive hypothesis remains to be conclusively proven.

Aminoglycoside drug interactions

Many drugs with potential nephrotoxicity of their own are used in combination with aminoglycosides and other antibacterials, particularly in very ill patients (Table 5). These may produce added or increased (synergism) nephrotoxicity. Methoxyflurane [92], cisplatin [93], amphotericin B [94], clindamycin [95], cephalosporins other than cephalotin (for example, methicillin or cephaloridine) [96] all have been reported as adding to the nephrotoxicity of aminoglycosides; but, they appear not to exhibit a synergistic action.

Concomitant use of radiographic contrast agents also should be suspected until proven to be unrelated. Loop diuretics increased nephrotoxicity in animal studies [58,60,97]; two clinical studies, however, could not find augmented toxicity [54,55]. In addition, loop diuretics given to healthy volunteers increased the renal clearance of gentamicin during the period of diuresis without influencing either the GFR or the distribution of gentamicin [98]. Nevertheless, because of the effect of volume contraction on aminoglycoside nephrotoxicity [56-58], it is necessary to use them carefully. Inhibition of prostaglandin synthesis with indomethacin increased aminoglycoside-induced nephrotoxicity in the rat. This finding suggests the possibility of a protective role for prostaglandins in this experimental model [99]. The consequences of giving nonsteroidal anti-inflammatory drugs to patients treated concomitantly with aminoglycosides are not knwon.

There is convincing clinical evidence that cephalotin in combination with aminoglycosides causes nephrotoxicity [1,47,96]. This was not seen when the combination was used in patients with mild infections [100]. In experimental animals, cephalotin did not influence [101] or protect from aminoglycoside nephrotoxicity [102,103]. It has recently been reported that significant renal failure can occur when gentamicin and cyclosporin A are used together in patients with bone marrow transplants [104]. When the two drugs were given simultaneously to rats, cyclosporin A induced a synergistic enhancement of gentamicin nephrotoxicity [105].

Unproven risk factors

Sex. Gentamicin nephrotoxicity is greater in male rats than in females of the Fischer 344 strain [106]. In the same strain of rat, gentamicin induced acute tubular necrosis in males and acute tubulo-interstitial infiltration in females [107]. We have been unable to confirm these observations in the Sprague-Dawley rat [108]. One prospective clinical study found no sex-related influences [54], while another reported a higher incidence in women [49].

Other. There is no conclusive clinical evidence that metabolic acidosis [109], prior aminoglycoside exposure or nephrotoxicity [3], and renal transplantation per se [3] constitute risk factors. There is no surprise that in patients with shock (usually secondary to severe gram negative sepsis) there is a greater frequency of aminoglycoside nephrotoxicity [49,51]. Only one study [49], however, has suggested shock as an independent risk factor. Further work is necessary to confirm the finding that concomitant administration of cationic amino acids to rabbits results in enhanced aminoglycoside nephrotoxicity [110]. The implications for patients receiving hyperalimentation and aminoglycosides are obvious.

Figure 3 illustrates a typical example of gentamicin-induced nephrotoxicity. The possible risk factors involved were overdosage, prolonged duration of therapy, failure to monitor serum aminoglycoside levels in the presence of increased risk, and a questionable role for the cephalosporins. The large majority of patients with aminoglycoside-induced acute renal failure recover. The prevention of aminoglycoside-induced nephrotoxicity follows the same general guidelines recommended for potentially toxic drugs (Table 6).

Table 6. General guidelines to prevent antibiotic-induced nephrotoxicity

1. Be aware of nephrotoxicity
2. Identify patients at risk (elderly, shock, liver disease)
3. Avoid dehydration maintaining an expanded extracellular fluid volume
4. Adjust dose of aminoglycoside to the continued changes in GFR (serum creatinine (Table 1), endogenous creatinine clearance). If possible,limit therapy to less than 10 days
5. Check frequently aminoglycoside serum levels, particularly in patients with severe infections and in patients with impaired renal function (gentamicin: peak not > 10 ug/ml; through not > 2 ug/ml).
6. Avoid or use with caution combination of drugs (other aminoglycosides, cephalosporins, methoxyflurane, furosemide, radiographic contrast media, chemotherapeutic agents, nonsteroidal anti-inflamatory drugs)
7. Be aware of the increased risk in elderly patients
8. Rational indication of potentially toxic antibiotic prescription

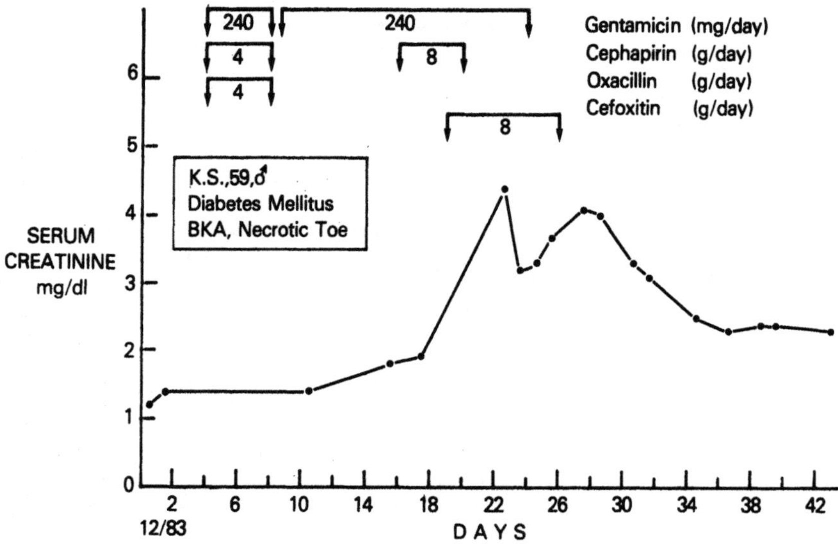

FIGURE 3. Risk factors in aminoglycoside-induced acute renal failure. A 59 year old patient with long standing type II diabetes mellitus and unilateral below the knee amputation was admitted to the Miami VA Medical Center because of a necrotic toe. He had a serum creatinine concentration during the first 10 days in the hospital of less than 1.3 mg/dl. He was started on full-dosage of gentamicin (80 mg every 8 hours) and he also received cephapirin and oxacillin (4 g/daily). Serum creatinine levels began to rise after 12 days of treatment and peaked at day 22, reaching a value of 4.5 mg/dl. At this time,he was seen by the nephrology service and the antibiotic treatment was discontinued. Subsequently renal failure improved slowly. Note (a) That serum creatinine in this patient increased definitively on the 12 day of treatment (a delayed onset of clinically apparent renal failure is common in gentamicin nephrotoxicity). (b) The serum creatinine levels, within the range of normal on admission, gave no assurance that this diabetic patient had a normal GFR. (c) Because of this, it is possible that at the onset he received a relatively large dose of gentamicin. Certaintly, this was the case after day 10, when GFR was decreasing progressively and he became overdosed in absolute terms. (d) Recovery of renal function remained incomplete after more than two weeks without antibiotic therapy (slow recovery is commonly seen in gentamicin acute renal failure, particularly in elderly patients). (e) The possibility that the concomitant administration of cephalosporin(s) might have adversely influenced the nephrotoxicity of gentamicin cannot be excluded.

RISK FACTORS IN ANTINEOPLASTIC DRUGS-INDUCED NEPHROTOXICITY

During the last two decades a number of antineoplastic drugs have received extensive clinical trials for the treatment of a variety of malignancies. Many of these agents have been shown to be associated with varying degrees of renal dysfunction and damage (Table 7). In addition to acute and chronic renal failure, prerenal azotemia, hypercalcemia, hyperuricemia, hyponatremia, hypocalcemia and hypomagnesemia have been described. Cyclophosphamide, for example, has been associated with the development of the syndrome of inappropriate antidiuretic hormone secretion, and acute renal failure has been reported following administration of methotrexate and streptozotocin.

Table 7. Renal dysfunction and body fluids abnormalities associated with antineoplasic agents

1. Severe and protracted ECF volume contraction (pre-renal azotemia)
   - Nausea and vomiting
     - Cisplatin *
     - Streptozotocin *
     - Dactinomycin
   - Diarrhea
     - Cisplatin *
     - 5-Fluoracil
     - Methotrexate

2. Hypercalcemia and hyperuricemia

3. Hyponatremia and fluid retention
   - Syndrome of inappropriate secretion of ADH
     - Cyclophosphamide *
     - Vincristine
     - Vinblastine

4. Acute renal failure
   - Cisplatin *
   - Nitrosoureas *
   - Methotrexate
   - Streptozotocin

5. Chronic renal failure
   - Cisplatin *
   - Nitrosoureas *
   - Mytomycin C

6. Other electrolyte abnormalities (cisplatin)
   - Magnesium depletion
   - Hypocalcemia
   - Hypokalemia
   - Salt wasting

* Clinically most important

The knowledge related to risk factors associated with antineoplastic drugs is more limited than that available for aminoglycosides or radiocontrast agents. We will only describe here cisplatin-induced acute renal failure.

Cisplatin is an inorganic platinum compound active against tumors, particularly testicular and ovarian, in addition to bladder, and head and neck carcinomas. The main limiting factor in the clinical use of the drug is the renal toxicity. Dose-related acute tubular necrosis has been described in a number of recent reports [111-115]

Dose. There is convincing evidence to indicate that the incidence of cisplatin-nephrotoxicity increases both with total dose (usually limited to less than 100 mg/m2, preferably 60 mg/m2, per treatment) and duration of treatment [114,116], and thus,with the total exposure to cisplatin. Chronic decreases in GFR have been reported in patients under treatment with cisplatin and followed for up to two years [117].

Age. It is generally assumed that elderly patients tolerate chemotherapy more poorly than younger patients, and thus, that their susceptibility to renal dysfunction may be increased. This is based in the known decrease of renal function with age. In addition, GFR may be overestimated in the elderly (see Introduction, Table 1). Furthermore, in patients with cancer and severe body wasting due to loss of lean body mass, the serum creatinine concentration may not be elevated despite a decreased GFR [117],because of the dependence of creatinine synthesis on the decreased muscle mass. Since this decreased renal function in the elderly limits the total dose of cisplatin that can be safely administered, and because it would appear beneficial to provide full-dose therapy regardless of age, to increase the chance of remission or cure, the recent study of Hrushesky et al [118] is of importance. These authors found a lack of age-dependent cisplatin nephrotoxicity. Older and younger patients with two kidneys had an equal, progressive, dose-related deterioration of renal function [118]. Of great interest, patients with only one kidney (uninephrectomy, total obstruction due to cancer) and lower pre-treatment GFR, did not show a further decline in renal function with cisplatin [118].

Pre-existent renal failure. There is very limited information on the effect of cisplatin in patients with pre-existent renal disease [114]. It has been assumed, however, that this is a risk factor,and perhaps a relative contraindication to cisplatin therapy, because the dose modification is not known [115]. The fact that cisplatin has been used with success in patients with obstructive uropathy secondary to ovarian carcinoma [119], and the findings described above [118], are however, reassuring.

Dehydration-hydration. There is substantial evidence that correction of preexistent dehydration, and administration of the drug with a vigorous hydration program diminishes cisplatin nephrotoxicity. Vigorous hydration has diminished both the indicence and severity of nephrotoxicity, without apparently affecting the therapeutic response, and, unfortunately, the extrarenal side-effects (severe nausea and vomiting) [120-122]. Hydration has been performed with saline, glucose, mannitol and diuretics in various combinations. Vogl et al, for example, have been able to reduce nephrotoxicity (which for the most part was mild) to 5% in 158 cancer patients treated with cisplatin, using a combination of hydration (2 liters of normal saline with glucose) and diuresis (mannitol) before and concomitantly with cisplatin [123]. Other regimens can be found in a recent review [124].

Of interest, is the protective effect of chloride-rich vehicles against cisplatin-nephrotoxicity. At equilibrium, the proportional distribution of total platinum between different complexes depends upon chloride concentration, and to a lesser extent, upon pH. Since low concentrations of chloride facilitate the conversion of cisplatin to cytotoxic species in aqueous solutions, the effect of hypertonic chloride solutions in protecting against cisplatin nephrotoxicity was tested in animals [125] and man [126]. Hypertonic saline provided protection against nephrotoxicity, without influencing the nonrenal toxicities of cisplatin in patients with testicular cancer treated with high-dose cisplatin (200 mg/m2) [126].

<u>Interaction with other nephrotoxins</u>. Cisplatin nephrotoxicity is enhanced by the simultaneous administration of other nephrotoxic agents ,such as gentamicin or other aminoglycosides [113,117,127]. Of particular importance appears to be the association of cisplatin with gentamicin and cephalothin. Four patients such treated developed severe and extensive acute tubular necrosis,which persisted until death occurring within few days to two weeks of this combination therapy [113].

It has been reported that probenecid could ameliorate cisplatin-induced nephrotoxicity in rats [128]. A recent report, however, urges caution in the use of such combination in patients, since the authors [129] found an enhanced nephrotoxicity in the rat with cisplatin plus probenecid. The decrease in renal function induced by cisplatin can influence also the toxicity of drugs excreted by the kidney, but without intrinsic nephrotoxicity. Cisplatin renal dysfunction was associated with an enhanced bleomycin-induced pulmonary toxicity [130].

Figure 4 illustrates a typical cisplatin-induced nephrotoxicity in a patient with metastatic laryngeal carcinoma. The possible risks factors in this patient are : (a) the severe wasting state, probably resulting in a low serum creatinine concentration, but within the range of normal in a patient with reduced GFR (data not available); (b) renal disease with nephrotic syndrome: biopsy-proven membranous glomerulopathy of unknown etiology; (c) the dose given was within the accepted therapeutic range, and it was administered with a vigorous hydration protocol.

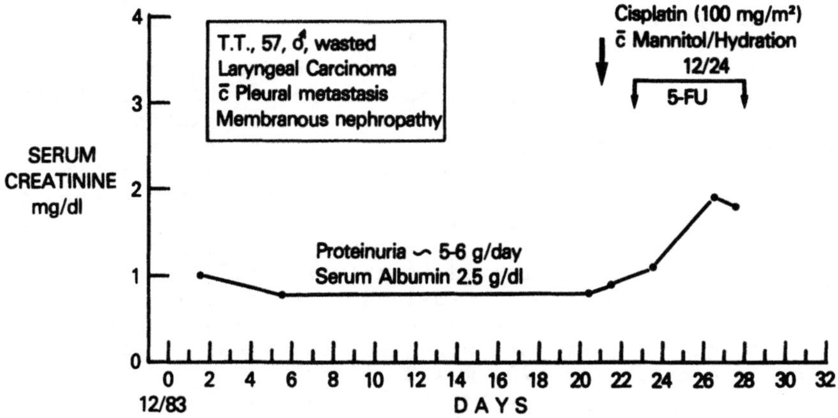

FIGURE 4. Risk factors in cisplatin nephrotoxicity. A 57 year old patient with metastatic laryngeal carcinoma was admitted to the Miami VA Medical Center for chemotherapy. He presented with severe muscular wasting. He had renal biopsy-proven membranous glomerulopathy with nephrotic syndrome (serum albumin was 2.5 g/dl and proteinuria 5 to 6 g per day). Note that during the first three weeks in the hospital his serum creatinine concentration was less than 1 mg/dl. However, because of the severity of his muscle loss and the presence of renal disease, these values (within the range of normal) overestimated the true reduction of his GFR. This is probable the reason for the rapid, but modest increase in serum creatinine following treatment with standard doses of cisplatin (100 mg/m2), given together with vigorous hydration with saline, glucose and mannitol during the 12 hours preceeding and 24 hours after the cisplatin infusion (12/24). It appears that 5-fluorouracil (5-FU), which he received for 5 days, is devoid of nephrotoxic effects. Thus, a relative overdose is the most likely explanation for the transient acute renal failure after cisplatin.

RISK FACTORS IN NONSTEROIDAL ANTI-INFLAMMATORY DRUGS (NSAIDs) NEPHROTOXICITY

The new category of drugs recently added to the enlarging list of nephrotoxins with clinical relevance are the NSAIDs. Few issues have raised more controversy than agreement on their safety or the true incidence of the renal abnormalities associated with their use. These drugs are used by an estimated 20 to 40 million persons in the USA [131,132].

It is generally agreed that the NSAIDs act by inhibiting renal prostaglandin synthesis [133,134]. Prostaglandin E2 (PGE2), a renal vasodilator and antagonist of the hydroosmotic effect of antidiuretic hormone,is synthesized in renal medullary interstitial cells. Prostacyclin or prostaglandin I2 (PGI2), a potent renal vasodilator, is synthesized in the walls of afferent arterioles and in the glomerulus. The kidney also forms small amounts of PGF2α, a PG with little intrinsic renal activity, and thromboxane A2, a potent vasoconstrictor [133, 134]. The NSAIDs appear to act primarily by inactivating the enzyme cyclo-oxigenase, decreasing the formation of PGH2 from arachidonic acid, and thus, subsequently of PGE2, PGF2α, etc.

Several types of renal abnormalities with important clinical implications have been described as resulting from prostaglandin inhibition (Table 8). The exact frequency of

Table 8. Potential renal abnormalities resulting from prostaglandin inhibition

1. Acute renal failure in disorders with decreased baseline renal blood flow secondary to enhanced renal vasoconstriction (hepatic cirrhosis, congestive heart failure, glomerulonephritis, shock, salt depletion or restriction).

2. Acute tubulo-interstitial nephropathy and glomerulonephritis (proteinuria, nephrotic syndrome) due to direct nephrotoxicity.

3. Hyperkalemia due to suppression of the renin-angiotensin-aldosterone system.

4. Sodium and water retention (with weight gain, hypertension, edema, hyponatremia) due to interference with the action of diuretics.

these abnormalities is unknown. Two major factors influencing the frequency of reports have been recognized: the population of patients at risk, and the physicians involved with the reporting. Nephrologists tend to see complicated, referral patients,and rheumatologists report on large number of patients with arthritis receiving NSAIDs. Many isolated reports of reversible acute renal failure [134-139], nephrotic syndrome and tubulo-interstitial nephropathy [134, 139-141], decreased renal function in edematous states [135,142], and hyperkalemia [134,143] have been attributed to the use of various NSAIDs.

The number of drugs in consideration is very large. In addition to sodium salicylate, aspirin and fenacetin, the following NSAIDs have been associated with nephrotoxicity: indomethacin, phenylbutazone, fenoprofen, ibuprofen, naproxen, sulindac, zomepirac, meclofenate, benoxaprofen, tolmetin, apazone, piroxicam, etc. Some, of course, are sold over-the-counter (aspirin). Recently the FDA has approved the over-the-counter-sale of ibuprofen in tablets of low dosage (200 mg) for the treatment of dysmenorrhea.

Controversy remains about the true clinical magnitude of NSAIDs nephrotoxicity. There is general agreeement, however, in foccusing the efforts of diagnosis and prevention to the patients populations at risk. Although, the later are incompletely defined, some groups have been identified (Table 9).

Table 9. Risk factors for developing renal abnormalities with the use of NSAIDs

<u>Patient-related factors</u>

1. Advanced age

2. Pre-existent renal disease (lupus, tubulo-interstitial nephropathy, diabetes, nephrosclerosis)

3. Rheumatoid diseases. Dysmenorrhea (?)

4. Clinical states associated with reduced effective blood volume (enhanced renin and angiotensin II levels) dependent on intact prostaglandin synthesis for maintenance of renal function
   (a) Volume depletion, shock states
   (b) Cirrhosis of the liver, congestive heart failure, nephrotic syndrome, glomerulonephritis
   (c) Salt loss due to diuretics

<u>Drug related factors</u>

1. Type of drug

2. Dose and duration of treatment

3. Association with other potential nephrotoxic drugs (aminoglycosides, radiocontrast, etc).

<u>Patient related factors</u>

<u>Elderly patients</u> are more likely to develop NSAIDs-induced nephrotoxicity because the general tendency to underestimate the lower GFR associated with aging (see introduction).

<u>Pre-existent renal disease</u>, particularly systemic lupus erythematosus (SLE), appears to be a risk factor for NSAIDs renal impairment [136,144]. Thirteen of 23 patients with SLE receiving aspirin for at least one week had significant decreases in Ccr [144]; this was also shown with ibuprofen, naproxen, and fenoprofen. The SLE patients with more severe

or active disease exhibited the largest (up to 58% of baseline) decreases. Likewise, even a single dose of aspirin (750 mg) decreased inulin clearance by 39 percent in patients with stable chronic renal failure and adequate sodium balance, whereas a placebo had no effect [137]. The mechanism(s) for this effect of NSAIDs in patients with renal disease may relate to the compensatory afferent arteriolar dilatation shown in experimental glomerulonephritis, and the possibility that this process may depend on locally produced PG [145].

Rheumatoid diseases. Patients with arthritis constitute the largest pool of patients consuming NSAIDs. The second one, probably, are women taking NSAIDs (mostly ibuprofen) for dysmenorrhea. The paucity of reports in this immense reservoir of patients may reflect the presence of minor renal functional changes, the absence of large controlled prospective studies, or most importantly, the absence of pathogenetic conditions resulting in enhanced renal (vasodilator) prostaglandin activity attempting to preserve renal functional homeostasis (see next).

Clinical states associated with reduced effective blood volume (hyperreninemic states). In these common clinical situations (volume depletion, shock states, cirrhosis, congestive heart failure, nephrotic syndrome, glomerulonephritis [134,135,142,146], renal functional homeostasis is dependent on a normal response of the renal prostaglandins to the renal vasconstrictive influences present (enhanced renin-angiotensin and adrenergic activity). Thus, NSAIDs by interfering with the synthesis of vasodilatory PG's may leave the renal vasoconstrictive influences unbalanced, and result in renal ischemia with decrease in GFR, and depending on circumstances, in the appearance of acute renal failure.

The use of diuretics in this background scenario should be emphasized [147]. Although in the absence of other risk factors diuretics given in association with NSAIDs are probably safe, renal impairment may appear when the above risk factors are present (see Fig. 5, Table 9).

Drug related factors

There is little information on the likelihood of the various different types of NSAIDs in producing nephrotoxicity. It appears that most of the tubulo-interstitial nephritis, nephrotic syndrome and hyperkalemia have been associated with the use of phenylpropionic acid (ibuprofen, fenoprofen, naproxen, etc) and indoleacetic acid (indomethacin, sulindac) derivatives.

Higher doses and prolonged treatment may be associated with a greater likelihood of toxicity.

The association of NSAIDs with other drugs known to have potential for renal damage (aminoglycosides, radiocontrast agents, cisplatin) should alert the physician,and enhance his level of clinical suspicion for nephrotoxicity, particularly in patients at risk.

Most of the renal abnormalities described with NSAIDs are reversible, although some may show a prolonged recovery period. Prevention of NSAIDs nephrotoxicity is directly related to the recognition of the risk factors (Table 9).

Table 10 illustrates the transient renal failure and hyperkalemia that developed in an elderly man with acute gouty arthritis, mild congestive heart failure and renal impairment treated with two NSAIDs of the indoleacetic acid derivative type (indomethacin and sulindac). Risk factors in this patient were: arthritis, age and pre-existent renal impairment, congestive heart failure and concomitant use of diuretics. Note that both NSAIDs have similar effects on renal function.

Table 10. Nonsteroidal anti-inflamatory drug nephrotoxicity

87 year old man with acute gouty arthritis (uric acid 11.5 mg/dl), mild congestive heart failure and renal impairment. Treatment included digoxin, furosemide, KCl supplementation and NSAIDs.

Miami VAMC 9/1980	Day 0	INDOMETHACIN * Rx 5 days Day 5	Day 8	SULINDAC * Rx 4 days Day 13	Day 14
Serum creatinine (mg/dl)	1.7	2.9	1.8	2.3	2.2
BUN (mg/dl)	38	72	50	63	63
Serum potassium (mEq/L)	3.7	6.1	4.1	6.2	5.3

* Indomethacin (Indocin®) was given for 5 days with the following dosage: day 1, 75 mg; day 2, 150 mg; day 3, 100 mg; and days 4 and 5, 75 mg. From day 6 to 9 he did not receive any NSAIDs. From day 10 through 13 he received sulindac (Clinoril®, 300 mg/day).

Figure 5 illustrates the reversible acute renal failure developing in a patient with congestive heart failure and mild arthritis. Risk factors in this patient were age (probably), congestive heart failure, hypertension and non-insulin dependent diabetes (pre-existent renal disease), the concomitant use of a thiazide diuretic, and the relative high dose of indomethacin used.

Physicians should be aware of the possibility of nephrotoxicity derived from the use of commonly prescribed drugs for therapeutic or diagnostic purposes. Aware physicians have no difficulty in recognizing drug-nephrotoxicity. Note that four of the five examples shown in this review to illustrate nephrotoxicity (figures 2 to 5), were personally observed by the author within the span of one month. Newer drugs should be considered potentially nephrotoxic until extensive and controlled experience proves the contrary. If drug-induced nephrotoxicity is to be avoided, specific patient populations at risk should be identified and preventive measures established. Finally, the possibility of nephrotoxicity should not deter the physician

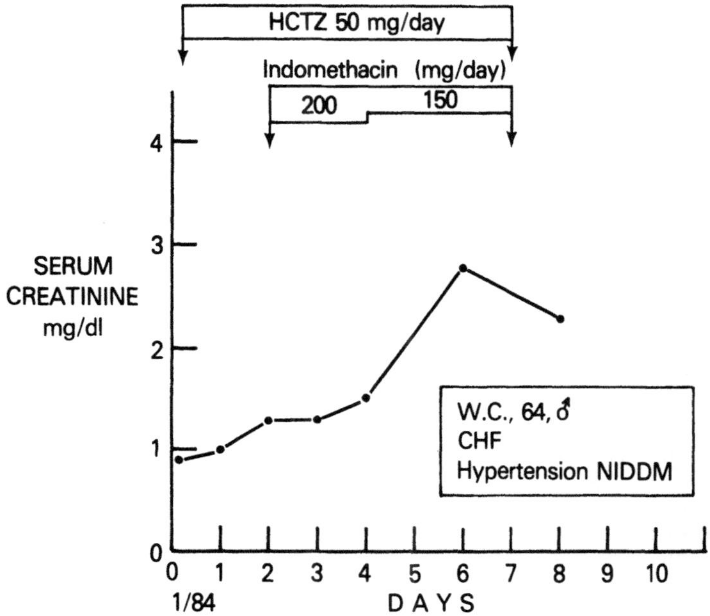

FIGURE 5. Risk factors in NSAIDs nephrotoxicity. A 64 year old man with compensated congestive heart failure, hypertension and non-insulin dependent diabetes (NIDDM) was admitted to the Miami VA Medical Center for mild arthritis. He was receiving hydrochlorothiazide 50 mg/day, and was edema free on admission. He developed transient impairment of renal function, without changes in serum potassium concentration, when indomethacin (indocin ®) was added for the minor symptoms of arthritis that he had.

from the rational indication of diagnostic procedures or the prescription of life-saving or necessary drugs.

Part of this work was aided by designated research funds from the Veterans Administration.

REFERENCES

1. Vaamonde, C.A.: Antibiotic-induced nephrotoxicity. In Nephrology, Volume 1, edited by Robinson, R.R., Proceedings IXth. International Congress of Nephrology, Los Angeles, CA, New York, Karger, S., 1984, pp 844-868.

2. Appel, G.B., Neu, H.C.: The nephrotoxicity of antimicrobial

agents (three parts). N. Engl. J. Med., 296:663, 1977.

3. Smith, T.R., Smith, C.R.: Risk factors for aminoglycoside nephrotoxicity. In The Aminoglycosides. Microbiology, Clinical Use, and Toxicology, edited by Whelton, A., Neu, H.C., New York, Marcel Dekker, 1982, pp 401-415.

4. Cockcroft, D., Gault, M.H.: Prediction of creatinine clearance from serum creatinine. Nephron 16:31, 1976.

5. Ehrnebo, M., Agurell, S., Jalling, B., Boreus, L.O.: Age differences in drug binding by plasma proteins: Studies on human foetuses, neonates and adults. Eur. J. Clin. Pharmacol., 3:189, 1971.

6. Krasner, J., Giacoia, G.P., Yaffe, S.F.:Drug-protein binding in the newborn infant. Ann. N.Y. Scad. Sci., 226:101, 1973.

7. Rane, A., Wilson, J.T.: Clinical pharmacokinetics in infants and children. Clin. Pharmacokinetics 1:2, 1976.

8. Cafruny, E.F.: Effects of drugs and toxins on the kidney. In Pediatric Kidney Disease, edited by Edelman, Jr., C.M., Boston, Little, Brown. Co., 1978, pp 935-939.

9. Shafi, T., Chou, S., Porush, J., Shapiro, W.B.: Infusion intravenous pyelography and renal function effects in patients with chronic renal insufficiency. Arch. Intern. Med., 138:1218, 1978.

10. Swartz, R.D., Rubin, J.E., Leeming, B.W., Silva, P.: Renal failure following major angiography. Am. J. Med., 65:31, 1978.

11. Van Zee, B.E., Hoy, W.E., Talley, T.E., Jaenike, J.R.: Renal injury associated with intravenous pyelography in non-diabetic and diabetic patients. Ann. Intern. Med., 89:51, 1978.

12. Heneghan, M.: Contrast-induced acute renal failure. Editorial. Am. J. Roentgenol., 131:1113, 1978.

13. Byrd, L., Sherman, R.L.: Radiocontrast-induced acute renal failure: A clinical and pathophysiological review. Medicine 58:270, 1979.

14. Canales, C.O., Smith, G.H., Robinson, J.C., Remmers, A.R., Sarles, H.E.: Acute renal failure after the administration of iopanoic acid as a cholecystographic agent. N. Engl. J. Med., 281:89, 1969.

15. Berezin, A.F.: Acute renal failure, diabetes mellitus, and scanning. Ann. Intern. Med., 86:829, 1977.

16. Hanaway, J., Black, J.: Renal failure following contrast injection for computerized tomography. J.A.M.A.,238:2056,1977.

17. Takazahura, E., Sawabu, N., Handa, A., Takada, A., Shinoda, A., Takeuchi, J.: Intrarenal vascular changes with age and disease. Kidney Int., 2:224, 1972.

18. Hollenberg, N.K., Adams, D.F., Solomon, H.S., Rashid, A., Abrams, H.L., Merrill, J.P.: Senescence and the renal vasculature in normal man. Circ. Res., 34:309, 1974.

19. Ansari, Z., Baldwin, D.S.: Acute renal failure due to radiocontrast agents. Nephron 17:28, 1976.

20. D'Elia, J.A., Gleason, R.E., Alday, M., Malarick, C., Godley, K., Warram, J., Kaldany, A., Weinrauch, L.A.: Nephrotoxicity from angiographic contrast material. A prospective study. Am. J. Med., 72:719, 1982.

21. Teruel, J.L., Marcén, R., Onaindía, J.M., Serrano, A., Quereda, C., Ortuño, J.: Renal impairment caused by intravenous urography. A prospective study. Arch. Intern. Med., 141:1271, 1981.

22. Coggins, C.H., Fang, L.S-T: Acute renal failure associated with antibiotics, anesthetic agents, and radiographic contrast agents. In. Acute Renal Failure, edited by Brenner, B.M., and Lazarus, J.M., Philadelphia, W.B. Saunders Co., 1983, pp 283-320.

23. Harkonen, S., Kjellstrand, K.M.: Exacerbation of diabetic renal failure following intravenous pyelography. Am.J.Med., 63:939, 1977.

24. Dudzinski, P.J., Petrone, A.F., Peroff, M., Callaghan, E.E.: Acute renal failure following high-dose excretory urography in dehydrated patients. J. Urol., 106:619, 1971.

25. Kamdar, A., Weidmann, P., Makoff, D.L., Massry, S.G.: Acute renal failure following intravenous use of radiographic contrast dyes in patients with diabetes mellitus. Diabetes 26:643, 1977.

26. Veseley, D.L., Mintz, D.H.: Acute renal failure in insulin-dependent diabetics. Episodes secondary to intravenous pyelography. Arch. Intern. Med., 138:1858, 1978.

27. Pillay, V.K., Robbins, P.C., Schwartz, F.D., Kark, R.M.: Acute renal failure following intravenous urography in patients with long-standing diabetes mellitus and azotemia. Radiology 95:633, 1970.

28. Barshay, M.E., Kay, J.H., Goldman, R., Coburn, J.W.: Acute renal failure in diabetic patients after infusion pyelography. Clin. Nephrol., 1:35, 1973.

29. Diaz-Buxo, J.A., Wagoner, R.D., Hattery, R.R., Palumbo, P.J.: Acute renal failure after excretory urography. Ann. Intern. Med., 83:155, 1975.

30. Shieh, S.D., Hirsch, S.R., Boshell, B.R., Pino, J.A., Alexander, L.J., Witten, D.M., Friedman, E.A.: Low risk of contrast media-induced acute renal failure in nonazotemic type 2 diabetes melliuts. Kidney Int., 21:739, 1982.

31. Mason, R.A., Arbeit, L.A., Giron, F.: Renal dysfunction after arteriography. J.A.M.A., 253:1001, 1985.

32. Teixeira, R.B., Kelley, J., Vaamonde, C.A.: Absence of sensitivity to the renal toxic effects of radiographic contrast material in the diabetic rat. Clin. Res., 30:464A, 1982.

33. Reed, J.R., Williams, R.H., Luke, R.G.: The renal hemodynamic response to diatrizoate in normal and diabetic rats. Invest. Radiol., 18:536, 1983.

34. DeFronzo, R.A., Humphrey, R.L., Wright, J.R., Cooke, C.R.: Acute renal failure in multiple myeloma. Medicine 54:209, 1975.

35. Cochran, S.T., Waisman, J., Pagani, J.J., Cahill, P.: Nephrotoxicity of epinephrine-assisted venography. Invest. Radiol., 17:583, 1982.

36. Fang, L.S., Sirota, R.A., Ebert, T.H., Lichtenstein, N.S.: Low fractional excretion of sodium with contrast media-induced acute renal failure. Arch. Intern. Med., 140:531, 1980

37. Avner, E.D., Ellis, D., Jaffe, R., Bowen, A'D.: Neonatal radiocontrast nephropathy simulating infantile polycystic kidney disease. J. Pediatrics 100:85, 1982.

38. Berdon, W.E., Schwartz, R.H., Becker, J., Baker, D.H.: Tamm-Horsfall proteinuria. Radiology 92:714, 1969.

39. Hayman, L.A., Evans, R.A., Fahr, L.M., Hinck, V.C.: Renal consequences of rapid high dose contrast CT: Am. J. Roent., 134:553, 1980.

40. Eisenberg, R.L., Bank, W.O., Hedgcock, M.W.: Renal failure after angiography. Am. J. Med., 68:43, 1980.

41. Rahimi, A., Edmondson, R.P.S., Jones, N.F.: Effect of radiocontrast media on kidneys of patients with renal disease. Br. J. Med., 282:1194, 1981.

42. Nicot, G.S., Merle, L.J., Charmes, J.P., Valette, J.P., Nouaille, Y.D., Lachâtre, G.F., Leroux-Robert, C.: Transient glomerular proteinuria, enzymuria, and nephrotoxic reaction induced by radiocontrast media. J.A. M.A., 252:2432, 1984.

43. Snyder, H.S., Killen, D.A., Foster, J.H.: The influence of mannitol in toxic reactions to contrast angiography. Surgery 64:640, 1968.

44. Old. C.S., Lehrner, L.M.: Prevention of radiocontrast-induced acute renal failure with mannitol. Lancet 1:885, 1980.

45. Anto, H.R., Chou, S-Y, Porush, J.G., Shapiro, W.B.: Mannitol prevention of acute renal failure associated with infusion intravenous pyelography. Clin. Res., 27:407A, 1979.

46. Lane, A.Z., Wright, G.E., Blair, D.C.: Ototoxicity and nephrotoxicity of amikacin. Am. J. Med., 62:911, 1977.

47. The EORTC International Antimicrobial Therapy Project Group: Three antibiotic regimens in the treatment of infection in febrile granulocytopenic patients with cancer. J. Infect. Dis., 137:14, 1978.

48. Lau, W.K., Young, L.S., Black, R.E., Winston, D.J., Linne, S.R., Weinstein, R.J., Hewitt, W.L.: Comparative efficacy and toxicity of amikacin/carbenicillin versus gentamicin/carbenicillin in leukopenic patients. Am. J. Med., 62:959, 1977.

49. Moore, R.D., Smith, C.R., Lipsky, J.J., Mellits, E.D., Lietman, P.S.: Risk factors for nephrotoxicity in patients treated with aminoglycosides. Ann. Intern. Med., 100:352, 1984.

50. Zakauddin, S., Adelman, R.: Urinary enzyme activity in neonates receiving gentamicin therapy. Clin. Res., 26:142A, 1978.

51. Cowan, R.H., Jukkola, A.F., Arant, B.S., Jr.: Pathophysiological evidence of gentamicin (G) nephrotoxicity in the neonatal puppy. Kidney Int., 14:628, 1978.

52. Marre, R., Tarara, N., Louton, T., Sack, K.: Age-dependent nephrotoxicity and the pharmacokinetics of gentamicin in rats. Eur. J. Pediatr., 133:25, 1980.

53. Karniski, L., Chonko, A., Stewart, R., Cuppage, F., Hodges, G.: The effects of gentamicin (G) on renal function in the sexually mature vs. sexually immature rabbits. Kidney Int., 14:726, 1978.

54. Smith, C.R., Maxwell, R.R., Edwards, C.G., Rogers, J.F., Lietman, P.S.: Nephrotoxicity induced by gentamicin and amikacin. Johns Hopkins Med. J., 142:85, 1978.

55. Reyman, M.T., Bradac, J.A., Cobbs, C.G., Dismukes, W.E.: Correlation of aminoglycoside dosage with serum concentration during therapy of serious gram-negative bacillary disease. Antimicrob. Agents Chemother.,16:353, 1979.

56. Bennett, W.M., Hartnett, M.N., Gilbert, D.N., Houghton, D., Porter, G.A.: Effect of sodium intake on gentamicin nephrotoxicity in the rat. Proc. Soc. Exp. Biol. Med.,

151:736, 1976.

57. Lecompte, J., Dumont, L., Hill, J., Souichi, P.D., Lelorier, J.: Effect of water deprivation and rehydration on gentamicin disposition in the rat. J. Pharmacol. Exp. Ther., 218:231, 1981.

58. Adelman, R.D.: Sodium depletion and diuretics in relation to aminoglycoside nephrotoxicity, In Nephrotoxicity, Ototoxicity of Drugs, edited by Fillastre, J.P., Rouen, Editions Inserm, 1982, pp 213-224.

59. Finn, W.F., Fernandez-Repollet, E.: Contribution of intravascular volume contraction to gentamicin nephrotoxicity. Kidney. Int., 21:217, 1982.

60. Kahn, T.: Effect of furosemide on gentamicin and netilmicin nephrotoxicity. Kidney. Int., 12:527, 1977.

61. DeRougemont, D., Oeschger, A., Konrad, L., Theil, G., Torhorst, J., Wenk, M., Wunderlich, P., Brunner, F.P.: Gentamicin-induced acute renal failure in the rat: Effect of dehydration, DOCA-saline and furosemide. Nephron 29:176, 1981.

62. Chiu, P.J.S., Miller, G.H., Long, J.F., Waitz, J.A.: Renal uptake and nephrotoxicity of gentamicin during urinary alkalinization in rats. Clin. Exp. Pharmacol. Physiol., 6:317, 1979.

63. Elliott, W.C., Parker, R.A., Houghton, D.C., Gilbert, D.N., Porter, G.A., Defehr, J., Bennett, W.M.: Effect of sodium bicarbonate and ammonium chloride ingestion in experimental gentamicin nephrotoxicity in rats. Res. Comm. Chem. Pathol. Pharmacol., 28:483, 1980.

64. Brinker, K.R., Bulger, R.E., Dobyan, D.C., Stacey, T.R., Southern, P.M., Henrich, W.L., Cronin, R.E.: Effect of potassium depletion on gentamicin nephrotoxicity. J. Lab. Clin. Med., 98:292, 1981.

65. Yarger, W.E.: Effect of potassium depletion on gentamicin-induced acute renal failure. Clin. Res., 26:806A, 1978.

66. Rankin, L.I., Krous, H., Fryer, A.W., Whang, R.: Enhancement of gentamicin nephrotoxicity by magnesium depletion in the rat. Min. Electr. Metab., 10:199, 1984.

67. Cabrera, J., Arroyo, V., Ballesta, A.M.: Aminoglycoside nephrotoxicity in cirrhosis: value of urinary beta 2 - microglobulin to discriminate functional renal failure from acute tubular damage. Gastroenterology 82:97, 1982.

68. Humes, H.D., Weinberg, J.M., Knauss, T.C.: Clinical and pathophysiologic aspects of aminoglycoside nephrotoxicity. Am. J. Kidney. Dis., 2:5, 1982.

69. Kaloyanides, G.J., Pastoriza-Munoz, E.: Aminoglycoside nephrotoxicity. Kidney. Int., 18:571, 1980.

70. Soberon, L., Bowman, R.L., Pastoriza-Munoz, E., Kaloyanides, G.J.: Comparative nephrotoxicities of gentamicin, netilmicin and tobramycin in the rat. J. Pharmacol. Exp. Ther.,210:334, 1979.

71. Senekjian, H.O., Knight, T.F., Weinman, E.J.: Micropuncture study of the handling of gentamicin by the rat kidney. Kidney. Int., 19:416, 1981.

72. Sheth, A.U., Senekjian, H.O., Babino, H., Knight, T.F., Weinman, E.J.: Renal handling of gentamicin by the Munich-Wistar rat. Am. J. Physiol., 10:F645, 1981.

73. Pastoriza-Munoz, E., Timmerman, D., Kaloyanides, G.J.: Renal transport of netilmicin in the rat. J. Pharmacol. Exp.Ther., 228:65, 1984.

74. Smith, C.R., Lietman, P.S.: Comparative clinical trials of aminoglycosides, In The Aminoglycosides. Microbiology, Clinical Use, and Toxicology, edited by Whelton, A., Neu, H.C., New York, Marcel Dekker, 1982, pp 497-509.

75. Walker, B.D., Gentry, L.O.: A randomized, comparative study of tobramycin and gentamicin in treatment of acute urinary infections. J. Infect. Dis., 134 (Suppl):S146, 1976.

76. Schentag, J.J., Plaut, M.E., Cerra, F.b., Wels, P.B., Walczak, P., Buckley, R.J.: Aminoglycoside nephrotoxicity in critically ill surgical patients. J. Surg. Res., 26:270, 1979.

77. Smith, C.R., Lipsky, J.J., Laskin, O.L., Hellman, D.B., Mellits, E.D., Longstreth, J., Lietman, P.S.: Double-blind comparison of the nephrotoxicity and auditory toxicity of gentamicin and tobramycin. N. Engl. J. Med., 302:1106, 1980.

78. Lerner, S.A., Seligsohn, R., Matz, G.J.: Comparative clinical studies of ototoxicity and nephrotoxicity of amikacin and gentamicin. Am. J. Med., 62:959, 1977.

79. Lerner, A.M., Cone, L.A., Jansen, W., Reyes, M.P., Blair, D.C., Wright, G.E., Lorber, R.R.: Randomized, controlled trial of the comparative efficacy, auditory toxicity, and nephrotoxicity of tobramycin and netilmicin. Lancet 1:1123, 1983.

80. Houghton, D.C., Plamp, C.E., DeFehr, J.M., Bennett, W.M., Porter, G.A., Gilbert, D.: Gentamicin and tobramycin nephrotoxicity. Am. J. Pathol., 93:137,1978.

81. Luft, F.C., Bloch, R., Sloan, R.S., Yum, M.N., Maxwell, D.R.: Comparative nephrotoxicity of aminoglycoside antibiotics in rats. J. Infect. Dis., 138:541, 1978.

82. Gilbert, D.N., Plamp, C.E., Starr, P., Bennett, W.M., Houghton, D.C., Porter, G.A.: Comparative nephrotoxicity of gentamicin and tobramycin in rats. Antimicrob. Agents Chemother.,13:34, 1978.

83. Ormsby, A.M., Parker, R.A., Plamp, C.E., Stevens, P., Houghton, D.C., Gilbert, D.N., Bennett, W.M.: Comparison of the nephrotoxic potential of gentamicin tobramycin and netilmicin in the rat. Curr.Therap. Res., 25:335,1979.

84. Houghton, D.C., Plamp, C.E., Gilbert, D.N., Kolhepp, S., Bennett, W.M., Porter, G.A., DeFehr, J., Webb, R.: Amikacin nephrotoxicity in the rat. J. Environ. Pathol. Toxicol., 4:227, 1980.

85. Luft, F.C., Yum, M.N., Kleit, S.A.: Comparative nephrotoxicity of netilmicin and gentamicin in rats. Antimicrob. Agents Chemother., 10:845, 1976.

86. Luft, F.C., Rankin, L.I., Sloan, R.S., Fineberg, N.S., Yun, M.N., Wong, L.: Comparative low-dose nephrotoxicity of dibekacin, gentamicin and tobramycin. J. Antimicrob. Chemother., 9:297, 1982.

87. Dalhgren, J.C., Anderson, E.T., Hewitt, W.L.: Gentamicin blood levels: a guide to nephrotoxicity. Antimicrob. Agents Chemother., 8:58, 1975.

88. Frame, P.T., Phair, J.P., Watanakunakorn, C., Bannister, T.W.P.: Pharmacologic factors associated with gentamicin nephrotoxicity in rabbits. J. Infect. Dis., 135:952, 1977.

89. Bennett, W.M., Plamp, C.E., Gilbert, D.N., Parker, R.A., Porter, G.A.: The influence of dosage regimen on experimental gentamicin nephrotoxicity:dissociation of peak serum levels from renal failure. J. Infect. Dis., 140:576, 1979.

90. Powell, S.H., Thompson, W.L., Luthe, M.A., Stern, R.C., Grossniklaus, D.A., Bloxham, D.D., Groden, D.L., Jacobs, M.R., DiScenna, A.O., Cash, H.A., Klinger, J.D.: Once-daily vs. continuous aminoglycoside dosing: Efficacy and toxicity in animal and clinical studies with gentamicin, netilmicin, and tobramycin. J. Inf. Dis., 147:918, 1983.

91. Schentag, J.J., Cumbo, T.J., Jusko, W.J., Plaut, M.E.: gentamicin tissue accumulation and nephrotoxic reactions. J.A.M.A., 240:2067, 1978.

92. Mazze, R.I., Coussins, M: Combined nephrotoxicity of gentamicin and methoxyflurane anesthesia in man. Br. J. Anaesth., 45:394, 1973.

93. Gonzalez-Vitale, J.C., Hayes, D.M., Cvitkovic, E., Sternberg, S.S.: Acute renal failure after Cis-Dichlorodiammineplatinum (II) and gentamicin-cephalothin

therapies. Cancer. Treat. Rep., 62:693, 1978.

94. Churchill, D.N., Seeley, J: Nephrotoxicity associated with combined gentamicin-amphotericin B therapy. Nephron 19:176, 1977.

95. Butkus, D.E., DeTorrente, A, Terman, D.S.: Renal failure following gentamicin in combination with clindamycin. Nephron 17:307, 1976.

96. Wade, J.C., Smith, C.R., Petty, B.G., Lipsky, J.J., Conrad, G., Ellner, J., Lietman, P.S.: Cephalothin plus an aminoglycoside is more nephrotoxic than methicillin plus an aminoglycoside. Lancet 2:604, 1978.

97. Lawson, D.H., Macadam, R.F., Singh, H., Garras, H., Hartz, S., Turnbull, D., Linton, A.L.: Effect of furosemide on antibiotic-induced renal damage in rats. J. Infect. Dis., 126:593, 1972.

98. Whiting, P.H., Barber, H.E., Petersen, J.: The effect of furosemide and piretamide on the renal clearance of gentamicin in man. Br. J. Clin. Pharmac., 12:795, 1981.

99. Higa, E.M.S., Schor, N., Boim, M.A., Ajzen, H., Ramos, O.L.: Prostaglandin inhibition in gentamicin and tobramycin nephrotoxicity. Clin. Res., 30:450A, 1982.

100. Giamarellou, H., Metzikoff, C., Parachristophorou, A.S., Dontas, A.S., Daikos, G.K.: Prospective comparative evaluation of gentamicin or gentamicin-plus cephalothin in the production of nephrotoxicity in man. J. Antimicrob. Chemother., 5:581, 1979.

101. Harrison, W.O., Silverblatt, F.J., Turck, M.: Gentamicin nephrotoxicity: failure of three cephalosporins to potentiate injury in rats. Antimicrob. Agents Chemother., 8:209, 1975.

102. Bloch, R., Luft, F.C., Rankin, L.I., Sloan, R.S., Yum, M.N., Maxwell, D.R.: Protection from gentamicin nephrotoxicity by cephalothin and carbenicillin. Antimicrob. Agents Chemother., 15:46, 1979.

103. Barza, M., Pinn, V., Tanguay, P., Murray, T.: Nephrotoxicity of newer cephalosporins and aminoglycosides alone and in combination in a rat model. J. Antimicrob. Chemother., 4 (Suppl A):59, 1978.

104. Hows, J.M., Palmer, S., Want, S., Dearden, C., Gordon-Smith, E.C.: Serum levels of cyclosporin A and nephrotoxicity in bone marrow transplant patients. Lancet 2:145, 1981.

105. Whiting, P.H., Simpson, J.G.: The enhancement of cyclosporin A-induced nephrotoxicity of gentamicin. Biochem. Pharmacol., 32:2025, 1983.

106.Bennett, W.M., Parker, R.A., Elliott, W.C., Gilbert, D.N., Houghton, D.C.: Sex-related differences in the susceptibility of rats to gentamicin nephrotoxicity. J. Infect. Dis., 145:370, 1982.

107.Kourilsky, O., Solez, K., Morel-Maroger, L., Whelton, A., Duhoux, P., Sraer, J.D.: The pathology of acute renal failure due to interstitial nephritis in man with comments on the role of interstitial inflammation and sex in gentamicin nephrotoxicity. Medicine (Baltimore) 61:258, 1982.

108.Vaamonde, C.A., Gouvea, W., Owens, B., Alpert, H.C.: Sex does not influence the protection against gentamicin nephrotoxicity in the diabetic rat. Kidney. Int., 25:238, 1984.

109.Hsu, C.H., Kurtz, T.W., Easterling, R.E., Weller, J.M.: Potentiation of gentamicin nephrotoxicity by metabolic acidosis. Proc. Soc. Exp. Biol. Med., 146:894, 1974.

110.Solez, K., Silvia, C.B., Craig, T., Stout, R., Whelton, A.: Adverse effect of amino acid mixtures in experimental aminoglycoside toxicity. Clin. Res., 28:462A, 1980.

111.Hardaker, W.T., Jr., Stone, R.A., McCoy, R.: Platinum nephrotoxicity. Cancer 34:1030, 1974.

112.Gonzalez-Vitale, J.C., Hayes, D.M., Cvitkovic, E., Sternberg, S.S.: The renal pathology in clinical trials of Cis-platinum (II) diamminedichloride. Cancer 39:1362, 1977.

113.Gonzalez-Vitale, J.C., Hayes, D.M., Cvitkovic, E., Sternberg, S.S.: Acute renal failure after Cis-Dichlorodiammineplatinum (II) and gentamicin-cephalothin therapies. Cancer Treat. Rep., 62:693, 1978.

114.Blachley, J.D., Hill, J.B.: Renal and electrolyte disturbances associated with cisplatin. Ann. Intern. Med., 95:628, 1981.

115.Editorial: Cisplatin. Lancet 1:374, 1982.

116.Rossof, A.H., Slayton, R.E., Perlia, C.P.: Preliminary clinical experience with cis-diamminedichloro-platinum (II) (NSC 119875, CACP). cancer 30: 1451, 1972.

117.Dentino, M., Luft, F.C., Yum, M.N., Williams, S.D., Einhorn, L.H.: Long term effect of Cis-diamminedichloride platinum (CDDP) on renal function and structure in man. Cancer 41:1274, 1978.

118.Hrushesky, W.J.M., Shimp, W., Kennedy, B.J.: Lack of age-dependent cisplatin nephrotoxicity. Am. J. Med., 76:579, 1984.

119.Pickering, D.G., Phillips, R.H., Ashford, R.F.: Cisplatin in obstructive uropathy. Lancet 2: 588, 1980.

120.Hayes, D.M., Cvitkovic, E., Goldberg, R.B., Sheiner, E., Helson, L., Krahoff, I.H.: High dose cis-platinum diammine dichloride: Amelioration of renal toxicity by mannitol diuresis. Cancer 39:1372, 1977.

121.Jacobs, C., Bertino, J.R., Goffinet, D.R.: 24-hour infusion of cis-platinum in head and neck cancers. Cancer 42:2135, 1978.

122.Stark, J.J., Howell, S.B.: Nephrotoxicity of cisplatinum (II) dichlorodiammine. Clin. Pharmacol. Therap., 23:461, 1978.

123.Vogl, S.E., Zavarinos, T. Kaplan, B.H.: Toxicity of Cis-diamminechloroplatinum II given in a two-hour outpatient regimen of diuresis and hydration. Cancer 45:11, 1980.

124.Garnick, M.B., Mayer, R.J., Abelson, H.T.: Acute renal failure associated with cancer treatment. In Acute Renal Failure, edited by Brenner, B.M., and Lazarus, J.M., Boston, Little, Brown, and Co., 1983, pp 527-554.

125.Earhart, R.H., Martin, P.A., Tutsch, K.D., Erturk, E., Wheeler, R.H., Bull, F.E.: Improvement in the therapeutic index of cisplatin (NSC 119875) by pharmacologically induced chloruresis in the rat. Cancer Res., 43:1187, 1983.

126.Ozols, R.F., Corden, B.J., Jacob, J., Wesley, M.N., Ostchega, Y., Young, R.C.: High-dose cisplatin in hypertonic saline. Ann. Intern. Med., 100:19, 1984.

127.Kawamura, J., Soeda, A., Yoshida, O.: Nephrotoxicity of cis-diamminedichloroplatinum (II) (cis-platinum) and the additive effect of antibiotics: morphological and functional observations in rats. Toxicol. Appl. Pharmacol., 58:475, 1981.

128.Ross, D.A., Gale, G.R.: Reduction of the renal toxicity of cis-dichlorodiammineplatinum (II) by probenecid. Cancer Treat. Rep., 63: 781, 1979.

129.Daley-Yates, P.T., McBrien, D.C.H.: Enhancement of cisplatin nephrotoxicity by probenecid. Cancer Treat. Rep., 68:445, 1984.

130.Van Barneveld, P.W.C., Sleiffer, D.T., Van der Mark, T.W., Mulder, N.H., Donker, A.J.M., Meijer, S., Schraffordt-Koops, H., Sluiter, H.J., Peset, R.: Influence of platinum-induced renal toxicity on bleomycin-induced pulmonary toxicity in patients with disseminated testicular carcinoma. Oncology 41:4, 1984.

131.Heinrich, W.L.: Nephrotoxicity of nonsteroidal anti-inflammatory agents. Am. J. Kidney. Dis., 2:478, 1983.

132. Calin, A.: In common clinical usage nonsteroidal anti-inflammatory drugs infrequently produce adverse effects on the kidney. Am. J. Kidney Dis., 2:485, 1983.

133. Levenson, D.J., Simmons, C.E., Jr., Brenner, B.M.: Arachidonic acid metabolism, prostaglandins and the kidney. Am. J. Med., 72:354, 1982.

134. Garella, S., Matarese, R.A.: Renal effects of prostaglandins and clinical adverse effects of nonsteroidal anti-inflammatory agents. Medicine 63:165, 1984.

135. Walshe, J.J., Venuto, R.C.: Acute oliguric renal failure induced by indomethacin: possible mechanism. Ann. Intern. Med., 91:47, 1979.

136. Kimberly, R.P., Gill, J.R., Bowden, R.E.: Elevated urinary prostaglandins and the effects of aspirin on renal function in lupus erithematosus. Ann. Intern. Med., 89:336, 1978.

137. Berg, K.F.: Acute effects of acetylsalicylic acid in patients with chronic renal failure. Europ. J. Clin. Pharmacol., 11:111, 1977.

138. Gary, N.E., Dodelson, R., Eisinger, R.P.: Indomethacin-induced acute renal failure. Am. J. Med., 69:135, 1980.

139. Brezin, J.H., Katz, S.M., Schwartz, A.B., Chinitz, F.L.: Reversible renal failure and nephrotic syndrome associated with nonsteroidal anti-inflammatory drugs. New. Engl. J. Med., 301:1271, 1979.

140. Katz, S.M., Capaldo, R., Everts, E.A., DiGregorio, J.G.: Tolmetin. Association with reversible renal failure and acute interstitial nephritis. J.A.M.A., 246: 243, 1981.

141. Bender, W.L., Whelton, A., Beschorner, W.E., Darwish, M.O., Hall-Craggs, M., Solez, K.: Interstitial nephritis, proteinuria, and renal failure caused by nonsteroidal anti-inflammatory drugs. Immunologic characterization of the inflammatory infiltrate. Am. J. Med., 76:1006, 1984.

142. Boyer, T.D., Zia, P., Reynolds, T.B.: Effect of indomethacin and prostaglandin A1 on renal function and plasma renin activity in alcoholic liver disease. Gastroenterology 77:215, 1979.

143. Tan, S.Y., Shapiro, R., Franco, R.: Indomethacin-induced prostaglandin inhibition with hyperkalemia. A reversible cause of hyporeninemic hypoaldosteronism. Ann. Intern. Med., 90: 783, 1979.

144. Kimberly, R.P., Plotz, P.H.: Aspirin induced depression of renal function. New Engl. J. Med., 296:418, 1977.

145. Stoff, J.S., Clive, D.M.: Role of prostaglandins in acute renal failure. In Acute renal Failure, edited by Brenner, B.M., Lazarus, G.M., Boston, Little, Brown, R. Co., 1983, pp 157-174.

146. Kleinknecht, C., Broyer, M., Gubler, M.C., Palcoux, J.B.: Irreversible renal failure after indomethacin in steroid-resistant nephrosis. New Engl. J. Med., 302:691, 1980.

147. Favre, L., Glasson, P., Vallotton, M.B.: Reversible acute renal failure from combined triamterene and indomethacin. A study in healthy subjects. Ann. Intern. Med., 96:317, 1982.

AMINOGLYCOSIDE NEPHROTOXICITY - CLINICAL AND EXPERIMENTAL OBSERVATIONS

Raymond D. Adelman, M.D.

The aminoglycoside antibiotics are widely used in the pediatric age population for the treatment of serious gram negative infections. The incidence of nephrotoxicity in patients receiving aminoglycosides varies according to the criteria defining nephrotoxicity, the aminoglycoside used, and the presence or absence of risk factors. One proposed risk factor is sodium depletion. Although clinical information is largely anecdotal, substantial experimental data support the influence of sodium balance on aminoglycoside nephrotoxicity.

EXPERIMENTAL

The effect of sodium balance on the course of nephrotoxin induced acute renal failure has been well described. When given 1% sodium chloride rather than tap water to drink, rats are protected against acute renal failure caused by such agents as glycerol (1), mercuric chloride (2), and uranyl nitrate (2,3). Hydropenic Munich Wistar rats receiving gentamicin and given 0.9% sodium chloride have higher whole kidney and single nephron glomerular filtration rates than rats on tap water alone (4). In contrast, sodium depletion enhances glycerol induced acute renal failure (5). Fischer 344 rats placed on a sodium-deficient diet and given gentamicin develop more severe renal failure than rats receiving a standard diet (6).

Modest changes in dietary sodium intake, such as those occurring in the rat during nocturnal feeding and daytime fasting, may also affect susceptibility to aminoglycosides (7). Male Fisher 344 rats injected with gentamicin in the morning after nocturnal feeding, a time of relative natriuresis (urinary sodium excretion = .074 mEq/hr) developed significantly less nephrotoxicity than rats injected in the evening, after abstention from feeding, a time of relative salt depletion (urinary sodium excretion = .040 mEq/hr) (Table 1).

TABLE 1.
Serum creatinine values in rats receiving gentamicin at 8 AM or 6 PM. (Ref. 7)

	8 AM (mg/dl)	6 PM (mg/dl)
Control	0.51 ± 0.01	0.47 ± 0.02
60 mg/kg	0.51 ± 0.02	0.58 ± 0.04
90 mg/kg	0.56 ± 0.02	0.98 ± 0.10*
120 mg/kg	0.93 ± 0.12	1.70 ± 0.07*

*p <.01 experimental AM vs experimental PM.

Volume depletion, by use of the potent diuretic furosemide, enhances the nephrotoxicity of several drugs (8). In our laboratory we have studied the effect of furosemide induced volume depletion in dogs receiving either gentamicin (9) or netilmicin (10) (Figure 1). Animals receiving gentamicin in a dosage of 10 mg/kg every 8 hours I.M. for 10 days developed a predictable rise in serum creatinine occurring by the 6th or 7th day. The onset of acute renal failure was associated histologically with hyaline droplet degeneration and focal tubular necrosis by light microscopy and with an increase in the number and size of lysozomes, many containing myelin-like figures, by electron microscopy. By the 9th to 12th day, severe diffuse acute renal tubular necrosis involving up to 70% of the tubular cells was demonstrated. Another group of animals was given the same dosage of gentamicin and, in addition, 2 mg/kg every 8 hours I.M. of furosemide, enough to cause a 5% reduction in body weight. Gentamicin nephrotoxicity was enhanced with earlier and steeper elevations in serum creatinine and blood urea nitrogen levels. Percutaneous renal biopsies on the 7th day of therapy showed widespread degeneration and necrosis of proximal tubular epithelial cells similar to that seen on the 12th day in dogs receiving gentamicin alone. Hence, furosemide induced volume depletion enhances the nephrotoxicity of gentamicin as demonstrated by changes in renal function and morphology.

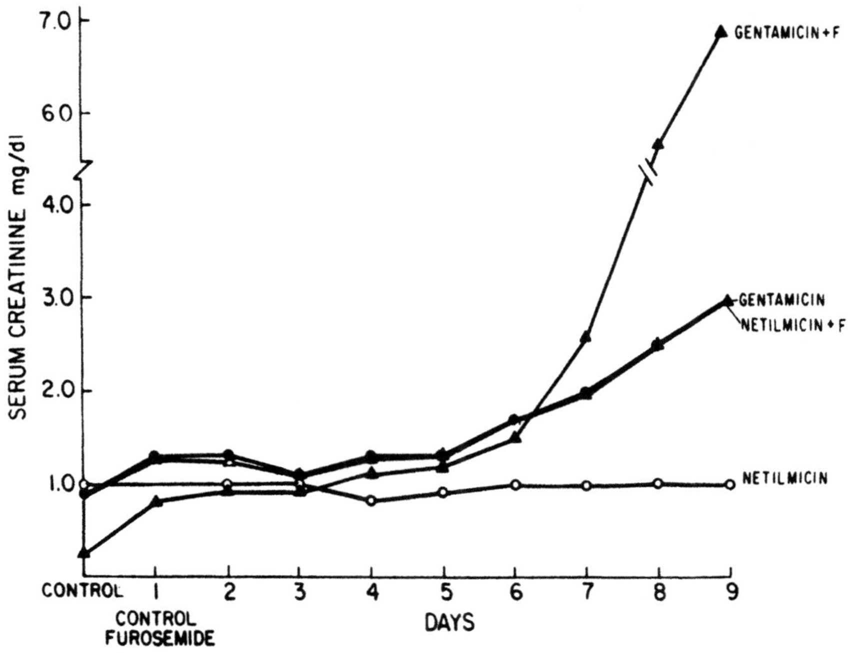

FIG. 1. Serum creatinine values in dogs receiving gentamicin alone or in combination with furosemide are compared to serum creatinine values in dogs receiving netilmicin alone or in combination with furosemide. (Ref.10)

A similar pattern occurred when dogs were given netilmicin alone and in conjunction with furosemide (Figure 1). Netilmicin given in dosages of 15 mg/kg every 8 hours for ten days led to no changes in serum creatinine or creatinine clearance, although urine osmolality fell significantly. Renal histology displayed diffuse severe hyaline droplet degeneration but only occasional foci of tubular necrosis. In contrast, dogs receiving netilmicin 15 mg/kg and furosemide 2 mg/kg every 8 hours had enhanced nephrotoxicity with serum creatinine values at day 9 rising to a level 3.0 mg/dl and with renal histology showing widespread and severe acute tubular necrosis. The most profound renal injury was present in furosemide treated animals with weight loss exceeding 5.5% of control body weight. The extent of volume depletion appeared to be the most important variable.

A final study compared dogs given netilmicin and furosemide with those given netilmicin, furosemide, and volume repletion by use of gavage. Gavage was instituted one hour after furosemide using a solution containing 75 mEq of sodium chloride and 40 mEq of potassium chloride per liter in a volume equal to 5% of body weight. Dogs receiving furosemide and netilmicin had significantly higher serum creatinine values than dogs receiving either furosemide or netilmicin alone. The volume repleted group, which received netilmicin, furosemide and gavage, maintained normal serum creatinine values throughout the experiment (11) (Table 2).

	Serum Creatinine (mg/dl)		
Day	0	3	10
Furosemide	.93	1.16	1.26
Netilmicin	.87	.75	.91
Netilmicin + Furosemide	.87	1.14	3.02*
Netilmicin + Furosemide + Gavage	.87	.81	1.02

*p <.01 compared to other groups

TABLE 2. Changes in serum creatinine values in dogs receiving furosemide, netilmicin, netilmicin + furosemide, and netilmicin + furosemide + volume repletion by gavage. (Ref. 11)

These data suggest that sodium balance has a significant impact upon aminoglycoside nephrotoxicity. Several clinical studies, however, have not identified diuretics as important risk factors in aminoglycoside nephrotoxicity. The impact of diuretics in our animal data appears mainly related to an effect on volume; patients receiving diuretics without substantial volume depletion would be unlikely to show enhancement of aminoglycoside nephrotoxicity. The possible influence on nephrotoxicity of parenteral or enteral sodium intake in patients receiving aminoglycosides has not been evaluated.

The mechanism by which sodium depletion enhances aminoglycoside nephrotoxicity is not clear. Volume depletion activates the renin angiotensin system as does hypokalemia, another consequence of diuretic therapy. This system has been implicated in a number of nephrotoxic acute renal failure models. Others have shown (2) that the effect of salt depletion can occur independent of the renin angiotensin system and that natriuresis per se confers protection. Our data in gentamicin treated rats similarly shows an inverse correlation between terminal serum creatinine values and urinary sodium excretion.

In summary, sodium depletion, due to decreased dietary sodium intake or increased sodium deficit after vigorous diuresis, enhances the nephrotoxicity of aminoglycosides in animal models. This enhancement is related to the degree of volume depletion and the extent of natriuresis and is associated with pronounced elevations in serum creatinine and severe alterations in renal morphology. Volume repletion to a significant extent protects against furosemide enhanced aminoglycoside nephrotoxicity.

CLINICAL

Significant elevations in serum creatinine occur in 1.5 - 25% of adults receiving aminoglycosides (12,13). 30% of adult cases of nonoliguric acute renal failure in one institution were due to aminoglycosides (14). Quoted figures may actually underestimate the true incidence of aminoglycoside nephrotoxicity since the diagnosis in most studies is based upon a significant elevation in serum creatinine, an insensitive marker of mild to moderate decreases in renal function. Keys, et al. (15) studied 27 patients who received aminoglycosides for 13 to 14 days. Only one patient had an elevation in serum creatinine >0.3 ml/dl; however, when glomerular filtration rate was measured with I^{125} iothalamate, 42% of patients had a significant decrease in glomerular filtration rate (range 15-49%) with a mean decrease of 23% in tobramycin treated and 26% in gentamicin treated patients. Trollfors, et al. (16) studied 36 patients receiving gentamicin for 10-14 days in whom trough gentamicin levels never exceeded 2 μg/ml. In 25 patients in whom the peak gentamicin level exceeded 4 μg/ml at least once (but never >6.8 μg/ml), no changes in serum creatinine were detected. However, glomerular filtration rate as determined by ^{51}Cr EDTA fell in 23 patients with a mean decrease of 17%.

Children have been thought to be less susceptible to drug induced acute renal failure. Indeed, in experimental animal models, age has been a significant variable with regard to nephrotoxicity. Pelayo (17) reported 1-2 week old puppies given uranyl nitrate had less morphological and functional renal injury than did 3-5 week old puppies. In contrast, Bidani (18) demonstrated a greater susceptibility of 3-4 week old rats to acute renal failure induced by either uranyl nitrate or mercuric chloride when compared to 7-8 week old rats. Conceivably, these differences may reflect a more rapid postnatal functional maturation in the rat compared to the puppy (19).

Experimental data on the impact of age on aminoglycoside treated animals is fairly consistent. Young rabbits, rats, and dogs appear less susceptible to aminoglycoside nephrotoxicity than older animals. Chonko (20) gave gentamicin 15 mg/kg/day to mature and immature rabbits; only the latter showed significant renal failure and tubular necrosis. Cowan, et al. (21) studied newborn puppies treated for 10, 20, or 30 days with gentamicin in a dosage of 5.0-7.5 mg/kg/day. Inulin clearance (ml/min) increased with age in control but not in gentamicin treated puppies. Inulin clearance (ml/min/grams of dry kidney weight) increased with age in control and decreased with age in gentamicin treated puppies. Tubular reabsorption of phosphate was also decreased with age in gentamicin puppies. While serum creatinine rose in older puppies and adult dogs given gentamicin, serum creatinine did not differ between control puppies and those receiving gentamicin for 10, 20 or 30 days. This failure to observe a rise in serum creatinine during gentamicin therapy despite changes in inulin clearance is not unexpected. As in the human infant, plasma creatinine at birth in puppies does not differ from that of the mother and decreases over the first month of life. Renal function, therefore, cannot be easily evaluated by monitoring changes in plasma creatinine during a time when plasma creatinine is normally falling and creatinine clearance is normally rising.

Cowan postulated that the relative tolerance of the neonate to gentamicin induced renal injury was due to changes in the distribution of renal blood flow during development from the juxtamedullary cortex to the outer cortex. During therapy injury to nephrons in the inner cortex would be offset by the subsequent contribution of outer cortical nephrons to overall renal function.

Clinical studies of aminoglycoside usage in children have primarily involved the neonate. Milner (22) and McCracken (23) reported virtually no nephrotoxicity in neonates treated with gentamicin. However, these conclusions were based on lack of changes in serum creatinine, an insensitive mark of renal injury, as already discussed. Others have looked at release of proximal tubular lysozymal or brush border enzymes as markers of nephrotoxicity and/or at disturbances in proximal tubular reabsorption of low molecular weight proteins such as β2 microglobulin. Tessin (24) reported increased levels of urinary alanine aminopeptidase without changes in blood urea nitrogen. Adelman and Zakauddin (25) reported increased activities of NAG, β-glucuronidase and muramidase (lysozyme) in full term and premature infants receiving gentamicin. Elinder (26) noted infants receiving gentamicin had an increased fractional excretion of β2 microglobulin and lower creatinine clearances following gentamicin therapy when compared to control infants. Feldman (27) analyzed creatinine kinetics in newborn infants receiving gentamicin. 7 of 22 treated infants had increases in plasma creatinine after day 5, well beyond the plasma creatinine levels found in infants receiving no drugs. Several infants more than doubled their plasma creatinine values. In the studies by Elinder and Feldman, no control population were included. However, the impact of coexisting illness on renal function was discounted. The authors noted there was usually an early improvement in renal function with therapy followed by deterioration toward the end of antibiotic therapy.

We have studied neonates randomized to receive amikacin or mezlocillin for treatment of neonatal sepsis (Table 3).

	Duration (d)		AAP (U/mg Cr.)	NAG (U/mg Cr.)	Creatinine Clearance (ml/min)
Mezlocillin (n=36)	6.4	Initial:	0.166	2518	0.62
		Treatment:	0.126	1640	0.69
Amikacin (n=36)	5.6	Initial:	0.248	2919	0.50
		Treatment:	0.265	2643	0.45

TABLE 3. Changes in renal function in neonates receiving mezlocillin or amikacin.

These data suggest mild amikacin nephrotoxicity. The activities of the urinary enzymes AAP and NAG tended to remain elevated during therapy with amikacin. Creatinine clearance rose during treatment with mezlocillin but declined during treatment with amikacin. Studies in adults in which nephrotoxicity was defined by a rise in serum creatinine and in infants comparing urinary NAG activities (28) suggest amikacin may be less nephrotoxic than gentamicin.

Although most studies of aminoglycoside nephrotoxicity emphasize changes in glomerular filtration rate, severe tubular dysfunction besides β_2-microglobulinuria can also occur. Cowan, et al (21) demonstrated decreased tubular reabsorption of phosphate in puppies given gentamicin. We have seen several cases of Fanconi syndrom (29) with severe hypokalemia, hyponatremia, and hypophosphatemia. Profound hypocalcemia can also occur unassociated with excess urinary losses of calcium and related to inappropriately low levels of parathormone.

In summary, clinical data do demonstrate changes in glomerular filtration rate and tubular function in infants and children receiving aminoglycosides. The exact incidence of aminoglycoside induced renal injury is not known. Clearly additional studies employing accurate methods for measuring glomerular filtration rates and proximal tubular function are needed to determine the incidence and extent of aminoglycoside nephrotoxicity in the pediatric population

REFERENCES

1. McDonald FD, Thiel G, Wilson DR, et al: The prevention of acute renal failure in the rat by long-term saline loading: A possible role of the renin-angiotensin axis. Proc. Soc. Exp. Biol. Med. 131:610, 1969.

2. Bidani A, Churchill P, and Fleischmann L: Sodium chloride induced protection in nephrotoxic acute renal failure: Independence from renin. Kid. Intl. 16:481, 1979.

3. Ryan R, McNeil JS, Flamenbaum W, Nogle R: Uranyl nitrate induced acute renal failure in the rat: Effect of varying doses and saline loading. Proc. Soc. Exp. Biol. Med. 143:289, 1973.

4. Schor N, Ichikawa I, Rennke HG, et al: Pathophysiology of altered glomerular function in aminoglycoside treated rats. Kid. Intl. 19:288, 1981.

5. Dibona GF and Sawin LE: The renin angiotensin system in acute renal failure in the rat. Lab Invest. 25:528, 1971.

6. Bennett WM, Hartnett MN, Gilbert D, et al: Effect of sodium intake on gentamicin nephrotoxicity in the rat. Proc. Soc. Exp. Biol. Med. 151:736, 1976.

7. Adelman RD and Wright J: "Natural" Na loading, a critical variable in experimental nephrotoxicity studies in the rat. Clinical Research 30:153A, 1982.

8. Lawson DH, Macadam RF, Singh H, et al: Effect of furosemide on antibiotic induced renal damage in rats. J. Infect. Dis. 126:593, 1972.

9. Adelman RD, Spangler WL, Beasom F, et al: Furosemide enhancement of experimental gentamicin nephrotoxicity: Comparison of functional and morphological changes with activities of urinary enzymes. J. Infect. Dis. 140:3, 1979.

10. Adelman RD, Spangler WL, Beasom F, and Ishizaki G: Furosemide enhancement of netilmicin nephrotoxicity in dogs. J. Antimicrob. Chemoth. 7:431, 1981.

11. Adelman RD, Spangler W , Thomson D, Beasom F: The role of volume depletion in furosemide enhanced aminoglycoside nephrotoxicity. Kid. Intl. 16:771(A), 1979.

12. Milman N: Renal failure associated with gentamicin therapy. Acta. Med. Scand. 196:87, 1974.

13. Smith CR, Lipsky JJ, Laskin OL, et al: Double blind comparison of the nephrotoxicity and auditory toxicity of gentamicin and tobramycin. NEJM 302:1106, 1980.

14. Anderson RJ and Schrier RW: Clinical spectrum of oliguric and nonoliguric renal failure in Acute Renal Failure, (Eds) Brenner BM and Stein JH. Churchill Livingston, New York, 1980.

15. Keys TF, Kurtz SB, Jones JD, et al: Renal toxicity during therapy with gentamicin or tobramycin. Mayo Clin. Proc. 56:556-559, 1981.

16. Trollfors B, Alestig K, Krantz I, et al: Quantative nephrotoxicity of gentamicin in nontoxic doses. J. of Infect. Dis. 141:3, 1980.

17. Pelayo JC, Andrews PM, Coffee AK, et al: The influence of age on acute renal toxicity of uranyl nitrate in the dog. Ped. Research 17:12, 1983.

18. Bidani A and Churchill P: Effects of sodium intake and nephrotoxin dose on acute renal failure in the young rat. Ped. Research 16:277, 1982.

19. McCrory WW: In Developmental Nephrology, Harvard University Press, Cambridge, 1972, p 94.

20. Chonko A, Savin V, Stewart R, et al: The effects of gentamicin on renal function in the mature versus immature rabbit. Proc. Am. Soc. Nephrol. 12:2A, 1979.

21. Cowan RH, Jukkola AF, Arant, Jr BS: Pathophysiologic evidence of gentamicin nephrotoxicity in neonatal puppies. Pediatr. Res. 14:1204-1211, 1980.

22. Milner RDG: Gentamicin in the newborn. Post Grad. Med. Journal 50:Sup. 7, 40-4, 1974.

23. McCracken GH, Jr. and Jones, LG: Gentamicin in the neonatal period. Am. J. Dis. Child. 120:524, 1970.

24. Tessin I, Bergmark J, Hiesche K, et al: Renal function of neonates during gentamicin treatment. Arch. Dis. in Child. 57:10, 758-760, 1982.

25. Adelman RD and Zakauddin S: Urinary enzyme activities in children and neonates receiving gentamicin therapy. Dev. Pharmacol. Ther. 1:325-332, 1980.

26. Elinder G and Aperia A: Development of glomerular filtration rate and excretion of β_2-microglobulin in neonates during gentamicin treatment. Acta Paediatr. Scand. 72:219-224, 1983.

27. Feldman H and Guignard JP: Plasma creatinine in the first month of life. Archives of Disease in Childhood 57:123-126, 1982.

28. Rajchgot P, Prober C, Klein J, et al: Aminoglycoside nephrotoxicity in premature neonates: Amikacin and gentamicin compared. Ped. Research 17:4, 154A, 1983.

29. Russo JC and Adelman RD: Gentamicin-induced Fanconi syndrome. J. of Ped. 96:151-153, 1980.

MANAGEMENT OF ACUTE RENAL FAILURE DUE TO NEPHROTOXIC AGENTS SORBENT HEMOPERFUSION

Charles L. Stewart, James F. Winchester and Pedro A. Jose

MANAGEMENT OF ACUTE RENAL FAILURE

Acute renal failure is a clinical syndrome that occurs when the homeostatic functions of the normal kidney are suddenly impaired. The causes of reduced renal function in the infant and young child as in the adult can be divided into: prerenal causes, usually due to hypoperfusion, post-renal causes related to obstuction, and intrinsic renal failure which may be due to congenital anomalies, vascular lesions, prolonged ischemia or nephrotoxic agents. Criteria for the diagnosis of acute renal failure used in the adult and older child, including oliguria and azotemia, may not be applicable to the newborn (1). The influence of factors such as gestational age, postnatal age, and concomitant disease on renal function frequently presents special problems in the diagnosis of renal failure in full and preterm infants. Acute renal failure is usually suspected when either oliguria, defined as urine flow less than 0.5 ml/kg/hour, or azotemia, defined as BUN greater than 20 mg/dl, is noted. As in the adult, acute renal failure can occur in newborns whose urine flow occurs at a normal rate. In adults the incidence of nonoliguric renal failure has been reported to be as high as 59% (2). In younger infants the incidence may be as high as 30% (3). A BUN higher than 20 mg/dl can occur in infants with normal renal function (4). Hypercatabolic states, sequestered bleeding, tissue necrosis, hemoconcentration, high protein intake, and inborn errors of urea excretion, may result in elevated blood urea levels despite normal renal function. In renal failure BUN rises approximately 5 mg/dl/day, with much greater increases in stressed infants (5). The rise in serum potassium is also much less in the newborn (0.25-0.50 mEq/L/day) compared to 1-2 mEq/L/day in adults. Moreover, the rise in serum phosphorus and magnesium, and fall in serum calcium associated with severe reduction in glomerular filtration rate is less rapid in the newborn than in adults. In general BUN may not rise until after a 50% reduction in glomerular filtration rate. Serum creatinine, on the other hand, increases linearly as glomerular filtration rate decreases and increases exponentially when filtration rate falls to below 30-40% of normal. Thus in older children, serum creatinine is an additional tool in assessing adequacy of renal function. In the newborn however, creatinine levels may not be as useful without first considering factors that influence levels. Creatinine is an end product of creatine metabolism and the serum creatinine level in steady state is related to muscle mass. In the newborn, serum creatinine is a consequence of maternal and fetal production so that neonatal levels approximate maternal values. High levels noted at birth usually decrease by 2 weeks of postnatal age (6, 7). A sustained rise in serum creatinine of 0.5 mg/dl/day is indicative of renal failure. Glomerular filtration rate can also be assessed from serum creatinine levels using the formula developed by Feld et al. They showed that glomerular filtration rate (ml/min/ $1.73m^2$) is equal to a constant K times the body length in cm divided by serum creatinine. The constant K is 0.4 in preterm infants, 0.45 in full term infants and 0.55 after one year (8).

The history, physical examination, urinalysis and other laboratory studies will usually be sufficient to categorize the cause of renal failure as prerenal, renal or obstructive etiology. Azotemia in the presence of normal urine flow is seen in non-oliguric renal failure, increased urea production, inborn errors of urea excretion, or prerenal failure coexisting with diuretic therapy. Azotemia in oliguric states may be seen in renal vascular disease, parenchymal disease, tubular necrosis or prerenal failure. Azotemia in anuric infants may be due to renal aplasia or agenesis, severe renal dysplasia, vascular accidents, cortical necrosis or complete obstruction. It must be noted, however, that 93% of infants void during the first 24 hours of life and 99% within 48 hours.

Laboratory aids have been used to help differentiate causes of renal failure in adults. The values are quantitatively different among preterm infants, full term infants, and adults. Table I lists some laboratory values for different parameters used in various forms of acute renal failure.

Table I. Laboratory values in various forms of acute renal failure (9).

	Pre-renal Oliguria		Oliguric Acute Tubular Necrosis	
	Adult	Infant*	Adult	Infant
Urina Na (mmol/L)	< 20	< 10	> 25	> 40
Urine Osmolality(mOsm/L)	> 500		< 350	
U/P Osmolality	> 2	> 2	< 1.1	< 1.1
U/P creatinine	> 40	> 20	< 10	< 10
U/P urea	> 20	> 5	< 10	< 10
FEx Na %	< 1	< 2	> 3	> 3**
Renal Failure Index (UNa/UCr/PCr)	< 1	< 2	> 1	> 3**
Urine sediment(Casts)	hyaline & granular		cellular	

*For infants > 32 weeks gestational age and preterm infants older than 2 weeks

** Values greater than 10 in 1 week old preterm infants < 32 weeks gestational age

In general, in prerenal failure the urine sodium concentration will be low while the urine (U) to plasma (P) ratios of osmolality, creatinine (Cr) and urea will be high, indicating a concentrated urine. In contrast, in oliguric tubular necrosis the urine sodium will be high while the urine osmolality and U/P ratios of osmolality, creatinine and urea will be low indicating defects in urinary concentrating ability. Recent studies have shown that the determination of the fractional sodium excretion (FEx Na) or renal failure index (UNa/UCr/PCr) to be highly accurate in distinguishing prerenal oliguria from oliguria due to acute tubular necrosis (10). A value less than 1 in adults and less than 2 in infants indicates prerenal failure while greater than 3 indicates acute tubular necrosis. This applies to adults and infants with gestational ages greater than 32 weeks. The fractional sodium excretion in newborn preterm infants less than 32 weeks is high and values for renal failure index greater than 10 have been reported (11). Sodium loss can be augmented in other conditions such as hypoxia, respiratory distress syndrome, hyperbilirubinemia, and the use of drugs including diuretics, theophylline, etc. In non oliguric renal failure use of these indices is of no particular value (12). The presence or absence of kidneys should be assessed using ultrasonography or radionuclide scanning methods.

The establishment of urine flow may be used as a diagnostic as well as a therapeutic maneuver to distinguish prerenal from oliguric acute tubular necrosis as a cause of renal failure. After determining the presence of urine in the bladder, the first step is to assure that there is adequate volume repletion, that there is no evidence of circulatory overload, and that the central venous pressure (if available) is not elevated. Then, a fluid challenge of 10% dextrose in water with 30 mM NaCl at 20 ml/kg over 1-2 hours may be undertaken. If adequate urine output is not established a trial of mannitol or furosemide or both may be initiated. In prerenal failure 60 ml/m^2/hour of 12.5% mannitol results in a urine output of at least 12 ml/m^2/hour within one hour of the in fusion (13). Intravenous furosemide 1-2 mg/kg can also be used. Once oliguric renal failure is established, fluid intake should be restricted to that required to replace insensible loss, urine output and any other extrarenal losses. Insensible water loss varies greatly depending upon gestational age and environmental conditions. Preterm infants weighing less than 1000 grams have insensible losses of approximately 2.8 ml/kg/hour. Infants weighing 1000-1250 grams have insensible losses of approximately 2.5 ml/kg/hour. These decrease to about 1.8 ml/kg/hour for infants between 1250 and 1500 grams. There is a further decrease to 1 ml/kg/hour for infants between 1500 and 1700 grams and 0.8 ml/kg/hour for those over 1750 grams. Radiant warmers and phototherapy for hyperbilirubinemia increase insensible loss by 30% (14). Nutritional status should be monitored carefully and maintained to provide a minimum of 50 kCal/kg/day. Electrolyte requirements must be adjusted accordingly. In the well managed patient hyperkalemia is rarely a problem. In the newborn a potassium level of 6.5 mEq/L is acceptable. Treatment of hyperkalemia can be achieved by several methods. Potassium can be removed by dialysis and exchange resins. Serum potassium can be shifted into intracellular fluids by the administration of glucose or bicarbonate. Some of the physiological effects of hyperkalemia can be blunted by calcium. The dosages of drugs with significant renal route of elimination must be carefully assessed and monitored to avoid potential toxic effects. In some instances of renal failure, dialysis may be a lifesaving therapeutic modality. Fluid can be ultrafiltered in cases of circulatory overload, congestive heart failure or pulmonary edema. Severe electrolyte disturbances, acidosis and uremia can usually be adequately controlled with dialytic therapy.

NEPHROTOXINS

One of the causes of acute renal failure is exposure to nephrotoxic agents which include heavy metals, glycols, organic solvents, salicylates, methoxychlorane, aminoglycosides, and amphotericin among others. There is abundant experimental evidence documenting nephrotoxin induced renal failure in adults (15-17). There is some clinical and experimental evidence suggesting that the immature kidney is more tolerant to the nephrotoxic effects of aminoglycosides than is its adult counterpart (18 19). It is well established that during the period of maturational growth developmental changes occur in perfusion of glomeruli, in distribution of filtration and blood flow, and in tubular transport. Age related differences in sensitivity to nephrotoxic agents could arise from normally occurring changes in renal function in the developing animal. Uranyl nitrate (UN) induced acute renal failure has been well documented in the mature animal. Pelayo et al. recently investigated the influence of age on UN induced acute renal failure in the immature dog (20). In these studies, mongrel puppies 1-2 weeks or 3-5 weeks of age were used. Renal function was studied 2 hours or 24 hours after giving 10 mg/kg of UN, a known nephrotoxin. Thereafter the kidneys were fixed in situ and prepared for light and electron microscopy. There were no differences in renal function between control and experimental groups 2 hours after UN at either age. At 24 hours younger puppies had a 60% decrease in glomerular filtration rate while glomerular filtration was almost zero in older puppies. Urine flow paralleled these changes in glomerular filtration rate. Two hours after UN, the fractional sodium excretion in younger puppies increased from 1.05% to 1.56% and increased further to 4.6% 24 hours after UN administration. These results were not statistically significant. In older puppies, however, the fractional sodium excretion increased from 0.49% in controls to 36.17% 24 hours after UN. Morphologic evidence corroborated the functional data. Two hours after UN administration in the younger puppies there appeared to be little if any morphologic effect. 24 hours after UN there were vacuoles in some of the more differentiated proximal tubules. In the older puppies, two hours after UN, large cytoplasmic vacuoles were seen in the more mature tubules. 24 hours after UN in the older puppies, there were populations of necrotic proximal tubules along with some normal appearing tubules. These findings substantiate the view that the early phase of developmental growth could provide a protective environment to the nephrotoxic effects of UN. These authors speculated that immaturity of both biologic systems regulating glomerular hemodynamics and uptake-transport processes by the renal tubule might have played a significant role in the amelioration of acute renal failure in the immature animals.

SORBENT HEMOPERFUSION

Infants and children are frequently exposed to agents which may be nephrotoxic poisons. In the United States there are approximately 2 million poisonings per year with at least 400 deaths in the pediatric age group (21). Thus efforts aimed at active drug removal should be initiated immediately following discovery of any significant ingestion in order to minimize organ damage and reduce morbidity and mortality. Various techniques such as vomiting, gastric lavage, oral antidotes, alkaline diuresis, and dialytic methods affect drug removal and prove useful in the management of severely poisoned patients. Sorbent hemoperfusion offers an alternative approach to the management of severely poisoned patients. Hemoperfusion is the direct passage of blood through adsorbing materials such as charcoal (carbon) or resins in order to remove toxic compounds from the circulatory system. The efficiency of hemoperfusion relies on the physical properties of drug adsorption and in many instances the clearances are better than that achieved with hemodialysis, peritoneal dialysis or forced diuresis. Factors that may affect the rate of adsorption include size of the carbon particles, temperature, pH and other physical factors (22). With the development of the various polymer coating techniques hemoperfusion has become a safer method for use in patients with toxic ingestion. The coating of the carbon may slightly decrease the rate of drug adsorption or blood clearance by the adsorbent column. This inhibition is determined by the molecular weight of the solute, lipid/water solubility, intercompartmental drug transfer rate, thickness and permeability of the polymer coating and biocompatibility of the coating surface (23). Other adsorbing agents such as the polystyrene amberlite compound XAD-4 have also been demonstrated to be clinically effective. They have been shown to be most effective in removing lipid soluble drugs with clearance rates from blood often exceeding those achieved by charcoal hemoperfusion (24).

The procedure for hemoperfusion involves the use of an arteriovenous shunt or suitable venous catheter to connect the patient to the hemoperfusion device by regular hemodialysis lines. In children, the extracorporeal circuit volume including blood lines must not exceed 10% of the estimated circulating blood volume. The column is rinsed before use with normal saline to remove any particles that may have been generated during shipping and handling of the perfusion device. The lines are then primed with normal saline containing heparin. Whole blood with heparin can be used instead of saline to prime the lines and the perfusion column in smaller patients. Manometers are placed before and after the hemoperfusion column; increasing pressure differential greater than 100 mm Hg indicates clotting of the column and the procedure should be terminated immediately. An air leak detector may be placed distal to the venous drip chamber. Blood is pumped from the patient through the hemoperfusion device at known flow rates using a roller pump. Heparin is administered at the start of the procedure at a loading dose of 100 U/kg as needed to maintain the clotting time 1½-2 times control. Hemoperfusion should be performed using relatively high blood flow rates to take advantage of the high rates of drug clearance by the adsorb-

Table II. NEPHROTOXIC DRUGS REMOVED WITH HEMOPERFUSION

ALCOHOLS
(ethanol)
(methanol)

ANALGESICS
Acetylsalicylic acid[*]
Methyl Salicylate
Phenylbutazone

ANTIDEPRESSANTS[+]
(amitriptyline)
amphetamine
(clomipramide)
imipramide
(nortriptyline)

ANTIMICROBIALS
amipcillin
erythromycin
gentamicin

BARBITURATES[*+]
amobarbital
barbital
butabarbital
hexabarbital
pentobarbital
phenobarbital
quinalbital
secobarbital
thiopental
vinalbital

CARDIOVASCULAR AGENTS[+]
N-acetylprocainamide
(digitoxin)
(digoxin)[*]
diisopyramide
methylproscillarin
procainamide
quinidine
quinine

NONBARBITUATE HYPNOTICS, SEDATIVES, AND TRANQ UILIZERS[+]
(acetamides)
carbromal
chloral hydrate
chlorpromazine
(diazepam)
diethyl pentenamide
diphenhydramine
ethchlorvynol[*]
glutethimide[*]
meprobamate
methaqualone[*]
methsuximide
methyprylon[*]
N-desmethsuximide
pentenamide
promazine
promethazine

PLANT/ANIMAL TOXINS, HERBICIDES/INSECTASIDES
Amanita phalloides[*+]
amanitin[+]
paraquat[*]
parathion
phalloidin[+]

SOLVENTS/GASES
carbon tetrachloride

MISCELLANEOUS
aminophylline[+]
angiotensin
dopamine
epinephrine
norepinephrine
oxalic acid
phencyclidine
phenols
(podophyllin)
theophylline[+]

* Extensively studied in vivo
\+ cause hypotension - acute renal failure not generally directly nephrotoxic

Drugs in parenthesis indicate hemoperfusion is ineffective or data are insufficient

ing columns. Blood flow rates generally range between 2-5 ml/kg/min with the total hemoperfusion time usually lasting between 3-5 hours depending upon the clinical status of the patient. Transfusion of fresh frozen plasma and platelet concentrate are used in patients with low platelet counts or other coagulopathies at the termination of the procedure (especially in hepatic failure patients). During hemoperfusion the patient must be monitored closely for complications. Appropriate cytologic and chemical determinations such as hematocrit, leukocyte and platelet counts, serum **calcium** and glucose as well as drug levels when indicated must be performed prior to, during, and at the termination of the hemoperfusion.

Complications of hemoperfusion include thrombocytopenia (30% ↓ with charcoal and 50% ↓ with XAD-4 hemoperfusion). The incidence of thrombocytopenia, charcoal embolization, leukopenia, hypocalcemia and low fibrinogen levels has been markedly reduced by the use of polymer coated charcoal. Eight children hemoperfused at Georgetown University Hospital exhibited only mild or moderate complications (28). Hemoperfusion is particularly effective in the removal of substances which are lipid soluble, highly protein bound and poorly distributed in plasma water. Such substances are not significantly removed by hemodialysis or peritoneal dialysis. The decision whether a patient should undergo active drug removal by extracorporeal dialysis or hemoperfusion is difficult and should be based on a careful assessment of the patient's clinical condition and a detailed knowledge of the metabolism and dialysis kinetics of the drug in question. Guidelines used for arriving at a decision have been advocated and a list of likely nephrotoxins **removable** by hemoperfusion is seen in Table II. (29)

References

1. Jose, P.A., Tina, L.U., Papadopoulou, Z.L., and Calcagno, P.L. Renal diseases. In Avery, G.B. (ed.) Neonatology. Pathophysiology and Management of the Newborn, 2nd edition, Philadelphia: J.B. Lippincott Co., 1981, p. 674.

2. Anderson, R.J., Linas, S.L., Berns, A.S., et al.: Non-oliguric renal failure. N. Engl. J. Med. 296: 1134, 1977.

3. Medani, C.R., Davitt, M.K., Huntington, D.F. et al.: Acute renal failure in the newborn. Contr. Nephrol. 15: 47, 1979.

4. Calcagno, P.L., and Lowe, C.U.: Substrate induced renal tubular maturation. J. Pediatr. 63: 851, 1963.

5. Williams, G.S., Klenk, E.L., and Winters, R.W.: Acute renal failure in pediatrics. In Winters, R.W. (ed.) The Body Fluid in Pediatrics. Boston: Little Brown and Co., 1973, p. 523.

6. Edelmann, C.M., Jr., Barnett, H.L., and Troupkou, V.: Renal concentrating mechanism in newborn infants. Effect of dietary protein content. Role of urea, and responsiveness to antidiuretic hormone. J. Clin. Invest. 39: 1062, 1960.

7. Greenhill, A., and Gruskin, A.B.: Laboratory evaluation of renal function. Pediatr. Clin. N. Amer. 23: 661, 1976.

8. Feld, L.G., Langford, D.J., Fleischman, A.R., and Schwartz, G.J.: A simple estimate of GFR in infants. Pediatr. Res. 17: 348A, 1983.

9. Jose, P.A.: Acute renal failure in the newborn. Neonatology Letter 1: 2, 1983.

10. Miller, T.R., Anderson, R.J., Linas, S.L., et al. Urinary diagnostic indices in acute renal failure. A prospective study. Ann. Int. Med. 89: 47, 1978.

11. Norman, M.E., and Asadi, F.K.: A prospective study of acute renal failure in the newborn infant. Pediatr. 63: 475, 1979.

12. Grylack, L., Medani, C., Hultzen, C., et al.: Non-oliguric renal failure in the newborn. A prospective evaluation of diagnostic indexes. Am. J. Dis. Child. 136:518, 1982.

13. Gordilla-Panigua, G., and Velasquez-Jones, L.: Acute renal failure. Pediatr. Clin. N. Amer. 23: 661, 1976.

14. Oh, W.: Fluid and electrolyte management. In Avery, G.A. (ed.) Neonatology. Pathophysiology and Management of the Newborn, 2nd edition, Philadelphia: J.B. Lippincott Co., 1981, p. 643.

15. Baylis, C., Rennke, H.R., and Brenner, B.M.: Mechanism of the defect in glomerular ultrafiltration associated with gentamicin administration. Kidney Int. 12: 344, 1977.

16. Eisner, G.M., Slotkoff, L.M., and Lilienfield, L.S.: Distribution volumes in the dog during anuria produced by uranyl nitrate. Am. J. Physiol. 214: 929, 1968.

17. Stein, J.S., Gottschalk, J., Osgood, R.W., and Ferris, T.F.: Pathophysiology of acute renal failure. Kidney Int. 8: 27, 1975.

18. Cowan, R.H., Jukkda, R.F., and Arant, B.D., Jr.: Pathophysiologic evidence of gentamicin nephrotoxicity in neonatal puppies. Pediatr. Res. 14: 1204, 1980.

19. McCraken, G.H., and Jones, L.G.: Gentamicin in the neonatal period. Am. J. Dis. Child. 120: 524, 1970.

20. Pelayo, J.C., Andrews, P.M., Coffey, A.K., et al. The influence of age on acute renal toxicity of uranyl nitrate in the dog. Pediatr. Res. 17: 985, 1983.

21. Arena, J.M.: Poisoning, Toxicology, Symptoms, Treatments. Springfield: Charles C. Thomas, 1974, p. 3.

22. Chang, T.M.S.: Removal of endogenous and exogenous toxins by microencapsulated adsorbent. Can. J. Physiol. Pharmacol. 47: 1403, 1969.

23. Denti, E., Luboz, M.P., and Tessori, V.: Adsorption characteristics of cellulose acetate coated charcoal. J. Biomed. Mater. Res. 9: 143, 1975.

24. Rosenbaum, J.L., Kramer, M.S., and Raja, R.: Resin hemoperfusion for acute drug intoxication. Arch. Intern. Med. 136: 263, 1976.

25. Papadopoulou, Z.L., and Novello, A.C.: The use of hemoperfusion in children. Pediatr. Clin. N. Amer. 29: 1039, 1982.

26. Winchester, J.F.: Haemostatic changes induced by adsorbent haemoperfusion. In Kenedi, R.M., Courtney, J.M., Gaylor, J.D.S., and Gilchrist, T. (eds.) Artificial Organs. London: MacMillan, 1977, p. 280.

27. Gelfand, M.C., Winchester, J.F., Knepshield, J.H., et al.: Charcoal hemoperfusion in severe drug overdosage. Trans. Am. Soc. Artif. Intern. Organs 23: 599, 1977.

28. Papadopoulou, Z.L., Novello, A.C., Gelfand, M.C., et al.: The use of charcoal hemoperfusion in children. Int. J. Pediatr. Nephrol. 1: 187, 1980.

29. Winchester, J.F. Acute methods for detoxification: oral sorbents, forced diuresis, hemoperfusion and hemodialysis in Clinical Management of Poisoning and Drug Overdose. Haddad, L.M., Winchester, J.F. (eds.), W.B. Saunders Co., Philadelphia, 1983, p. 140.

ACUTE DIALYSIS AND ULTRAFILTRATION IN THE NEWBORN

Carolyn Abitbol, M.D., Michael Freundlich, M.D., Gaston Zilleruelo, M.D. and Jose Strauss, M.D.

Dialytic treatment of the newborn infant is a complex issue. Many neonatologists are reticent to institute this type of therapy with the many technical complications and risks inherent in the procedure. Those infants who might be considered in need of dialytic treatment are usually so profoundly ill as to increase the relative risk of the procedure. In fact, from a second vantage, one might suppose that the high mortality of neonates treated with dialysis comes from the delay incurred while contemplating the risk.

Early peritoneal dialysis in lieu of mechanical ventilation was used quite successfully in the treatment of premature infants with severe hyaline membrane disease without renal failure by Boda et al. (1) of Hungary in 1971. They studied 92 infants in a controlled trial in which 50 were treated with peritoneal dialysis and 42 were treated with alkali and glucose infusions after the respiratory distress had progressed in severity. Mortality in the dialyzed patients was significantly less (58%) than in the non-dialyzed patients (83%).

Indications

Indications for acute dialysis in an infant cannot be governed by guidelines set forth for older children and adults. Fluid balance in the neonate is probably the single most critical issue in deciding when to institute dialysis. No adequate rate of urine flow can be arbitrarily chosen as being normal for a neonate whose fluid intake is determined by the need to deliver medications. When a critically ill infant develops decreased cardiac output, renal perfusion falls, resulting in lower urine flow. If urine volume does not respond proportionately to fluid administration, the result is a cascade of decompensations culminating in pulmonary edema, anasarca, and worsening cardiac failure. The risk of the dialysis procedure increases and the efficacy decreases when the infant has developed severe metabolic complications and poor peritoneal perfusion. Improved success might be forthcoming if the treatment could be started earlier in conjunction with the development of safer techniques.

Our recommended indications for beginning acute dialysis in the infant are shown in Table I. Inadequate urine flow would be consonant with low urine volume relative to fluid administration and accumulation of extracellular fluid. This may or may not be associated with azotemia or a rise in serum creatinine. Intractable acidosis is most often seen as severe lactic acidosis where the need of inordinate amounts of buffer require a large fluid vehicle. Dialysis can serve to administer buffer and remove excess fluid volume. Intractable hyperkalemia which is unresponsive to conservative measures or associated with life-threatening arrhythmias dictates urgent dialytic intervention. On the other hand, non-oliguric renal failure need not require dialysis unless associated with severe metabolic or neurologic aberrations. Drug intoxication, if responsive to dialysis is, of course, indication for such treatment.

Table I

INDICATIONS FOR DIALYSIS OF THE INFANT
Inadequate urine flow
Life-threatening edema
Intractable acidosis
Intractable hyperkalemia
Uremic or drug "intoxication"

Once dialysis is considered in the list of treatment options, the modality and associated risks must be weighed. Hemodialysis in the neonatal period is the more difficult technical procedure (2) and carries significant risk (3) if all professionals, including nurses and technicians, are not experienced in its use in the infant. The small infant and child are extremely susceptible to symptoms of disequilibrium (4) which results in cerebral edema and cardiovascular instability that may be life-threatening. Therefore, by far, the first option in most institutions is peritoneal dialysis.

Complications

Major complications of peritoneal dialysis are shown in Table II. Perforation of an abdominal viscus is seen mostly with very hard non-flexible catheters that have to be inserted by the trocar technique. Accumulation of extracellular fluid in the subcutaneous, pleural or pericardial space is seen most frequently when the patient has poor splanchnic blood flow. This leads to poor ultrafiltration with accumulation of more interstitial fluid. Extravasation of dialysate may occur if the catheter is pulled back so that the perforations are in the subcutaneous space allowing the infusion of dialysate subcutaneously. Peritonitis is always a risk with a catheter indwelling in the peritoneum; there seems to be some association of increased risk when the tube requires increased manipulation such as reinsertion or if there is leakage at the exit site. Bleeding is most frequently associated with hard catheters, especially with the trocar insertion.

Table II

MAJOR COMPLICATIONS OF PEDIATRIC PERITONEAL DIALYSIS
Bleeding
Perforation of Viscus
Hydrothorax
Subcutaneous extravasation of dialysate
Infection

Catheter Types

Basically, two types of catheters have been used in acute peritoneal dialysis in the neonate. The pediatric Trocath® (Travenol) is a relatively non-flexible plastic catheter which is inserted by a trocar technique. It differs from the adult type catheter in that the perforations extend only 2 1/2 to 3 cms. from the tip. This allows less of a possibility of subcutaneous extravasation due to dislodgement of the catheter into the subcutaneous space. Recently, some centers have used the Tenckhoff® catheter for acute peritoneal dialysis in the neonate (5). This offers the tremendous advantage of a soft catheter which can remain indwelling for longer periods of time. The main disadvantage of this catheter is that it is not inserted at the bedside in most institutions and, therefore, requires surgical insertion which delays treatment. In most instances, the pediatric Trocath® was used at the initiation of the peritoneal dialysis and the Tenckhoff® was placed subsequently.

The soft Argyle® chest tube catheter can be used effectively as a peritoneal dialysis catheter. It offers the advantage of immediate insertion at the bedside with a small trocar. This catheter is as flexible as the Tenckhoff® catheter and can remain indwelling for long periods of time if necessary. It is also radio-opaque, allowing radiographic confirmation of its placement. In 14 neonatal patients and 16 peritoneal dialyses, it has not been associated with bleeding or perforation of viscus (6). This was in contradistinction to the use of the Trocath® catheter in nine neonates during which four patients suffered major complications including three viscus perforations and four episodes of bleeding.

Technique

The acute peritoneal dialysis system has been well described (7). Some suggestions in altering the technique will be made here. The traditional placement of the catheter in the midline 1/3 the distance below the umbilicus is not optimal in the infant. Rather, the placement of the peritoneal catheter is preferably done in the left lower quadrant 1/3 the distance from the iliac prominence to the umbilicus. This position allows for greater stability, avoids the frequently enlarged liver and spleen, and allows for a greater length of the catheter to be inserted into the peritoneal cavity.

The dialysate for the neonate may be altered to contain bicarbonate rather than lactate as the buffer. This avoids administration of large quantities of lactate which may not be metabolized as rapidly in an hypoxic neonate (8). The suggested concentration of the solutes are listed in Table III. Heparin is sometimes added to avoid the accumulation of fibrin in the peritoneal catheter, although this has not been necessary when using the Argyle® catheter. Ultrafiltration can be enhanced by adding increased concentrations of dextrose, mannitol or salt-poor albumin. The albumin is added in a concentration of 5 g/dl to the dialysate; it seems most efficacious in the hypoproteinemic patient. Problems with hyperglycemia do arise in the sick neonate, probably related to unpredictable variations in insulin response. When this occurs, we do not infuse insulin intravenously but rather add insulin to the dialysate in a concentration of one unit per 5 grams of dextrose.

Table III

CONCENTRATION OF SOLUTES IN PERITONEAL DIALYSATE

Dextrose (g/L)	15 - 25 - 42.5		
Ions	mEq/L	Salts	mg/dl
Sodium	131	NaCl	567
Calcium	3.5	$NaHCO_3$	292
Magnesium	1.5	$CaCl_2$	25.7
Chloride	102	$MgCl_2$	15.2
Bicarbonate	35		

Hemo-Ultrafiltration

There is a separate procedure which also uses a dialytic membrane but does not perform dialysis per se. It is hemo-ultrafiltration and has been used for a number of years in the treatment of severe edema in chronic dialysis patients, both in children and adults (9). It has also been used in non-dialyzed patients, adult patients with chronic congestive heart failure (10) and in some children with nephrotic syndrome (11). We have had the opportunity to use the procedure in a few very ill neonates (12).

The indications for ultrafiltration are limited and include situations of life threatening edema, which are, specifically, pulmonary edema, cardiac failure, and cerebral edema.

It is an extra-corporeal system and involves the passage of blood across a semi-permeable membrane while positive and/or negative pressure is being exerted across that membrane with the generation of a transmembrane pressure. An ultrafiltrate of plasma is removed and collected in a cannister. The whole system is primed preferably with fresh whole blood, or with washed packed cells reconstituted with plasma. Blood flow rates are very slow, as low as 10 ml/min. The low blood flow rate as well as the increased metabolism of heparin in the neonate (13) require high doses of heparin to prevent clotting of the system. Access to the circulation can be obtained through the umbilical vessels or through cannulation of the saphenous or jugular vein.

The ultrafiltrate of plasma, as shown in Table IV, appears to be plasma water. Essentially no albumin is removed in the ultrafiltrate. As shown by the pre- and post-ultrafiltration plasma values in one neonate (Table IV), the low pre-ultrafiltration plasma albumin was corrected to normal by the ultrafiltration procedure.

Table IV

COMPONENTS OF PLASMA AND ULTRAFILTRATE

		PLASMA		ULTRAFILTRATE
		BEFORE	AFTER	
Sodium	mEq/L	136	140	144
Potassium	"	3.0	2.4	2.4
Chloride	"	109	103	110
Bicarbonate	"	17	22	15
Total protein	g%	2.4	5.2	0.95
Albumin	"	2.1	3.9	0
Hb	"	10.1	15.5	
Hct %		30.1	46.0	
Platelets/cmm		150,000	107,000	

Physiologic mechanisms called into play during ultrafiltration are, as yet, not fully explained; this is particularly true relative to the removal of large volumes of ultrafiltrate without compromise in hemodynamic stability in small patients. The physical factors involved may be postulated in the equation for movement of interstitial water (Fig. 1) (14). Edema formation is favored when intracapillary hydrostatic pressure exceeds that of the interstitium and when intracapillary oncotic pressure is less than that of the interstitium.

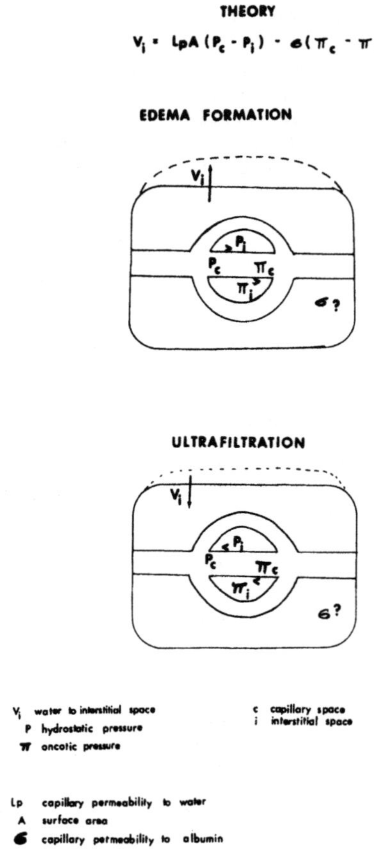

Figure 1. Diagram of factors influencing water movement to the interstitial space.

During ultrafiltration, the negative pressure exerted across the filtering membrane tends to decrease the intracapillary hydrostatic pressure. At the same time, removal of plasma water without albumin tends to increase the intracapillary oncotic pressure. Both these alterations favor the movement of fluid from the interstitial space to the intravascular space resulting in rapid mobilization of interstitial fluid and maintenance of intravascular volume during the ultrafiltration procedure. This remains conjecture, but certainly further investigation will allow us to define the situations in which ultrafiltration of the neonate would be a safe and expeditious procedure for removal of life-threatening edema.

Until more experience is gained, the procedure of ultrafiltration in the neonate remains an extremely grave undertaking which must be weighed with the risk of sudden death. It seems wise to caution particularly against its use in situations where there is low peripheral vascular resistance as a result of peripheral vasodilators or septic shock.

CONCLUSION

In summary, techniques of peritoneal dialysis in the neonate have improved considerably and may now be applied with minimal risk and improved outcome as long as treatment is instituted early.

Hemo-ultrafiltration, as hemodialysis in the infant, remains an extremely difficult technical procedure with a high risk margin. Although its application is limited, it certainly should be pursued as a potentially valuable treatment modality for some clinical circumstances.

REFERENCES

1. Boda, D., Muryani, L., Altorjay, I., et al.: Peritoneal dialysis in the treatment of hyaline membrane disease of the newborn premature infants. Acta Pediatr. Scand. 60:90, 1971.

2. Kjellstrand. C., Shideman, J., Santiago, E., et al.: Technical advances in hemodialysis of very small pediatric patients. Proc. Dial. Transplant Forum 1:124, 1971.

3. Kjellstrand, C., Mauer, S., Buselmeier, T., et al.: Hemodialysis of premature and newborn babies. Proc. Eur. Dial. Transplant Assoc. 10:349, 1973.

4. Peterson, H. and Swanson, A.: Acute encephalopathy occurring during hemodialysis. The reverse use effect. Arch. Intern. Med. 113:877, 1964.

5. Yahav, J., Barzilay A., Aladjem, M., et al.: Acute peritoneal dialysis in children. Int. J. Ped. Neph. 2:33, 1981.

6. Personal experience.

7. Manley, G., and Collipp, P.: Renal failure in the newborn: Treatment with peritoneal dialysis. Am. J. Dis. Child. 115:107, 1968.

8. Branning, W.S.: The acid base balance of premature infants. J. Clin. Invest. 21:101, 1942.

9. Bergstrom, J.: Ultrafiltration without dialysis for removal of fluid and solutes in uremia. Clin. Nephrology 9:156, 1978.

10. Kramer, P., Wigger, W., Rieger, J., et al.: Arteriovenous hemofiltration: a new and single method for treatment of overhydrated patients resistant to diuretics. Klin. Wochenschr. 55:1121, 1977.

11. Abitbol, C.L., Green, M., Grurzner, P., et al.: Treatment of critical neonatal edema with hemo-ultrafiltration. Int. J. Pediatr. Nephr. 5:163, 1984.

12. Widstan-Attorps, U., Asaba, H., Bergstrom, J., et al.: Successful use of extracorporeal ultrafiltration in treatment of therapy-resistant nephrosis. Int. J. Pediatr. Neph. 2:61, 1981.

13. McDonald, M. and Hathaway, W.: Anticoagulant therapy by continuous heparinization in newborn and older infants. J.Pediatr. 101:451, 1982.

14. Auckland, K. and Nicolaysen, G.: Interstitial fluid volume: Local regulatory mechanisms. Phys. Review 61: 556, 1981.

PANEL DISCUSSION

Jose Strauss, M.D., Moderator

COMMENT: Very nice work. I admire that. We also have had some use of both peritoneal and hemodialysis in very small children. My choice of a peritoneal catheter has verted to a single cuff Tenckhoff. On request, Quinton will provide you with a catheter that is even smaller than their neonatal model which allows the cuff to be buried even in very small babies. I prefer it because you never know how long you are going to need to dialyze. Because of the occasional repetitive nature of peritoneal dialysis and my feeling, in the adult patients anyway, that it has cut down a significant amount on the risk of peritonitis, I hope that we will transfer this experience to pediatric patients. Installation of the catheter is really not a problem. I usually have a surgeon do it but it can be done at the bedside. My second comment is that I agree wholeheartedly that in the mainstay, if you have the time, peritoneal dialysis is the best way to go in the neonate. But there are occasions when the hyperkalemia is very severe and refractory and arrhythmias appear to be present in imminently moribund patients. We have hemodialysed infants as small as 800 grams using umbilical artery catheters successfully; so, I wouldn't exclude that in the acutely ill neonate but I would emphasize that it is much safer to do peritoneal dialysis if you have the time for it.

COMMENT-REPLY: I appreciate your comments, especially about the Tenckhoff catheter. I, too, think that the Tenckhoff catheter can be used acutely. It seems, however, that circumstances arise in hospitals when it isn't available. Ingenuity should make it possible for you to use an alternate but if I were in the best of circumstances, and had the Tenckhoff available to me to use acutely, I would certainly use that above the Argyle. I would do that not only for the niceness in the cuff of the catheter but also for the flow effect. I didn't mention that the Argyle is not a suitable catheter for use in children out of the neonatal period, mainly because it also has some positional problems. I've had difficulties in back-flow from that catheter. It's not so much that it is dangerous; it just doesn't work as well. So, I wouldn't use it out of the neonatal period. Again, I guess, I've developed a lot of prejudices against hemodialysis in the newborn. I like to be technically excellent at a procedure when I offer it to a patient and I've repeatedly run into difficulties with hemodialysis. It is not, obviously, that I am afraid to use a procedure, I feel schooled in hemodialysis but I don't think I could offer it to the neonate.

COMMENT: We've also had a fair amount of experience with peritoneal dialysis in newborns and I would echo the sentiments of others that the Tenckhoff, in my experience, has been much easier to use, fewer complications, a much softer catheter and a generally more efficient fluid removal. One of the problems with peritoneal dialysis in the newborn, especially with regard to the premature, is that it is very, very difficult in the very small infant to get adequate volume removal. Often, they are terribly sensitive to the volumes that you infuse. In fact, if you give over 20-30 ml/kg they get acute respiratory compromise. So, you are dealing with a situation where your dialysis is going to be inefficient; it's going to be less efficient if you are dealing with a shocky baby with a decreased perfusion of the peritoneal cavity. That does represent a problem. You are sometimes forced to use very high glucose concentrations in the dialysate media; that can cause a life-threatening hyperglycemia. In that situation, one must monitor blood-glucose levels very carefully and give insulin when required. I noticed in the slides shown that there continues to be an extremely high mortality with the very low birth weight infants. That has been our experience as well. When we get to dialyze a 3 kg full term baby, I am usually quite optimistic. But when we dialyze someone who is 600 grams or 800 grams, we continue to be beset by a very high mortality. I think there are two reasons for this. One is the inefficiency of the dialysis; the other is the tendency to use the pediatric nephrologist and the Tenckhoff catheter or any other catheter as elements of last rites. It is terribly important when one has a neonate in acute renal failure, that dialysis be considered early. One is most efficacious if one starts that modality earlier. I would also like to mention that there is one modality which I think will become available to the pediatric population in a few years. That is hemofiltration using the Amicon filter. This is an extremely effective way of removing volume very quickly and also removing potassium and other solutes as well. I look forward to that as perhaps one of the answers to handling acute renal failure in the small premature.

COMMENT: I was interested in the comment about the continuous intravenous ultrafiltration. We use this in adults in specific situations. I should warn you that it is so effective that you have to watch the hemodynamics on the spot. You can put a patient into shock by removing too much fluid too fast. The Amicon filters are extremely effective for ultrafiltration. It is a welcome advancement but I think it must be used with great care.

COMMENT: First of all, I would echo the comments that there is no doubt that the single cuff Tenckhoff is the safest, most efficient catheter to use if you have the time to put it in properly. I am not so sure that "putting them in properly" means putting them in at the bedside. One loses certain advantages. We have gotten completely away from using a trocar for acute dialysis and to a technique which was described in an abstract about 1975. That is to use the same technique we use for putting femoral vein (Angiocath) catheters followed by a wire, followed by an eight French catheter that's used for hemodialysis. The advantage of this is that it can be done very quickly, very safely. No trocar ever has to enter the abdomen. The disadvantage is that one doesn't quite get the flow, especially the outflow, that one would like. But it can be very easily and safely put into a 600 gram baby. I could describe that at the blackboard if anyone would be interested.

MODERATOR: Anyone interested? Yes. Why don't you do that?

DESCRIPTION: This is the child's abdominal wall. A small incision is made. The Angiocath (16 gauge) is placed in, a wire is then inserted through the Angiocath and directed to the area of the abdomen where you want to place the catheter, usually the right lower quadrant. The Angiocath is then removed, the wire is left in place, and an eight French catheter is slipped over the wire into the area you desire the catheter to be. The wire is then removed and that eight French catheter is hooked up for dialysis. As I said, because of the small bore of the catheter, you don't get fast outflows; whereas you may be able to drain an abdomen in five minutes with a Tenckhoff, this might take 15. The other disadvantage is that this is a small catheter which has small holes very prone to getting plugged. But the beauty of it is that if you do get the catheter plugged, thereby obstructing outflow, you just go back in, put the wire back into the catheter, take that catheter out, and then you put a new eight French catheter in over the top of the wire. In this way you do not have to repuncture the abdomen.

QUESTION: What kind of French catheter?

RESPONSE: It has one small hole at the end and multiple side holes, just like the Tenckhoff would have, really, except that it is smaller. It is also reasonably flexible; it is not rigid. That whole set-up comes in one tray.

COMMENT: It is called Argon Hemodialysis Tray Number Three. It has everything you need in there to place the catheter or what we use it for, peritoneal dialysis.

MODERATOR: Would you have any other comment on what has been discussed? Experiences? Choices?

COMMENT: As a nurse, I feel comfortable using the tray as described simply because we can get it in fast. I don't like to walk into a situation and perform dialysis on a child who should have been started 8 hours before. Using this technique, I know that we can safely get this catheter in and replace it as fast as we need to.

MODERATOR: Regarding hemoperfusion and hemodialysis, we have had several proponents at these Seminars throughout the years. Dr. Kjellstrand was here and described his successful hemodialysis technique in neonates. So, maybe it cannot be generalized that it is not a tool that should be or can be applied to the neonate. It may be that you need certain expertise and maybe it should be applied with caution; but, again, other people are using it effectively. Therefore, it may not be necessary to rule it out.

COMMENT: The only advantage I can see in doing hemodialysis over peritoneal dialysis in a neonate is really a theoretical one--for ultrafiltration. Peritoneal dialysis for ultrafiltration depends upon whether or not the fluid can be mobilized from the interstitium and into the vascular space; this depends on the permeability of the theoretical peritoneal membrane. In most situations in which the fluid is in the interstitium, if you can't mobilize it into the circulation you can't ultrafiltrate it any better with hemodialysis than you can with peritoneal dialysis. It would depend upon a relative decrease in the vascular space to increase the protein concentration, the hematocrit and whatever other forces might be mobilized. But, at the same time, you would produce vasoconstriction and very well may decrease the movement of fluid from the interstitium into the vascular space. So, although some people still hold to the use of hemodialysis in the newborn, that is their experience and they have been reluctant to move away from something they are comfortable with and technically competent to do. But, in my opinion, I don't think that it has served me any better - and it certainly is better on my coronary circulation - to watch peritoneal dialysis in progress than the constant agonizing over an 800 or 1000 gram baby or even a 2000 grammer on hemodialysis. I don't see all the advantage. It is a theoretical advantage and it depends upon what you are comfortable with. I am going to do what I am best at doing and I think if I have the opportunity to begin it early, almost prospectively with the need rather than as last rites, as was mentioned, then I think that peritoneal dialysis will serve us well and it is something that more of us can do than hemodialysis.

MODERATOR: Yes, but I think that it is important to point out that it is not a universal statement. In other words, the point I am making is that here we are sharing thoughts and opinions, and since there is a group that has other good experiences, I think that we shouldn't say that theirs is an untenable procedure; you prefer to do something else. But you should not rule out the other procedure which in competent hands for that procedure, is working well. It's the same thing as percutaneous kidney biopsy. In competent hands, with people who use it often, it is a very safe procedure. Others who don't use it often do surgical biopsies. That doesn't mean that there is only one way of doing a biopsy. Similarly, there is not only one way of dialyzing a baby. In a baby who doesn't ultrafiltrate well with the regular schedule and composition of peritoneal dialysis, some would go to hemodialysis, others would increase the glucose concentration of the peritoneal dialysis solution, and still others would increase the frequency of the exchanges from every four hours to every two or even one hour.

COMMENT: This is not a critical statement of the way some people prefer hemodialysis; this is my personal opinion. There would have to be a practical advantage to doing hemodialysis in any situation that would make it preferable over peritoneal dialysis. All I can see is a theoretical one as far as the principles are concerned. If someone is better at doing hemodialysis than at peritoneal dialysis, or just as competent - in other words the outcome or morbidity is no different - then, it is a matter of choice but I wouldn't advocate it. For me, the morbidity would be greater with hemodialysis. I have done it, and I don't like to do it.

MODERATOR: Your point is well taken. I want you to know that in practice, our approach is similar to yours.

COMMENT-QUESTION: I'm not in disagreement; that I prefer peritoneal dialysis should be no question. I strongly prefer peritoneal dialysis; however, occasionally I have had infants who developed hyperkalemia and severe acidosis so quickly that in my judgement they would not survive for peritoneal dialysis to correct the biochemical abnormalities. In those instances, especially if umbilical catheters are already in, it's not very much more difficult than what we have heard about ultrafiltration, to do a short - couple of hours - hemodialysis.

One other comment. I was intrigued by and had a thought about your ultrafiltration and the cardiac arrests that you had going on. It has been my practice when I have tried hemodialysis, if I didn't have fresh blood available, to prime the system with bank blood; but then, I dialyze that circuit for a few minutes before I hook up the patient. I wonder, since you prime the system, whether or not the citrate and other things in the bank blood might not be part of the problem you had.

RESPONSE: Yes, of course we try to analyze all our mistakes. I did consider that as a possibility. In fact, in priming the system, no dialysate was used at all and it was bank blood. Just some exchanges; also, with the Reye's Syndrome, we had similar problems. It may very well be related to that because at autopsy of the Reye's Syndrome patient, we found some abnormal pigments in the liver. The other thing is that in the two patients who had cardiac arrest at initiation, those patients were the ones to whom you could administer the last rites before ultrafiltration. They really were moribund at the time and probably the procedure should not even have been attempted.

QUESTIONS: Two questions. One is related to the infant with a tense, shiny abdomen or a gastroschisis. When the nephrologist is called - again probably for the last rites - he is asked to do something. Peritoneal dialysis seems almost unfeasible in this circumstance. Perhaps this would be an indication for hemo. Does the panel have comments on that? My second question is a technical one related to the ultrafiltration procedure. What flow rate do you use? What rate of fluid removal do you aim for?

RESPONSE: I'll start with the first. Again, I hate to be so hardheaded about it but this may be a circumstance where an extracorporeal system should be used, particularly the ultrafiltration with infusions going on at the same time; in other words, the diafiltration that was referred to earlier may be beneficial under these circumstances. I feel very strongly about the hemodynamic instability during hemodialysis. At the beginning, I used to ultrafiltrate them a little and then I would let the dialysate run by and try to get a little dialysis in and then I would go back to the ultrafiltration. As soon as the dialysate started to flow, the patient became hemodynamically unstable. But, once I started the ultrafiltration again, the patient stabilized. So, I feel that something about the solute shifts with the hemodialysis is what makes hemodialysis more dangerous. One of the advantages of ultrafiltration is that it is very effective at very low blood flows. Really, with the Amicon you only need a mean pressure of 30 mmHg and it is propelled by the patient's own arterial mean pressure. With ultrafiltration we have used a blood pump and we have hand pumped it at flows as low as 5-10 ml/min; by the way, that requires large amounts of heparin.

QUESTION: Out of curiosity, to the Panel, do you use bicarbonate dialysis at all? We use it in adults when they have instability during dialysis. Do you use bicarbonate dialysis regularly in small children?

RESPONSE: We switched to bicarbonate dialysis for all our hemodialysis patients, both chronic and acute, about two years ago.

RESPONSE: We also have used it for hemodynamically unstable children and prefer it.

RESPONSE: In the newborn period, for peritoneal dialysis, we make a peritoneal bath using bicarbonate.

COMMENT: May I make one comment about that? Again, switching back to peritoneal dialysis in the neonate, one of the common problems we run into is lactic acidosis. I think one should be prepared to use a lactate free dialysate unless one has absolutely confirmed that the patient's lactate level is normal and unlikely to rise.

QUESTION: Is this lactic acidosis or are you talking about lactic acidemia? At least in the adult, we frequently see elevation of serum lactate. If you use a lot of glucose you will get it, too. I wonder if we are talking about just pure lactic acidemia or the syndrome we call lactic acidosis because they are very different.

RESPONSE: These children frequently have lactic acidosis even before dialysis, in absolutely extraordinary amounts. We are talking about levels of 20 to 30 and 40. They also have significant acidosis which is usually a combination of both respiratory and metabolic acidosis. We have seen some children who were placed on lactate-containing dialysate solutions who did poorly.

MODERATOR: Coming back to ultrafiltration, would you recommend its use? Do you think it is an experimental approach? Should we go from here and start using it as routine treatment? What is routine treatment in the neonate? As we were talking yesterday about using drugs that are approved for adults, as we apply adult procedures to the neonate, we may be making a number of assumptions, not necessarily correct. What would be your medico-legal, scientific, old-man wisdom type of statement?

RESPONSE: I would say that I see an interesting use for ultrafiltration in the neonate, being used more often to remove fluid, to improve perhaps fluid overload, to remove fluid that has been administered in excess and has not been excreted by the kidney. There are two situations in which it might be effective. One is prior to the time when we are able to limit fluid administration to the right amount, whatever that happens to be. The other is related to the use of peritoneal dialysis on patients in Hungary; those were babies with respiratory distress syndrome and showed an improved outcome. You have to remember that this therapy was applied because there were no ventilators in Hungary. So, treatment of respiratory distress was by distressed physicians wanting to do something other than throw these children away. Combine that with the popular, new treatment which I don't agree with: the use of furosemide in the treatment of respiratory distress syndrome to induce diuresis. Again, that's an effort to correct a problem that has been created, in my opinion. But, if you can't get it out by the urinary tract and you've given it through the vascular system and the fluid resides in the interstitium of the lung, one way to get it out would be by ultrafiltration. That is, using an in-system non-dialyzed way of removing fluid from the vascular space, assuming that that fluid can be mobilized from the interstitium and into the vascular space. I guess a study really ought to be done before somebody goes back and begins to treat respiratory distress syndrome with this. I think it makes as much sense as the use of furosemide. A comparable study of ultrafiltration versus furosemide needs to be done. I think there is an appropriate place for ultrafiltration and I would hope that we would never have to use furosemide or ultrafiltration, but if we get into that circumstance, I see a particular use for ultrafiltration and it has theoretical advantages. I'd like to see it used experimentally and a study done, before it is used in a widespread clinical manner.

QUESTION: I'd like to ask a question about a clinical situation that arose not too long ago that has dwelled on my mind terribly. First of all, there is a patient who is extremely ill, nephrotic, and we have been asked to ultrafilter. Of course, he has just about 10 liters of interstitium fluid; he is in recurrent pulmonary edema, and his albumin is 1.2 g/dl. The question is, how to prime the system. We got into a little bit of a debate about whether or not it is beneficial to give recurrent doses of 25% albumin. I would like to know what your opinion would be of giving large doses of 25% albumin and then ultrafiltering, not continuously, but just after that dose of albumin.

RESPONSE: If the patient has a normal GFR, does not have parenchymal disease with nephrotic syndrome, then with the use of albumin you can eventually use the kidney to ultrafilter. The problem is mobilizing that fluid into the vascular space. If you mobilize it sufficiently, then you will be able to excrete it in the urine with or without diuretic therapy; usually, we use a combination of either single or double diuretics to augment that diuresis. If it is someone with pulmonary edema, who is overloaded, that patient is compromised; then, I would say that because of the rapidity with which you could remove fluid with ultrafiltration - without the use of diuretics - that you could theoretically improve the cardio-respiratory status of this patient much more readily with ultrafiltration. So, I see a role for it. I don't remember being in a situation in which I haven't been able to solve that just with repeated albumin and diuretic therapy; but, I do it very carefully. I'm afraid to leave the patient because people who have seen me or other people use albumin and diuretic therapy, may think "this is easy - I can do it myself!" Former residents go out in private practice and have that situation and they just order the albumin infusion and order the diuretic to be given at a certain time. A general pediatrician, a former resident, was totally surprised when pulmonary edema and cardio-respiratory arrest, difficult resuscitation, brain damage and law suit came after the casual approach to the nephrotic with this therapy. I always say that if you are going to do it, you'd better hang around, you'd better do it very carefully. The same would apply to ultrafiltration if I had it available and we agreed that we should use it. I have just not thought about it but I'm glad you brought it up.

COMMENT-QUESTION: I would like to underline the statement that was just made. That is, one can acutely expand the vascular volume of a nephrotic patient with large doses of albumin and precipitate congestive heart failure. So, one has to use it cautiously, gradually, and with a careful eye on the patient. Second, furosemide may have to be used in somewhat larger dosages in the nephrotic because furosemide binds to protein. It, in fact, binds to the protein that is present in the urine and that renders it less accessible to its site of action. Some of the studies out of Minnesota suggest that furosemide in a nephrotic might in fact be less effective for that reason. I would also like to underline my concern about the use of furosemide in the newborn. We have seen a lot of children with significant hypercalciuria and with nephrocalcinosis due to the chronic use of extremely high doses of furosemide. I have never quite understood why it is being used and why so much. A controlled study is warranted.

I would like to ask a question about Acute Renal Failure in infants. Often the diagnosis is made because of a decrease in urine output. I feel rather uncomfortable with this almost religious reverence to ml/kg/hr which in fact I find the house officers using even more when dealing with a 40 kg child in the pediatric intensive care unit - a situation which is even more irrelevant. Obviously, there are two problems here. One is the output which depends to some extent on input and second, patients can have a non-oliguric acute renal failure with adequate urine output and still have renal failure. Also, I would like to make a comment on the Renal Failure Index in the premature with Acute Renal Failure. Although we do use this and we use fractional excretion of sodium and we do use urine to plasma creatinine ratios, there is a rather large overlap. Frequently, I am left in the position of trying to explain why two out of three point in one direction and one out of three point in another direction. Finally, I'd like to ask about the fluid challenge: some use a challenge of 30 mEq/L of sodium chloride as saline; others have recommended fluid challenges of D_5W. I personally prefer isotonic saline. I am wondering whether there are certain circumstances in the neonate which would suggest use of a hypertonic solution. Finally, I wonder whether or not there has been any success with low dose dopamine infusion in the neonate with Acute Renal Failure.

RESPONSE: Now let me see. It's a tall order. One question was the definition of renal failure. The second one, the indices. On the definition: those are just criteria to determine if there is the possibility of renal failure. They are not meant to indicate that once the patient has those variables, he is in renal failure. If the urine output is decreasing, obviously something is happening. Maybe it is appropriate for the patient but, by the same token, maybe you are giving too little fluid, or indeed the patient is going into renal failure, bearing in mind of course that from 30 to 50% of patients with renal failure may not be oliguric.

The use of the indices in the very pre-term infant could be misleading especially when the infant is seen at the point where he already has had a fluid challenge, he's already gotten this and that medication, is on this and that drug. Of course, under the circumstances, it is very difficult to interpret any results. But assuming that you have a patient who has not been receiving any of these drugs, there are some studies to indicate that certain parameters are better in predicting the possibility of honest to goodness renal failure than others. One that Dr. Gordillo has used is the osmolality ratio. According to him if the ratio is less than 1.1 it is predictive of Acute Renal Failure. That was a retrospective study, as I recall, in the Pediatric Clinics of North America. In the adult population, a prospective study showed that the fractional sodium excretion and the Renal Failure Index could be of a highly predictive value. The problem in the pre-term infant, as you know, is that normally the fractional sodium excretion could be very high especially if you give a lot of sodium and water. So, one may not be able to make a distinction between one type of renal failure and another, just by using the renal failure indices. Then, how does one arrive at a diagnosis of renal failure in these newborns? It would have to be with the use of a constellation of history, physical examination, and some of these indices and see which one would point in the right direction.

The reason that fluid challenge was chosen, (30 milimols of sodium chloride), is because some of these patients may already be fluid overloaded to begin with; in those cases, the sodium situation is different. That's why it was chosen to be that way. If you give normal saline and the other parameters of adequate volume depletion do not give you the real story, then you will have overloaded them with sodium. With the use of dopamine, I have not really done that sort of study. There was a paper, I think from San Diego, which reported that low doses of dopamine were given and the effect on renal function. That was presented initially as an abstract at the San Antonio meetings several years ago. By that time, what they had was about six patients. Two of them had increase in renal function; one didn't change, and two actually decreased. My comment at that time was that that was a very honest assessment of dopamine infusion in newborns. I don't know of any prospective study showing that dopamine improves renal function or that it ameliorates renal failure in any way.

COMMENT: Regarding the use of the indices of renal failure in adults, I think that it's important to remember that we have to be careful in basing the diagnosis on a number. The clinical setting in which this occurs and all the things that happen between the patient's arrival, the time of consultation to the Renal Service, interfere with the use of these tests. There was an Editorial in The American Journal of Medicine within the last two years making an important point: in using the fractional excretion of sodium, it has to be understood that there is a gray zone between the normal of < 1 and the clearly abnormal > 3, The clinical circumstances (contrast medium administration, edematous states, etc.) modify the interpretation of those indices. Maybe a challenge with diuretics will help clarify this problem.

COMMENT: I would like to make a comment on the urine flow rate. Somewhere along the line, neonatologists have adopted this approach and it is now a thorn in my side! It has theoretical bases which I object to. If one applies this to a 26 week 600-700 g infant, for a urine flow rate of 1 cc/kg/hr this infant may have a GFR of 0.1 to 0.2 ml/min, or somewhere between 6 and 12 ml/min/1.73m^2. To excrete 1 ml/kg/hr of urine, that means that the infant has to reject 10 to 20% of what he filters in order to qualify and escape the diagnosis of Acute Renal Failure. If you apply that to a term infant or even carrying that up to the 60 kg adult with a GFR of 125 ml/min, you are asking him still to excrete less than 1% of what he filters to have an adequate urine flow rate. Now, why does a 600 grammer have to reject 17 to 20% of his glomerular filtrate to escape the diagnosis of Acute Renal Failure? This is beyond me! Why can't he also be allowed to reject only 1% or 2% of his glomerular filtrate? Well, that would make us kind of nervous because we wouldn't be able to measure it! We would have to dust off the bladder from time to time! So, it makes us uncomfortable. Somehow we are lulled into this false sense of security when we see urine coming out. I would like to remind you that urine that comes into the bladder is the end product of renal function. It is not renal function. It is not a measure of renal function. It is only a balm that we apply to ourselves as we try to treat these babies.

Regarding the comment about the fractional excretion of sodium and the indices in the newborn infant who already has a fractional excretion of sodium > 3% under 30 weeks of gestation, a single dose of furosemide 1 mg/kg I.V. (the standard dose) will increase the fractional excretion of sodium from 1 to 12-15%; and because the 1/2 life of furosemide in the very pre-term infant may be up to 18 or 24 hours, perhaps even longer, one dose of furosemide 24 hours before may make you unable to use those indices in any meaningful fashion. The fluid challenge in the studies of others and of ours in puppies, show that even giving isotonic saline, less tha 5% of that remains in the vascular space of the fetus or the newborn. It goes into the interstitium. So, if you say that you gave 10 ml or 20 ml/kg normal saline and very little urine came out, it may be because only a few mls of the infusate (1-2 ml/kg) actually remained in the vascular space and were circulated to the kidney for excretion and part of it may have been reabsorbed. So, that may not be a valid test and there is some argument for a fluid challenge with plasma or something which will expand the vascular space. We have already talked of what happens or what can happen when you use colloid to expand the vascular space: you may produce vasodilatation and result in a decreased cardiac output and effective arterial blood volume, which will result in a decrease in urine flow rate. So, you have to think about what you are doing and what the physiological response is in the animal, be it four legged or two legged, that you are studying. Just because it sounds good, it is not sufficient.

COMMENT: I think that you have to be careful with the albumin, because the capillaries of the pre-term infant are very permeable to albumin and it might just go into the lungs and you will have more problems.

COMMENT: I was not recommending albumin. I was saying that it has a theoretical advantage of keeping more of the volume in the vascular space to prompt the diuresis; if that is as far as you are able to think in terms of renal function, if urine flow rate is your end point in assessing the patient. But, the capillaries are leaky and permeable to protein, and what you will do in giving albumin is that that albumin will go into the interstitium and raise the oncotic pressure of the interstitial fluid thus retaining that fluid in the interstitial space and preventing the fluid from re-entering the circulation. The only way it will get back usually is through the lymphatic circulation.

QUESTION: Have you ever had any success using sodium modelling to mobilize interstitial fluids? Have you employed sodium modelling at all?

RESPONSE: No. I have no experience with that. I haven't used it. I would be interested in hearing about it.

COMMENT-QUESTION: I know it is employed in the adult population. I was curious to know whether you had used it or any other select solutes as water transport media or to maintain equilibrium.

RESPONSE: No.

QUESTION: What is that again? I didn't get it.

RESPONSE: Sodium modelling. Do you ever use high sodium at the onset of dialysis or while tapering off to bring the patient out of dialysis with normal serum sodium? Some people have been successful in mobilizing fluids from the intracellular and interstitial spaces with this approach.

RESPONSE: That would have a theoretical disadvantage. We would be dealing with two problems: using a hypertonic sodium containing solution and losing water. Most infants would be cared for under the usual Sahara technique of drying fruit (radiant warmers). So, you have an evaporative loss of water. It becomes almost an impending disaster to give hypertonic sodium containing solutions in the face of high insensible water losses. You would have hypernatremia and hyperosmolality and it would be difficult to get rid of it. The adult has a much better buffering capacity in his interstitial fluid to handle that small amount of hypertonic saline. I think we would get into difficulty with the premature infant, at least the way we understand it now.

COMMENT: I think I would echo that. If I recall some studies correctly, what was done was to produce hypernatremia in kittens and they did develop cerebral hemmorrhages. Since that is a problem in the premature infant (increased osmolalities associated with intra-ventricular hemorrhage), infusing hypertonic solutions in the pre-term infant would be unwise.

MODERATOR: It has been shown that intraventricular hemorrhages can be induced also with the infustion of albumin; these were studies performed here in Miami by the Neonatology group of Dr. Bancalari.

COMMENT: This brings up the issue of fluid and electrolytes balance in the neonate. I am astonished at the number of times that those experiments in kittens are repeated in our nursery every day and how these, infants ever come out able to look straight, let alone get through school. Absolutely extraordinary oscillations in serum sodium take place over relatively short periods of time. I would urge you, as I urge our Neonatologists, not only to pay attention to the serum sodium but to make sure that correction of hyper- and hyponatremia is done in a gradual and gentle manner, unless there is a medical necessity for more rapid correction.

MODERATOR: Actually, we did some studies with albumin trying to see what happens with GFR. About 25 years ago Bill Silverman had asked me the question: "What happens with the GFR when one infuses albumin into a hypoalbuminemic neonate?". I didn't have the answer since nobody had the data. If you followed Homer Smith's reasoning you would think that the GFR would decrease because the oncotic pressure increases; in fact, what happened is that the blood pressure increased and with that, the GFR also increased probably due to a greater effect of the hydrostatic pressure increase that that of the oncotic pressure increase. Presumably, under those circumstances, there is a greater tendency for the prematurely born neonate to bleed in his head.

QUESTION: I have a question regarding aminoglycoside toxicity in the newborn. Aminoglycosides are used in our nursery in 75-80% of the critically ill newborns. It was very interesting to see the morphologic and biochemical abnormalities that were shown here. Does this have much clinical relevance? Have you followed any of these infants? Are there any long-term renal problems? We have not seen those changes. We usually monitor serum values very religiously and we tend to use much lower glycoside levels than is usually recommended. Do you have any thoughts on why we do not see those changes?

RESPONSE-COMMENT: That is a two part question. In reference to the latter comment, a lot of neonates you see with aminoglycosides do have very high trough levels; in the premature the dosage interval probably needs to be lengthened because of the persistence of the antibiotic over a longer period of time. As for seeing much nephrotoxicity, I guess it depends upon how much you search for it. It is quite difficult to determine nephrotoxicity in neonates by monitoring serum creatinine alone because of three problems: the significant decrease in GFR that must occur before serum creatinine rises, the difficulty in detecting significant changes in serum creatinine in the newborn (simply because we may be starting at very low levels) and, finally, the fact that during the first week to one month of life, plasma creatinine is declining and creatinine clearance is improving, thus making it difficult to detect a "true" decrease in GFR. That has to be used as a background against following plasma creatinine with regard to nephrotoxicity. It would be interesting for somebody to do studies of inulin, iodothalamate or creatinine clearance to see what the true incidence is. The other problem is, obviously, that in dealing with any neonatal population, you are dealing with at least a hundred variables. You would have to be able to control the study so that all the other problems, acidosis, hypoxia, hypotension, concommitant use of other nephrotoxic agents, ventilatory therapy, etc. are taken into consideration. Obviously, we have seen elevated serum creatinines in renal failure. We have been unwilling to ascribe that strictly to aminoglycosides because of everything else that was going on. What we have seen that may be related to aminoglycosides is the presence of Fanconi Syndrome. We have seen some infants with significant sodium and bicarbonate wasting which we feel may represent a proximal tubular syndrome related to aminoglycoside therapy and is associated with lysozymuria. We really don't know what is its incidence.

QUESTION: On the same topic, have you looked at your animals long term to see if there are any residual morphologic changes?

RESPONSE: We have not; others have. There is evidence that with a variety of nephrotoxic models, including the aminoglycoside model, several years out one may develop a tubulo-interstitial nephritis. I don't know that there have been clinical studies in adults who received large doses of aminoglycosides without apparent nephrotoxicity but who were studied years later to see if they had tubulo-interstitial nephritis.

COMMENT: This is a very interesting point because the question is: "Is there a chronic syndrome from aminoglycoside nephrotoxicity?" I think it is fair to say that despite what is in the literature on experimental data, I would say that there is not such a situation in patients. Clinically, I would say that there is no proof that it exists; one could also say that there is no proof that it doesn't exist. In other words, the studies have not been done. There is a group at a famous institution in this country who has been pushing the idea that it does exist. But, if you look carefully at its data (which include some clinical data) where they saw a male to female ratio, where they find that the males had more intense ATN and the females much less intense ATN (a tendency to develop interstitial nephritis of "low-grade"), you question their results and interpretation. I showed their paper and their microphotographs to the pathologist who works with us in aminoglycoside nephrotoxicity; he said, "Well, you cannot say anything. These immunofluorescence studies to me are background immunofluorescence". I am not sure. There are two papers in the world literature saying that there is a chronic lesion resulting from acute interstitial nephritis but I don't think this has been shown to be the case. The only group that's pushing this--and I think not based on solid data, not like you would like to have before accepting this--is the group I mentioned before. In other species we find no difference related to gender, either. We were going to embark on a study with long range follow-up and repeated administrations of gentamicin for several months to see if we really could get chronic changes. You say, "Well, not many patients will get aminoglycosides every two or three months". As agressive as medicine is these days, if you are in the Intensive Care Unit more than once, you will get them.

Some workers in Portland looked into one of the other pertinent questions. They performed experiments where they injected rats with the usual dose of aminoglycoside for two weeks. Then they continued and they got the usual renal failure, the high output renal failure. By the end of the second week most of the animals had recovered. Then, they continued the administration for two more weeks, a total of a month and nothing happened during the second wave. So, this is another area to be questioned. Does an episode of acute renal failure prevent you from another episode when you are in the recovery phase? But I'm not sure that people have shown that there is a chronic lesion from aminoglycoside nephrotoxicity.

COMMENT: Two points. First, we are looking at a newborn population to see whether or not recurrent courses of aminoglycoside therapy are a high risk item. So far, we don't see that as well but that's very preliminary. The question of chronic tubulo-interstitial nephritis secondary to aminoglycosides is actually interesting beyond the world of aminoglycosides because it indicates that we are not necessarily dealing with a simple, unifaceted approach to renal disease. There have been a number of animal models suggesting that exposure to one kind of toxin makes one more susceptible when exposed to another kind of toxin. We talked earlier about the combination of antibiotics--for example, some of the cephalosporins enhancing the nephrotoxicity of the aminoglycosides. That also has been reported with cyclosporine which may or may not become popular over the next year or so. There are studies in animals showing that exposure to mercuric chloride or exposure to some of the diphenyl compounds, exposure to lead, may make the animal population more susceptible when it is exposed to other potentially nephrotoxic agents like aminoglycosides. It may be that some of the differences that are seen in clinical studies with regard to incidence of nephrotoxicity are the reasons why some patients with all the risk factors don't get it and others do get it. This may relate to a previous clinically subtle--undetectable--insult to the kidney from a variety of causes. So, it may be that we are dealing with some cumulative problems. I would agree, though, that the data are not strong right now for chronic tubulo-interstitial nephritis due to aminoglycosides in humans.

COMMENT: I think that we need to go back and look carefully at the studies that were done prior to the recommendation of aminoglycoside therapy for premature infants: usually 2.5 mg/kg given every 12 hours for the first week of life and then automatically increased after the first week of life on the assumption that GFR increases after the first week of life. Well, we talked about it here; that just does not happen. Also, the four babies in the study in the early 70's which made those recommendations, had urine collections and creatinine clearances which were not accurately timed. In addition, they were done in infants that were not what we call very low birth weight prematures--probably the greatest precentage of those who get the medications. Now, some of you still will follow those recommendations. They are ironclad. I fight them almost daily because the studies that have been done in human infants, looking at half-life of aminoglycosides, show that prior to 34 weeks of conceptional age, the time when we and others have shown that GFR does increase, the half-life of aminoglycosides is quite prolonged even after several weeks of post-natal life. We're talking about half-life of 18 to 24 hours, not two to four hours. So, first of all, the recommendation for the doses--both the total amount and the interval--as far as I am concerned, is inappropriate for a week old, very low birth weight, premature infant. Secondly, if you follow the recommendations of the infectious disease people in getting frequent peak and trough levels, they don't understand what peak and trough levels mean. The trough levels for the aminoglycosides don't increase. Usually, in an older individual, the creatinine will rise or certainly the GFR will decrease before your trough levels begin to increase. Following the recommendation of 2.5 per kilo and getting a trough level after an IV dose of one hour, we are seeing peak levels in these babies of greater than 20. And trough levels that rise, don't come down very quickly. From our studies in the dog, gentamicin does not accumulate in any other organ but the kidney. I mean, the kidney is the sink. Gentamicin leaves the body either in a renal tubular cell or free in the urine, one way or the other. If the kidney is not filtering, the level of aminoglycoside will not decrease. It has a prolonged half-life. We have to rethink the dose of aminoglycoside according to the conceptional age of the baby, and we should follow the studies of those who have done the proper pharmacokinetic measurements, showing that we cannot adjust the dose until the baby has reached a conceptional age of at least 36 weeks. I think those aspects of the problem are very important. The kidney is going to be protected because of its unique blood flow distribution. I am not worried about long term nephrotoxicity. We've done some studies in puppies to see what the lesions look like three to six months later. We can't find the lesion but we can still find some aminoglycoside in tissues but we can't find the lysosomal changes. I'm concerned about the ototoxicity and the other changes which occur with these extremely high levels; they not only peak at 24 mcg/ml but 24 to 48 hours later, they still are around 18. In most situations, the babies would already have received four more doses of the drug.

MODERATOR: In terms of the renal damage that we have heard about today, leading to Acute Renal Failure, you just mentioned the lysosomal changes. What about the mitochondrial changes seen in hypoxic Acute Renal Failure? The group from Boston presented at the International Society of Oxygen Transport to Tissues, some fascinating changes in the ascending limb of the loop of Henle which would go along with some of the findings in terms of excessive loss of sodium in the urine. Is that a universal lesion or is that something peculiar to hypoxia? Does it not happen with aminoglycosides or other toxics?

COMMENT - RESPONSE: As you know, the group at Ann Arbor has done a number of studies which were originally done in France several years ago. They concluded that indeed there are mitochondrial abnormalities in stage three and four of gentamicin nephrotoxicity, in which hypoxia at least was not induced experimentally. If this is a primary event or not, we don't know. The interpretation depends on what you believe to be the mechanism for the so-called lysosomal phospholipidosis which occurs with gentamicin administration. It is a matter of quantity and of other things that we are completely missing. There are reports of mitochondrial changes; whether these are primary or secondary, I don't think we know.

MODERATOR: How persistent are these changes? When do we talk of a real problem for the patient? What is the meaning of the enzyme changes in the urine or a creatinine increase in the blood? Are we talking about esoteric findings that are nice to enter in the chart or talk about in Miami at a Seminar but no more than that? Do they truly carry a significance? If they do, when do they carry that significance? When do we need to start worrying?

RESPONSE-COMMENT: Indeed they are important. One of the problems alluded to before is the polypharmacy. We practice agressive medicine not only with drugs but with procedures. Many times people say, "What's the problem even if the GFR drops 30%?" What is that? If you are normal at 120, you are not going to notice a GFR of 90 or 95. Not even 60. People say, "What is the clinical relevance of this?" I think there is a lot to say about this because if you transfer this question to a medical-surgical or coronary care or a neonatal unit, then you have the multiplying effect. The patient is dehydrated, so the GFR drops a certain point. Then his renin-angiotensin system is activated. Somebody gives him aspirin which blocks the synthesis of prostaglandin and a salutory vasodilator intrarenal mechanism is blocked; now, vasoconstriction predominates. Somebody gives him an aminoglycoside. It's a Gram negative sepsis so they combine it with a cephalosporin; all those drugs may have interaction with each other. You say, "You are really making a drama out of the case". Not really. The patient may have a cancer and he is receiving cis-platinum or methotrexate or may have in the future an immunological disorder and he gets cyclosporine or he needs a radiological study and he gets contrast material. I am simply describing polypharmacy and polyprocedures. Are you surprised now that the patient develops Acute Renal Failure? I'm not.

MODERATOR: I just wanted, for the record, to put a clinical touch. We are seeing a patient with diabetes who has had a CT scan with contrast material and developed renal failure, was dialyzed and transplanted. So, it is important. I am glad to be able to stir the panel up in order to get answers to some touchy questions.

COMMENT: One example of the polypharmacy is gentamicin ototoxicity. Lots of these infants are receiving very large doses of furosemide and it is accumulating in the face of decreased renal function. We caution the neonatologists to try and give the gentamicin and furosemide at different times. There is some relationship between the gentamicin peak dosages and the ototoxicity. Regarding the question if urinary enzymes are too sensitive and if they are of any clinical relevance, we have noted marked enzymuria--predominately the enzymes located in the lysosomes which manage to store most of the aminoglycosides. We've noted these in patients who receive aminoglycosides but frankly have not found those to be clinically useful in detecting the patients who are going to have subsequent elevations in serum creatinine. We haven't looked at it with regard to creatinine clearance. It may be that patients will show changes in creatinine clearance or inulin clearance and we may be able to predict that by the amount of enzymuria. Of patients we have studied, most have marked elevations in these enzymes even before they are started on aminoglycosides because they are sick and they may already have some tubular cell injury antedating the use of the aminoglycoside. The one enzyme that we have found helpful clinically has been the lysozyme. The lysozyme and $Beta_2$ microglobulin are reabsorbed by the proximal tubule. When there is significant proximal tubule dysfunction, there are increased levels of either lysozyme or $Beta_2$ microglobulin in the urine. We found that when those levels start to rise, we often get elevations in serum creatinine subsequently. So, the changes that occur in the proximal tubule cells with aminoglycosides are very interesting, very striking, but there is a lot of debate as to their relevance in the genesis and maintenance of Acute Renal Failure. It would require a three day symposium just to discuss that. A significant lysozyme enzymuria we have seen in gentamicin treated dogs but, despite high doses and prolonged administration, we can't induce Acute Renal Failure. So, regarding those particular changes, I think the ballot is still uncertain as to their relevance to Acute Renal Failure. The mitochondrial changes do occur and are quite striking. The questions are how and why they occur. Virtually all the studies looking at aminoglycoside uptake and deposition inside the proximal tubules indicate that labeled gentamicin is bound very tightly and in very high concentrations in the lysosomes and it is very hard to find a lot of free gentamicin, especially exposed to mitochondria and enough to cause mitochondrial injury. It may be that gentamicin affects calcium metabolism which in turn plays a role in the mitochondrial dysfunction and subsequent Acute Renal Failure.

QUESTION-COMMENT: What you are mentioning might go along with what last year was mentioned or proposed here: the concept of tubular memory. Patients who had received aminoglycosides would have the tendency to develop nephrotoxicity even if they received subsequent doses 6, 8, 10 months later. I don't know if that is a separate concept but I would like your reaction to that proposition.

RESPONSE: That's the first I have heard of that. But I would not agree with that, at least from my observations.

COMMENT: I support what was just said.

QUESTION: A question and a comment. First, your method of administration of aminoglycosides; was it by IV push or by slow IV administration? We have certainly seen--because of the very small volume of the drug, especially with the very small premature--that people tend to give it very quickly. We monitor drug levels now, usually after the first dose, daily or at least twice daily afterwards, and find that if you give an IV push, you tend to get much higher peak levels. We all must be extremely careful about the method of administration. It should be given slowly, within 30 minutes to an hour. I certainly agree with the comment that the pharmacokinetics in the small sick premature infant are different from those in the larger or healthier babies, and need to be taken into consideration.

COMMENT: Absolutely, I have nothing to add to these comments except to echo them. What I have found is that when you say "Give an IV push", it is pushed right in. When you say, "Give it slowly", it's given over three minutes. That's not the way I would do it; that's the way I watch it happen. That's the way people seem to interpret it but I think a slow infusion would be better and perhaps we would be better off giving it intramuscularly if we don't have time to infuse it slowly. The high peak levels are extremely important.

COMMENT: An article just came out in the Journal of Pediatrics showing that the method of IV administration may also be important. Certain routes produce more delayed peaks than others.

MODERATOR: We must stop here because of time limitations. If there are any further questions or comments that you want to make, please get them to me and we will review them at another time. Thank you.

EDITOR'S COMMENTS:

This Panel Discussion was "juicy" and full of practical as well as theoretical questions-information. The subjects discussed included techniques of peritoneal dialysis, hemodialysis, hemoperfusion, continuous I.V. ultrafiltration, use of bank blood and bicarbonate vs lactate and the related subject of lactic acidosis, pitfalls in the diagnosis of Acute Renal Failure by urine flow and other methods, interstitial fluid and intravenous fluid administration including sodium and albumin, and aminoglycoside nephrotoxicity as it relates to specific agents, cumulative problems, association with other agents and hypoxia, and rate of administration. In keeping with the Seminar theme, all subjects referred to the neonate. An overriding tone of self-questioning was evident in the exchanges, with emphasis on the possible rights and wrongs or even more, whether or not we know how to differentiate them. It was noted that there are different approaches, all of which may be right for certain situations, and that maybe we need to temper our criticisms or praises of one approach - diagnostic or therapeutic - versus another.

III

CONGENITAL DISORDERS

SYNDROMES WITH RENAL MALFORMATIONS

P.J. Benke, M.D., Ph.D., A. Feuer, M.S., R. Fojaco, M.D.,
J. Misiewicz, M.D. and M.E. Carlin, M.D.

The term syndrome is derived from a greek word that means things that travel together. A syndrome describes a grouping of signs and symptoms of an entity that may or may not have a known underlying etiology. Renal anomalies are frequently part of a pattern, so the nephrologist should look for other malformations when renal anomalies are identified. Making a syndrome diagnosis where none was known does more than establish a diagnostic coup. Definition of a syndrome: 1) helps families appreciate that there is a name for the problem, 2) helps define the outcome, and 3) is useful in genetic counselling and recurrence risk, even when no therapy is possible. No renal anomaly is specific for a given syndrome, but a good nephrologist can look at the rest of the patient and define anomalies, group findings, and entertain a syndrome diagnosis.

POTTER'S SYNDROME

This is the premier pediatric dysmorphic syndrome with renal anomalies.[1-5] These children have redundant, dehydrated skin with multiple folds, ocular hypertelorism, epicanthal folds, a flattened nasal bridge with a flat nasal tip, a small chin that frequently has a transverse crease, large, poorly lobulated, low-set and flattened ears, and a short neck. Congenital limb contractures and club feet are frequently found. The anomalies are secondary to oligohydramnios. Amnion nodosum and low birth weight are common. An infant with Potter's Syndrome is shown in Figure 1.

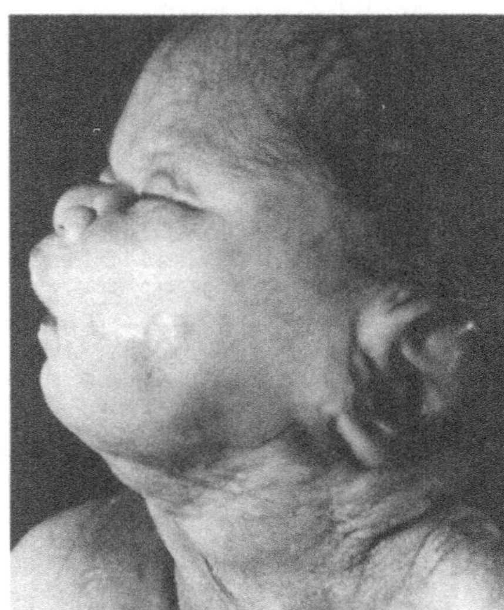

Figure 1. A child with Potter's Syndrome.

The syndrome is universally fatal. Forty percent of these infants are stillborn and most others live only a few hours because of severe lung hypoplasia, absence of surfactant and resulting respiratory insufficiency. In the rare case that survives a day or two, death results from renal failure.

The lower urinary tract frequently has hypoplastic or absent ureters and/or bladder on pathological examination. The uterus and vagina can be absent in females while the vas deferens and seminal vesicles may be affected in males. Sometimes a cloaca or a urinary tract fistula remains. Other associated malformations may include anal atresia, absent sigmoid colon or rectum, esophageal and/or duodenal atresia, cleft palate, terminal limb anomalies, and caudal regression (sirenomelia).

The frequency is 1/5,000-1/10,000 births. The incidence in males is three times more frequent than in females; and recurrence risk is 2-3%. Twins are usually discordant. Since the oligohydramnios is not as severe in twins, facial features are less marked. The alpha-fetoprotein is elevated in some cases and there is an increased rate of open neural tube defects in siblings of Potter's Syndrome infants.

We have reviewed all cases of Potter's Syndrome at two large South Florida hospitals from 1979-83 and found an excess of affected males in Potter's Syndrome type IA and type II. Congenital heart disease was present in 5 of 30 patients, with upper extremity anomalies (Holt-Oram Syndrome) seen in 2 of these patients. Other associated anomalies are shown in Table 1.

Table 1. Anomalies observed in cases of Potter's Syndrome at two Florida Hospitals.

	Male (Number)	Female (Number)	Additional renal findings		Associated Anomalies	
Type IA Renal Aplasia	9	3	Hypoplastic bladder	3/12	Accessory spleen	1/12
			Ureteral agenesis and/or hypoplasia	2/12	Adrenal anomalies	3/12
					Annular pancreas	1/12
					Cataracts	1/12
					Cleft palate	1/12
					Club foot	2/12
					CNS anomalies	1/12
					Coarctation of aorta	1/12
					Hypoplastic nails	1/12
					Incomplete bowel rotation	1/12
					Simian crease	1/12
					Ventricular fibroelastosis	1/12
Type IB Renal Dysplasia	2	3	Hypoplastic bladder	1/5	Accessory spleen	1/5
			Dilated bladder and urinary tract	1/5	Arthrogryposis	1/5
					Bicornate uterus	1/5
					Patent anus	1/5
Type II Polycystic Dysplastic Kidneys	7	4	Hypoplastic bladder	2/11	Accessory or abnormal spleen	3/11
			Hypoplasia or atresia of ureters	8/11	Cataracts	1/11
			Horseshoe kidney	3/11	Club foot	2/11
			Dilated kidney and/or urinary tract	1/11	Diaphragmatic hernia	2/11
					Holt-Oram (truncus arteriosus)	2/11
					Hypoplastic nails	1/11
					Hypoplastic prostate	1/11
					Patent anus	1/11
					Patent ductus arteriosus	1/11
					Simian crease	3/11
					Ventricular hypertrophy	1/11
					Wormian bone	1/11
Mixed Polycystic Kidney and Absent Kidney	0	2	Atresia or agenesis of ureter	2/2	Adrenal anomalies	1/2
			Absent bladder	1/2	Atrial septal defect	1/2
					Choanal atresia	1/2
					Esophageal anomalies	1/2
					Incomplete bowel rotation	1/2
					Sirenomelia	1/2

FETAL ALCOHOL SYNDROME

Characteristic dysmorphic features in the fetal alcohol syndrome include: arched eyebrows, narrow palpebral fissures, epicanthal folds, anti-mongoloid slant, esotropia, ptosis, broadened flattened nasal bridge, long flattened philtrum, micrognathia, low-set ears often with a typical "railroad track" appearance, thin lips, short fifth fingers with clinodactly and generalized short terminal phalanges often with nail hypoplasia. Neurological immaturity with both gross and fine motor delay as well as hypotonia are typical. Congenital heart disease, especially atrial and ventricular septal defects, and cleft palate are common while radio-ulnar synostosis is seen rarely. A child with fetal alcohol syndrome is shown in Figure 2.

Many patients have pre- and postnatal growth failure, microcephaly and neurological and cognitive delays. Not all exposed infants develop the syndrome and it is unclear exactly how much alcohol is necessary to cause such effects. Consumption of alcohol in the first trimester is more detrimental than consumption in the last two trimesters. Renal anomalies are frequent enough in the fetal alcohol syndrome to justify ultrasound of the kidney in each suspected case. Although there is little mention of renal anomalies in the fetal hydantoin syndrome, both alcohol and hydantoins have growth suppressant effects in the fetus, both may lead to children with similar physical features, and both may lead to renal anomalies. Anomalies associated with the fetal alcohol syndrome are shown in Table 2.

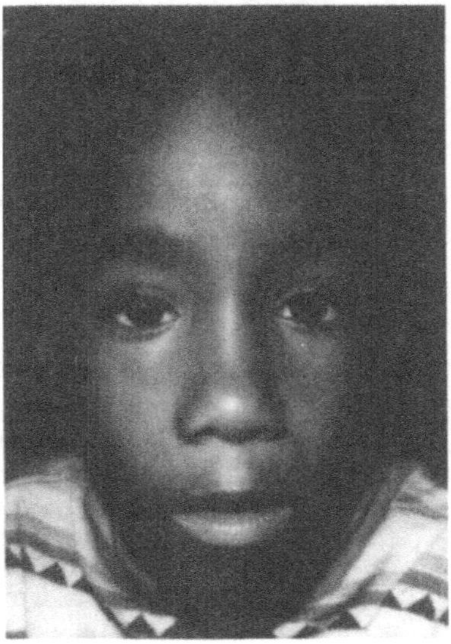

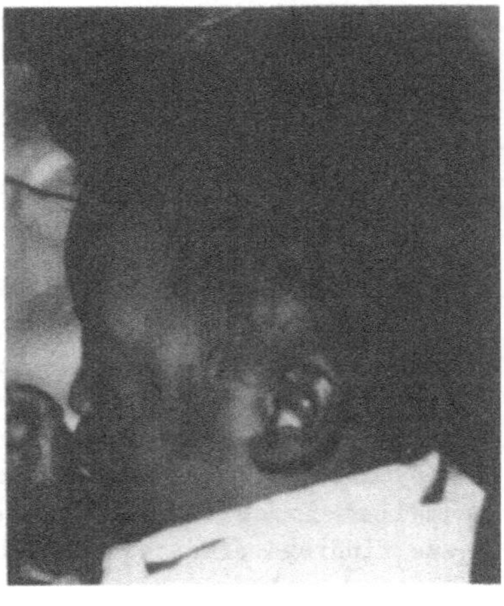

Figure 2. Two children with fetal alcohol syndrome. Note short palpebral fissures, epicanthal folds, and long philtrum in top photo. Lower photo illustrates railroad tract ear anomaly.

Table 2. Features of renal anomalies in published accounts of the fetal alcohol syndrome.

REFERENCE	FREQUENCY OF RENAL ANOMALIES + TYPE OF PATIENTS DESCRIBED	SPECIFIC RENAL ANOMALIES MENTIONED
Debeukelaer, et al., 1977 (6)	No frequency estimated Describes 1 black male	Single hypoplastic kidney with poor function, normal calyceal pattern.
Dunigan & Werlin, 1981 (7)	No frequency estimated Describes 1 female	Enlarged liver, portal system, and right kidney, small left kidney, calyceal blunting,cirrhosis, normal collecting system, portal fibrosis, and extrahepatic biliary atresia.
Habbick, et al., 1979 (8)	1/3 American Indian females described was affected (33%)	Renal tubular ectasia;large kidneys with cystic tubules,liver fibrosis.
Qazi, et al., 1979 (9)	Overall estimate from published cases: 3% of all cases have renal anomalies. Describes 6 black children	Horseshoe kidney with third ureter; poorly functioning hypoplastic kidneys or unilateral hypoplasia with hypertrophied kidney; renal pelviectasis with superior calyectasis; malrotated enlarged kidneys. Also reports crossed fused ectopia, hydronephrosis, and ureteropelvic junction obstruction.
Smith, et al., 1979 (10)	Estimates 30% have renal anomalies	Mild ureteropelvic junction obstruction and renal hypoplasia.
Smith, 1982 (11)		Occasional renal malformations. Similar anomalies noted in fetal hydantoin and fetal trimethadione syndromes.

MALFORMATION SYNDROMES WITH FREQUENT RENAL ANOMALIES

Children with Williams Syndrome (elfin facies, congenital heart disease, neonatal hypercalcemia); overgrowth syndromes (Hemihypertrophy, Beckwith-Wiedemann); Noonan Syndrome (low set ears, antimongoloid slant, ptosis, pectus, congenital heart disease, short stature, delayed speech, and occasional mental delay); and Klippel-Feil Syndrome (12) have renal anomalies in sufficient frequency to justify study of the kidneys. These findings are shown in Table 3.

Table 3. Features of specific syndromes.

SYNDROME	RENAL FINDINGS
Williams	Renal artery stenosis
Hemihypertrophy	Wilm's tumor
Beckwith-Wiedemann	Wilm's tumor
Aniridia, retardation	Wilm's tumor
Noonan	Duplication of collecting system, renal hypoplasia
Klippel-Feil	Solitary, fused, pelvic kidneys (20%)

Children with single umbilical artery and ear anomalies, particularly low-set ears or ear pits, should have ultrasound or IVP examination of the kidneys. Ear pits, with or without branchial arch cysts and renal anomalies may be part of the B.O.R. (branchio-oto-renal) Syndrome (13) which is dominantly inherited. A child with this syndrome is shown in Figure 3, and his IVP is shown in Figure 4.

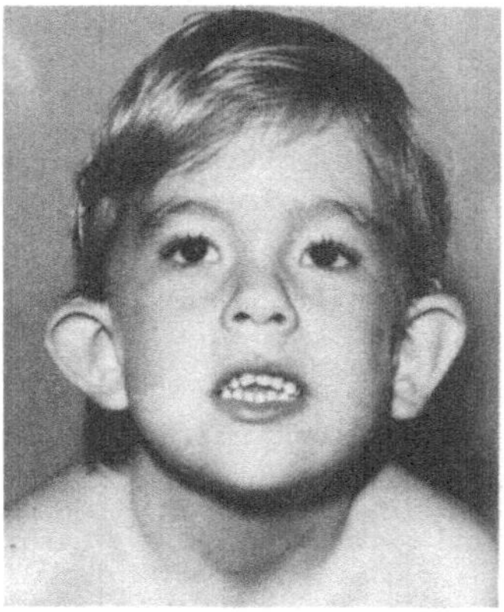

Figure 3. A child with the B.O.R. Syndrome. Note low ears and left neck scar from the branchial arch cyst.

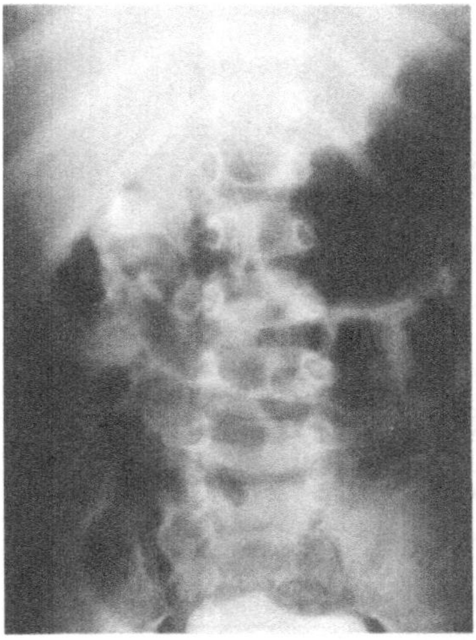

Figure 4. Single kidney in a child with the B.O.R. Syndrome.

Established malformation syndromes with renal anomalies are shown in Table 4. Table 5 compares some of the newest malformation syndromes with renal anomalies.

CHROMOSOME SYNDROMES WITH RENAL ANOMALIES

Added or deleted chromosome material interferes with morphogenesis and organ formation so it is not surprising that many chromosome disorders are associated with renal anomalies. In practical terms, it is important to note that renal anomalies are at least 50% in Trisomy 13, trisomy 18 and Turner's Syndrome, and definition of these anomalies frequently serves a useful purpose. Thus, all children with these syndromes should have an ultrasound or an IVP. A renal ultrasound is of use in Down's Syndrome because the risk of anomalies is at least 5%. Chromosomal problems that have been associated with renal anomalies are delineated in Table 6.

Table 4. Partial listing of other non-chromosomal syndromes with renal anomalies.

SYNDROME	RENAL AGENESIS	RENAL DYSPLASIA	RENAL HYPOPLASIA	RENAL HYPERPLASIA	RENAL ECTOPIA	RENAL CYSTS	OTHER RENAL, HEPATIC AND BLADDER FINDINGS	EXTREMITIES
MECKEL SYNDROME [100% have renal anomalies]		Bi	Y	Y		100% Y	Hepatic hyperplasia with enlarged portal tracts, hepatic fibrosis, and some cysts. Prominent extramedullary hematopoiesis hypoplastic bladder and ureters.	postaxial polydactyly (55-70%), some short limbed dwarfism, talipes, simian crease
B.O.R. SYNDROME (BRANCHIO-OTO-RENAL) [>90% have renal anomalies, 6% have renal failure]	Bi or Uni	66% Bi	Bi		crossed	Y	Partial duplication of renal pelvis, bifid or absent ureters, blunted malrotated calyceal system, absent bladder, nephrophthisis.	talipes, hands sometimes coarse, spade-like
V.A.C.T.E.R.L. SYNDROME (VERTEBRAL-ANAL-CARDIO-T-E FISTULA-RENAL/RADIAL-LIMB) [53-82% have renal anomalies]	30% Y	Y	Uni		Uni	22% Y	18% have obstructive lesions.	agenesis of thumbs, pre-axial polydactyly, bones small or absent
ROBERTS SYNDROME					horse-shoe kidney	poly-cystic		phocomelia, bones rudimentary/absent, bowing talipes, syndactyly
ZELLWEGER SYNDROME (CEREBROHEPATORENAL)		Y			horse-shoe kidney	>50% have glomerular micro-cysts	Hepatomegaly, tubular ectasia.	camptodactyly, simian crease 43%, clinodactyly 53%, overlapped toes 54%, talipes
RUBENSTEIN-TAYBI SYNDROME [50% have renal anomalies]	Uni					hydro-neph-rosis	Duplication of kidney and ureters.	broad thumb and hallux tips 100%, broad fingertips 72%
PRUNE BELLY SYNDROME		Bi			Bi	hydro-neph-rosis	Malrotation, urethral atresia and hydroureters.	talipes
ROKITANSKY (KUSTER-HAUSER) SYNDROME (MULLERIAN APLASIA) [30-50% have renal anomalies]	Bi or Uni		Y				Double ureters.	syndactyly, distal limb defects

References 11-31. Uni = unilateral Bi = bilateral Y = present

FACIAL/NECK	HEART	OTHER ASSOCIATED OR OCCASIONAL ANOMALIES	POPULATION FREQUENCY	HETEROZYGOTE EXPRESSION	ASSOCIATED PROBLEMS AND MISCELLANEOUS
microcphaly, cataracts, oral clefts 30%, retinal dysplasia, micrognathia, microphthalmia, absent olfactory lobes, sloping forehead, coloboma	some congenital disease	encephalocele/occip. meningocele 63-80%, hydrocephalus 15%, anencephaly 10%, lung hypoplasia, accessory spleen, ambiguous genitalia, absent pituitary gland, NTD's	Yemenite Jews affected in higher frequencies than general population.	Sibs have triad of features 2/3 of time.	Often confused with trisomy 13. AFP has been elevated in all prenatal diagnoses reported (probable cause is renal lesion).
bilateral pre-auricular pits & sinuses, some"lop" hypoplastic posteriorly rotated low-set ears, lachrimal duct stenosis, saddle nose		hearing deficit, malformed cochlea, stapes fixation, cleft fistulas, occasional branchial cysts, hypoplastic lungs		Severe renal dysplasia in 6% of heterozygotes.	
oral clefts 18%, abnormal pinna	VSD 30%, PDA 26%, ASD 20%	vertebral anoms 36%, anal atresia 40%, TE fistula 24%, esophageal atresia, malrotated small bowel, single umbilical artery	Cauc males affected most frequently. Overall rate= 1.63/10,000 liveborn.	Parents had bi- & tri-furcation of renal pelvis (in one family)	Assoc. w/trisomies 13 & 18, 5p- del., extrophy of cloaca anomalad, conjoined twins, sirenomelia, & amniotic bands.
often severe oral clefts, microcephaly, silvery hair, ocular proptosis, and lenticular opacities, hypoplastic nasal alae, facial hemangiomata	congenital disease	lumbar spina bifida, enlarged genitalia, cryptorchidism			May be the same as the pseudothalidomide syndrome.
brachyturricephaly, high forehead, rounded face, hypertelorism, mongoloid slant, epicanthal folds, micrognathia, retinopathy, corneal clouding, ptosis, nystagmus, high arched palate, odd ear helices	VSD, PDA, patent foramen ovale	hypotonia, severe MR cryptorchidism, hypoplastic thymus, clitoromegaly, delayed skeletal maturation, hyperplastic islet cells	Females affected almost 2X as often as males. In Australia, 1/100,000 livebirths.		
microcephaly 97%, high-arched palate 96%, anti-mongoloid slant 94%, broad beaked nose 87%, hypertelorism 87%, strabismus 76%	murmurs 31%	vertebral anoms 62%, short stature 77%, MR 100%, hirsuitism 64%, low bone age 87% rib anomalies 56%			
microcephaly		abdominal muscles deficient, pulmonary hypoplasia, cryptorchidism			20-38% have Turners (XO) Syndrome.
conductive deafness	some anomalies	vertebral anoms 10%, no vagina, malformed uterus & bladder	Only females affected.		Associated with Klippel-Feil malformations.

Table 5. New Renal Malformation Syndromes.

SYNDROME	RENAL	EXTREMITIES	FACIAL/NECK	OTHER ANOMALIES
RENAL DYSPLASIA/ MESOMELIA/RADIO-HUMERAL FUSION SYNDROME	Bilateral hypoplasia, atypical dysplasia (normal nephrons scattered through the kidney)	short forearms & metacar-pals, talipes	beaked nose w/depressed nasal root, mild micro-gnathia, high palate, long thin vermillion lips	long thin ribs, anterior rounding of lumbar vertebrae & short stature
ACRO-RENAL-OCULAR SYNDROME	Unilateral hypoplasia, crossed ectopia or unilateral sacral ectopia, malrotation of bladder diverticula	preaxial polydactyly thumb hypoplasia, convex nail	brachycephaly, nystagmus, ptosis, eye coloboma, pre-auricular tag, Duane anomaly	pulmonic stenosis, choanal atresia
SCHINZEL-GIEDION SYNDROME	Some bilateral hyperplasia and hydronephrosis	post-axial polydactyly hyperconvex nails, short forearms (ulnar), talipes	coarse facies, midface retraction, frontal bos-sing, short upturned nose macroglossia, malformed ears, redundant neck skin facial hemangiomata, hypertelorism	ASD, skeletal dysplasia, wide open cranial sutures, hyper-trichosis, hypo-plastic nipples & dermal ridges, choanal stenosis, simian crease, hypospadius
RADIAL RAY APLASIA AND RENAL ANOMALIES SYNDROME	Unilateral agenesis, crossed ectopia	angular talipomanus absent radius & thumbs	auricular malformations	short stature
NEUROFACIODIGI-TORENAL (NFDR) SYNDROME	Unilateral agenesis	triphalan-gism, broad halluces, long thumb, flat feet, hyperexten-sible elbow	brachycephaly, high fore-head, nose groove, lowset poseriorly rotated ears w/short auricles & ante-verted lobules, hyperte-lorism, short neck, slight anti-mongoloid slant	megalencephaly, severe mental retardation, short stature, cryptorchidism
LYMPHEDEMA/HY-PERPARATHYROID-ISM/NEPHROPATHY SYNDROME	Bilateral hypoplastic kidneys with inadequate function	lymphedema of forearms hands &legs short nail beds	brachydactyly, cataracts, conjunctival edema, broad nasal bridge, mild ptosis medial flare of eyebrows, facial hypertrichosis	systolic murmur, itchy dry skin, increased carrying angle, scrotal lymphedema
ACRO-RENAL-MANDIBULAR SYNDROME	Bilateral agenesis & dysplasia, absent ure-ters, cysts, & uterus unicornis or didelphys	bilateral split hand split foot	hypoplastic mandible, low interorbital distance, small tongue	pectus carinatum, a few pulmonary cysts, vertebral anomalies
ACRORENAL SYNDROME	Unilateral agenesis, bilateral hypoplasia, hypoplastic ureters, & hydronephrosis	split hand split foot	minor facial anomalies	some VSD, coarc-tation of aorta, minor skeletal anomalies
FRASER (CRYPTO-PHTHALMOS) SYNDROME	Bilateral agenesis	partial cutaneous syndactyly	cryptophthalmos, "pinched" nose, hypoplastic nares, forehead hair, cupped ears	laryngeal, anal & vaginal atresia, lung hypoplasia, cystic ovaries
UPPER LIMB/RENAL MALFORMATIONS SYNDROME	Crossed-fused renal ectopia, caliectasis, vesico-ureteral reflux, hyperplastic dysplastic kidneys, hydronephrosis	absent thumbs, small or absent arm bones & fingers		short stature, T-E fistula, duodenal atresia, heart murmur, VSD

References 11, 25, 32-44

Table 6. Chromosome disorders with renal malformations. See references 45 and 46.

GENETIC CHANGE		RENAL AND GENITO/URINARY ANOMALIES MENTIONED	INCIDENCE
I. ADDITIONAL GENETIC MATERIAL	1q23 trisomy	multiple renal anomalies	rare
	3q2 trisomy	polycystic, aplastic, or accessory kidney	frequent
	4p trisomy	multiple renal anomalies	rare
	4q2+3 trisomy	horseshoe kidney, renal hypoplasia, dilated ureters	frequent
	7p	V-U reflux, hydronephrosis	
	7q3 trisomy	multiple renal anomalies	common
	8 trisomy	renal and ureteral malformations	infrequent
	8q2 trisomy	hydronephrosis with hydroureter	1/16
	8p trisomy	ureteral stenosis, absent bladder	rare
	9p tetrosomy	multiple renal anomalies	frequent
	9q3 trisomy	hydroureter	infrequent
	9 trisomy	multiple renal anomalies	frequent
	10q2 trisomy	multiple renal anomalies	common
	10p trisomy	polycystic, aplastic, or double kidneys, rotation anomalies and aplasia of ureter	common
	11q2 trisomy	urogenital malformations (often in 11;22 transloc.)	frequent
	12q2 trisomy	hydronephrosis with ureterocele, ectopia	infrequent
	13 trisomy	polycystic hydronephrotic kidneys, duplication of ureters and/or kidneys	30-60% [45] 60-80% [46]
	13q2+3 trisomy	multiple renal anomalies	infrequent
	17q2 trisomy	urinary tract malformations	freq; 4/4
	18 trisomy	ectopic or horseshoe kidney, megaloureter or double ureter, hydronephrosis	frequent; 70%
	18q2 trisomy	multiple renal anomalies	rare; 1/11
	18p+q1 trisomy	ectopic or polycystic kidneys	infrequent
	20p trisomy	multiple renal anomalies	rare
	21 trisomy	agenesis, hypoplasia, horseshoe kidney	3-7%
	22p ->q2 trisomy	multiple renal anomalies	rare
	47,XXY and other Klinefelters	hypospadius	infrequent
	XXXXY	hydronephrosis	10%
	Tri- & Tetraploidy	renal dysplasia, hydronephrosis, urinary anomalies	common
II. DELETED GENETIC MATERIAL	1q4 monosomy	single kidney	1/4
	4p monosomy	multiple renal anomalies	infreq [45] or 33% [46]
	4q3 monosomy	multiple renal anomalies	frequent
	5p monosomy	multiple renal anomalies	rare
	11q2 monosomy	multiple renal anomalies	infrequent
	11p13 monosomy	WAGR ASSOCIATION: Malrotated kidneys assoc. with aniridia, mental and growth retardation, ambiguous genitalia, and Wilm's tumor or gonadoblastoma	frequent 6/11 have tumor
	13q3 monosomy	hypoplastic kidneys	common
	16q23-26	absent or horseshoe kidney	
	18q-	multiple renal anomalies	common;40%
	ring 18	hydronephrosis, tubular dilation	20%
	ring 21	renal agenesis, ureteral anomaly	common
	21q monosomy	multiple renal anomalies	common
	45,X	horseshoe kidney, hypoplasia, agenesis, rotational malformations, hydronephrosis, bifid ureters	40-60% [45] 60-80% [46]

SYNDROME IDENTIFICATION

There are basically 3 ways that a syndrome can be identified:

1) Comparison to previous personally observed cases;
2) Establishing a "gestalt" of a case and comparing it to reference pictures or material; and
3) Listing anomalies and looking up a differential diagnosis of an anomaly in a text like Smith (11).

Careful observation of the head, neck, hands and heart are important when dealing with an individual with anomalies. Appreciating that other findings are present, and listing all the findings are the first steps in identifying a syndrome. If specific renal anomalies were associated with specific syndromes this task would be easier. Except for the syndromes in Table 3, this is rarely the case. Although the path to a syndrome diagnosis may be difficult, practice makes it easier. Like the turtle, progress in syndrome identification can only be made by sticking one's neck out.

Blood should be drawn for chromosome studies from all children with multiple anomalies or renal anomalies and developmental delay.

ACKNOWLEDGEMENTS

We thank Nicole Oncin for help with the preparation of this manuscript.

REFERENCES

1. Schmidt, W., Schroeder, T.M., Buchinger, G. and Kubli, F.: Genetics, pathoanatomy and prenatal diagnosis of Potter I syndrome and other urogenital tract diseases. Clin. Genet. 22: 105, 1982.
2. Marras, A., Mereu, G., Dessi, C. and Macciotta, A.: Oligohydramnios and extrarenal abnormalities in Potter syndrome. J. Pediatr. 102: 597, 1983.
3. Wright, J.C.Y. Jr. and Christopher, C.R.: Sirenomelia, Potter's syndrome and their relationship to monozygotic twinning. A case report and discussion. J. Repro. Med. 27: 291, 1982.
4. Cote', G.B.: Potter's syndrome and chromosomal anomalies. Hum. Genet. 58: 220, 1981.
5. Chappard, D., Lauras, B., Fargier, P. and Knopf, J.F.: Sirenomelie et dysplasie renale multikystique. J. Genet. Hum. 31: 403, 1983.
6. Debeukelaer, M.M., Randall, C.L. and Stroud, D.R.: Renal anomalies in the fetal alcohol syndrome. J. Pediatr. 91: 759, 1977.
7. Dunigan, T.H. and Werlin, S.L.: Extrahepatic biliary atresia and renal anomalies in fetal alcohol syndrome. Am. J. Dis. Child. 135: 1067, 1981.
8. Habbick, B.F., Zaleski, W.A., Casey, R. and Murphy, F.: Liver abnormalities in three patients with fetal alcohol syndrome. Lancet i: 580, 1979.
9. Qazi, Q., Masakawa, A., Milman, D. et al.: Renal anomalies in fetal alcohol syndrome. Pediatrics 63: 886, 1979.
10. Smith, D.F., Wood, B. and P. MacLeod: Skeletal and renal alterations in the foetal alcohol syndrome. Abstract presented at Chicago Birth Defects Conference, June 24-27, 1979.
11. Smith, D.W.: Recognizable Patterns of Human Malformation, 3rd edition. Philadelphia: W.B. Saunders Co., 1982.
12. Duncan, P.A.: Embryologic pathogenesis of renal agenesis associated with cervical vertebral anomalies (Klippel-Feil phenotype). Birth Defects XIII (3D): 91, 1977.

13. Melnick, M., Hodes, M.E., Nance, W.E., et al.: Branchio-oto-renal dysplasia and branchio-oto dysplasia: Two distinct autosomal dominant disorders. Clin. Genet. 13: 425, 1978.
14. Gorlin, R.J., Pindborg, J.J. and Cohen, M.M.: Syndromes of the Head and Neck. New York: McGraw-Hill, 1976.
15. Khoury, M.J., Cordero, J.F., Greenberg, F., et al.: A population study of the VACTERL association: Evidence for its etiologic heterogeneity. Pediatrics 71: 815, 1983.
16. Hsia, Y.E., Appadorai, V., Breg, W.R. and Howard, R.O.: Chromosomal abnormality (46,XX,3p+) in a case of the Meckel syndrome. Birth Defects X (8): 19, 1974.
17. Pagon, R.A., Smith, D.W. and Shepard, T.H.: Urethral obstruction malformation complex: A cause of abdominal muscle deficiency and the "prune belly". J. Pediatr. 94: 900, 1979.
18. Kaffe, S., Rose, J.S., Godmilow, L., et al.: Prenatal diagnosis of renal anomalies. Am. J. Med. Genet. 1: 241, 1977.
19. Kelley, R.I.: Review: The cerebrohepatorenal syndrome of Zellweger, morphologic and metabolic aspects. Am. J. Med. Genet. 16: 503, 1983.
20. Melnick, M. and Myrianthopoulos, N.C.: External ear malformations: Epidemiology, genetics, and natural history. Birth Defects XV (9): 19, 1979.
21. Dusdieker, L.B., Means, L., Bull, M.J., et al.: VATER association-Severe manifestations in an affected patient. Birth Defects XIV (6B): 369, 1978.
22. Fournier, J.L., Jacquemin, J., Farriaux, J., et al.: L'association V.A.T.E.R. et ses limites. J. Genet. Hum. 27: 265, 1979.
23. Kaufman, R.L., McAlister, W.H., Ho, C-K, and Hartmann, A.F.: Family studies in congenital heart disease VI: The association of severe obstructive left heart lesions, vertebral and renal anomalies; a second family. Birth Defects X (7): 93, 1974.
24. Schiavulli, E. and Liberatore, G.: La sindrome V.A.T.E.R.. Minerva Pediatrica 34: 821, 1982.
25. Bergsma, D.: Birth Defects Compendium, 2nd edition. The National Foundation, March of Dimes. New York: Alan R. Liss, Inc., 1979.
26. Temtomy S. and McKusick, V.A.: The genetics of hand malformations. Birth Defects XIV (3): 133, 1978.
27. Goodman, R.M. and Gorlin, R.S.: The Malformed Infant and Child. New York: Oxford University Press, 1983.
28. Sarto, G.E. and Simpson, J.L.: Abnormalities of the mullerian and wollfian duct systems. Birth Defects XIV (6c): 37, 1978.
29. Pinsky, L.: A community of human malformation syndromes involving the mullerian ducts, distal extremities, urinary tract and ears. Teratology 9: 65, 1974.
30. Shokeir, M.H.K.: Aplasia of the mullerian system: Evidence for probable sex-limited autosomal dominant inheritance. Birth Defects XIV (6C): 147, 1978.
31. Park, I.J. and Jones, H.W.Jr.: A new syndrome in two unrelated females. Birth Defects VII (6): 311, 1971.
32. Ulbright, C.E., Hodes, M.E. and Ulbright, T.M.: New syndrome: Renal dysplasia, mesomelia, and radiohumeral fusion. Am. J. Med. Genet. 17: 667, 1984.
33. Halal, F., Homsy, M. and Perreault, G.: Acro-renal-ocular syndrome: Autosomal dominant thumb hypoplasia, renal ectopia, and eye defect. Am. J. Med. Genet. 17: 753, 1984.

34. Kelley, R.I., Zackai, E.H. and Charney, E.B.: Congenital hydronephrosis, skeletal dysplasia, and severe developmental retardation: The Schinzel-Giedion syndrome. J. Pediatr. 100: 943, 1982.
35. Schinzel, A. and Giedion, A.: A syndrome of severe midface retraction, multiple skull anomalies, clubfeet, and cardiac and renal malformations in sibs. Am. J. Med. Genet. 1: 361, 1978.
36. Donnai, D. and Harris, R.: A further case of a new syndrome including midface retraction, hypertrichosis, and skeletal anomalies. J. Med. Genet. 16: 483, 1979.
37. Schinzel, A.: A syndrome of midface retraction, multiple radiological anomalies, renal malformations and hypertrichosis. Hum. Genet. 62: 382, 1982.
38. Sofer, S., Bar-Ziv, J. and Abeliovich, D.: Radial ray aplasia and renal anomalies in father and son: A new syndrome. Am. J. Med. Genet. 14: 151, 1983.
39. Freire-Maia, N., Pinheiro, M. and Opitz, J.M.: The Neurofaciodigitorenal (NFDR) Syndrome. Am. J. Med. Genet. 11: 329, 1982.
40. Dahlberg, P.J., Borere, W.Z., Newcomer, K.L. and Yutuc, W.R.: Autosomal or X-linked recessive syndrome of congenital lymphedema, hypoparathyroidism, nephropathy, prolapsing mitral valve, and brachytelephalangy. Am. J. Med. Genet. 16: 99, 1983.
41. Halal, F., Desgranges, M-F., Leduc, B., et al.: Acro-renal-mandibular syndrome. Am. J. Med. Genet. 5: 277, 1980.
42. Miltenyi, M., Balogh, L., Schmidt, K., et al.: A new variant of the acrorenal syndrome associated with bilateral oligomeganephronic hypoplasia. Eur. J. Pediatr. 142: 40, 1984.
43. Burn, J. and Marwood, R.P.: Fraser syndrome presenting as bilateral renal agenesis in three sibs. J. Med. Genet. 19: 360, 1982.
44. Siegler, R.L., Larsen, P. and Buehler, B.A.: Upper limb anomalies and renal disease. Clin Genet. 17: 117, 1980.
45. deGrouchy, J. and Turleau, C.: Clinical Atlas of Human Chromosomes, 2nd edition. New York: John Wiley & Sons, 1984.
46. Zonana, J. and Di Liberti, J.H.: Congenital and hereditary urinary tract disorders. In: Principles and Practice of Medical Genetics. A.E.H. Emery and D.L. Rimoin, Eds., New York: Chruchill Livingstone, 1983, p. 987.

NATURAL HISTORY OF CONGENITAL ANOMALIES OF THE KIDNEY AND URINARY TRACT

Gaston Zilleruelo, M.D., Michael Freundlich, M.D., Carolyn Abitbol, M.D., Nuria Dominguez, M.D., Brenda Montane, M.D. and Jose Strauss, M.D.

Many times the pediatrician or the neonatologist is confronted with a newborn who is found to have a congenital anomaly of the kidney or the urinary tract. This clinical situation usually raises several questions. Among them are, what are the most common types of malformations? What is the usual outcome? Does an early diagnosis and intervention modify the outcome of these patients? And finally, what are the alternatives for management? It is difficult to discuss the natural history of these anomalies since most of them are modified by some type of procedure as soon as they are detected. Therefore, we shall focus here on the "unnatural" history of these congenital anomalies and various new methods of evaluation and management which have substantially modified their prognosis.

A traditional concept for many years has been that significant obstruction to the outflow of urine, if unrelieved, causes inexorable damage to the kidneys and ultimately renal failure and death (1). However, the outcome of these patients has changed in recent years, mainly because of our increased awareness and ability to detect and correct early in life (even during intrauterine life) some of these malformations and also our ability to preserve life with chronic peritoneal dialysis started in the neonatal period. The development of newer techniques of imaging of the kidney and urinary tract has made it possible to diagnose these anomalies with precision and attempt their correction with various urological procedures (2, 3).

The opportunity to salvage functioning renal tissue and to preserve the potential for future renal growth by relief of obstruction has been considered great if corrective surgery was performed during the first years of life. One study concluded that surgical intervention prior to one year of age was necessary in order to achieve lasting improvement of renal function in children with obstructive uropathy and chronic renal failure (4). Figure 1 presents the outcome of 12 children who had corrective surgery under one year of age; those who were operated upon after two years of age are presented in Figure 2. Though the differences seem obvious, mean follow-up for the total group, however, was less than five years.

Review of the experience in children with chronic renal failure from some centers, including ours, has shown that congenital anomalies of the kidneys and urinary tract even today constitute the vast majority of causes of chronic renal failure (CRF) in children (5, 6). Table I presents the most common types of congenital anomalies in our Medical Center. Among the obstructive uropathies, posterior urethral valves and

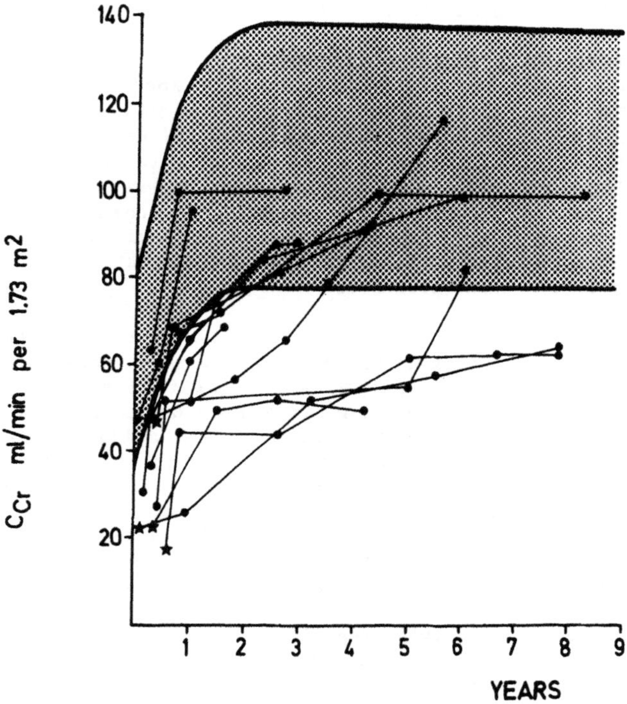

Figure 1. Changes in GFR following surgical treatment of hydronephrosis in 12 children operated upon before one year of age. Solid-line curve and cross-hatched area, range of normal variation of creatinine clearance in children. Stars, measurements of renal function done before surgical treatment. Solid circles, measurements of renal function performed after surgery. Reproduced with permission from Mayor, G., Genton, N., Torrado, A., et al.: Renal function in obstructive nephropathy: Long term effect of reconstructive surgery. Pediatrics 56:740, 1975.

TABLE I COMMON TYPES OF MALFORMATION IN 50 CHILDREN WITH CRF UNIVERSITY OF MIAMI, 1973-1982

TYPE OF MALFORMATION	SEX		TOTAL
	M	F	
OBSTRUCTIVE UROPATHIES	27	8	35
Posterior urethral valves	11	0	11
Primary v-u reflux	5	4	9
Prune-belly syndrome	5	0	5
UP junction obstruction	2	2	4
UV junction obstruction	2	2	4
Neurogenic bladder	2	0	2
RENAL MALFORMATIONS	5	10	15
Hypoplasia/dysplasia	1	8	9
Cystic diseases	4	2	6

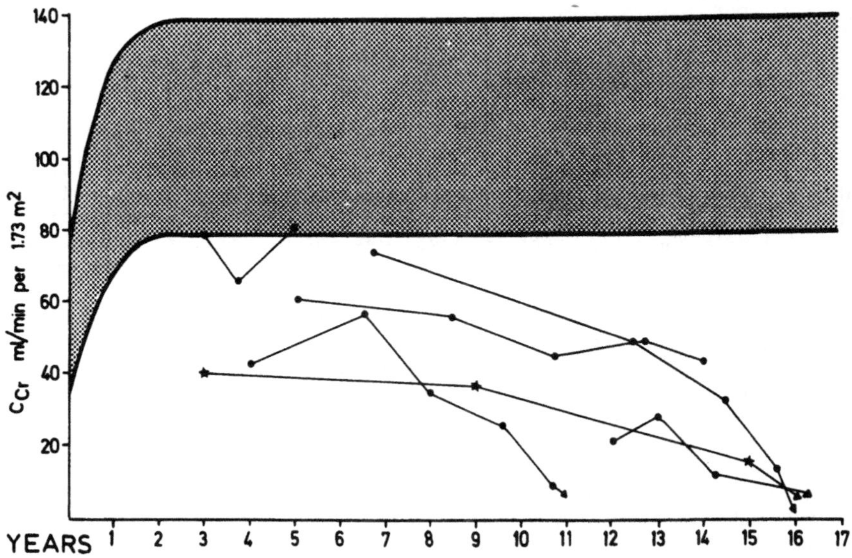

Figure 2. Changes in GFR following surgical treatment of hydronephrosis in six children operated upon after two years of age. Solid-line curve and cross-hatched area, range of normal variation of creatinine clearance in children. Stars, measurements of renal function done before surgical treatment. Solid circles, measurements of renal function performed after surgery. Reproduced with permission from Mayor, G., Genton, N., Torrado, A., et al.: Renal function in obstructive nephropathy: long term effect of reconstructive surgery. Pediatrics 56:740, 1975.

primary vesicoureteral reflux were the most commonly found anomalies. In the renal malformations group, the hypoplasias, dysplasias, and cystic diseases were the most common anomalies. When we analyzed the rate of progression from CRF to end-stage renal disease (ESRD), we found a mean time interval of several years (Table II), suggesting that meaningful conclusions may not be reached unless follow-up is at least five years. An unexpected finding was the fact that in spite of early corrective surgery, many of these children continued with progressive deterioration in renal function.

TABLE II

RATE OF RENAL FUNCTION DETERIORATION X AGE (RANGE) YEARS

DIAGNOSIS	AGE AT APPARENT CLINICAL ONSET	ONSET CRF	CRF ESRD
Obstructive Uropathies	1.1 (0.08-15)	3.1 (0.16-11)	5.5 (0.7-12)
Renal Malformations	3.9 (0.08-16)	7.0 (0.16-16)	1.7 (0.08-4)

A recent report analyzed the time interval between the initial urinary diversion or surgical reconstruction and the institution of dialysis in three groups of children based upon age at time of the initial procedure (7). The interval was not significantly different between patients treated during the first year of life and those treated between one and 8 years of life (time interval 10 years vs 9 years, respectively). It is possible that the degree of obstruction and dysplasia present in the children under one year of age was more severe than that occurring in the older children and that this more severe lesion led both to early detection and early onset of ESRD. On the other hand, surgical intervention after 8 years of age was associated with a significantly shortened time interval prior to the need for dialysis (three years) (Figure 3). In our experience, patients with obstructive uropathy and congenital anomalies of the kidneys progressed to CRF and ESRD at widely variable rates (6). Still, mean time interval to reach ESRD was 8 6/12 years in our series (Table II) and up to 10 10/12 years in that of others (8). Therefore, a prolonged follow-up period is needed to assess the ultimate outcome of renal function in these patients. It seems that we should temper our enthusiasm regarding the ability of surgical correction to prevent progression to ESRD until more time has elapsed from the recent past with an interventionist approach. Table III presents the final outcome observed in our experience. After a mean follow-up period of five years, about half of the patients with obstructive uropathy and two-thirds of the patients with congenital anomalies had either reached ESRD or died.

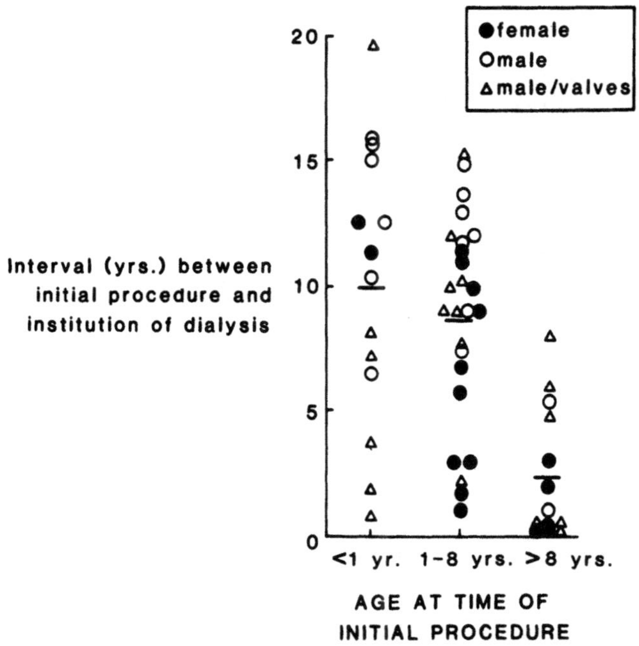

Figure 3. Interval between the initial urinary diversion or surgical reconstruction and the institution of dialysis in three groups, based upon the age at the time of initial procedure. Reproduced with permission from Warshaw, B.L., Edelbrook, H.H., Ettenger, R.B., et al.: Progression to end-stage renal disease in children with obstructive uropathy. J Pediatr 100:183, 1982.

TABLE III

OUTCOME IN 50 CHILDREN WITH CRF SECONDARY TO CONGENITAL RENAL/URINARY ANOMALIES

UNIVERSITY OF MIAMI, 1973-1982

DIAGNOSIS (N)	FOLLOW-UP	CURRENT STATUS (N)				
	X (RANGE) YEARS	CRF	HD	CAPD	TX	DEATH
Obstructive Uropathies (35)	5 (1-10)	17	6	1	7	4
Renal malformations (15)	4.6 (1-10)	5	4	0	6	0

Why does this progression still occur? Why is chronic parenchymal deterioration still progressing despite early intervention and despite adequate relief of obstruction? Several factors which might affect the progression or the reversibility of obstructive damage are presented in Table IV. Duration and degree of obstruction probably are the most important of these factors (1). However, other mechanisms of nephron injury may be present. Progressive glomerulosclerosis has been observed in rats with partial (5/6) nephrectomy (9). A sustained increase in renal plasma flow and glomerular capillary pressure occurs in this model and may lead to glomerulosclerosis in the remnant kidney (9, 10). The reduction in nephron population of this experimental model is similar to that of the hypoplastic-dysplastic kidney and a similar mechanism may account for the progressive renal damage in both situations. This would go along with the recent theory proposed by Brenner of the glomerular mesangial overload as a contributing factor to progression of ESRD (11).

TABLE IV

OBSTRUCTIVE UROPATHY

FACTORS THAT AFFECT RECOVERABILITY OF RENAL FUNCTION

Magnitude of intrapelvic pressure
Degree of obstruction
Duration of obstruction
Stage of renal development
Unilateral or bilateral obstruction
Associated renal disease (dysplasia)
Presence or absence of infection
Extrarenal vs. intrarenal pelvis

In patients with vesicoureteral reflux who develop glomerulosclerosis and proteinuria, a significant correlation was reported between degree of proteinuria and decline in renal function (12). This could be related to autologous immune complex glomerulonephritis with antibodies to tubular epithelium antigen (13). Finally, hyperparathyroidism and hyperlipidemia which develop as a result of CRF, may induce further renal damage (14, 15).

From the above, we can conclude that surgical correction in extrauterine life will always be too late for some patients. Would correction of these anomalies early in life (even intrauterine life) be more effective? Fetal intervention for congenital hydronephrosis has been a matter of controversy due to the difficult medical and ethical questions raised when the fetus is found to have a fluid filled mass in the abdomen (16-18). Figure 4 presents one possible approach to the management of a fetus with urinary tract malformations based on prenatal sonographic assessment of the urinary tract anatomy and functions (18). However, this approach seems to oversimplify the current status of fetal hydronephrosis. There are problems in the diagnosis and management of these situations. There are several unsolved questions, including those regarding accuracy in prenatal ultrasonography in the diagnosis of obstructive hydronephrosis. Not all large, sonoluscent, retroperitoneal masses in the fetal abdomen are the result of obstructive uropathy. Therefore, the fetus with presumed hydronephrosis should have repeated studies with real time ultrasonography in order to confirm or modify the initial finding (3, 16). Dilatation of the collecting system may be transient and may resolve before delivery. Overt distention of the bladder may produce intermittent hydronephrosis that disappears after the fetus voids. Thus, it is important to obtain ultrasound studies at several phases of bladder filling (3). Several diagnostic errors of presumed uropathy have occurred especially when ultrasonography was performed by inexperienced people. Recent studies showed that up to 60% of patients with proven obstructive uropathy at birth had an incorrect diagnosis by prenatal ultrasonography (16). We also have found diagnoses in utero that are not documented after birth.

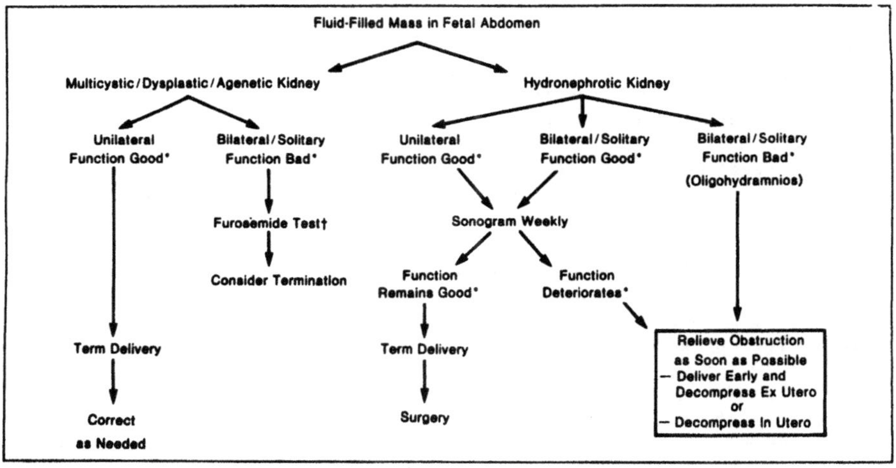

Figure 4. Suggested treatment of fetus with urinary tract malformation based on prenatal sonographic assessment of urinary tract anatomy and function: asterisk, renal function inferred from volume of amniotic fluid and volume of urine in fetal bladder; dagger, sonographic assessment of fetal urine production (bladder-filling, amniotic fluid volume) after giving furosemide to mother. Reproduced with permission from Diament, M.J., Fine R.N., Ehrlich, R., et al.: Fetal hydronephrosis: Problems in diagnosis and management. J Pediatr 103:435, 1983.

The fundamental distinction that must be made in the evaluation of a fetus with suspected renal abnormalities is between unilateral and bilateral disease. No intervention is justified on unilateral disease with contralateral normal kidney. The second most common problem is the differentiation between multicystic kidney and hydronephrosis due to uretero-pelvic junction obstruction or vesico-ureteral reflux. Other diagnostic problems include low pressure hydronephrosis due to vesico-ureteral reflux, lower urinary tract obstruction due to posterior urethral valves (usually present with large bladder and large ureters), and obstruction at the low uretero-vesical junction.

Another item of discussion is the assessment of fetal renal function and the persistent decrease after a certain (unknown) period of obstruction. The question then would be: "What is the minimum period of GU obstruction after which renal function becomes irreversibly decreased?" The best single guide to fetal renal function, although imperfect, is the volume of amniotic fluid (15). Observation of fetal bladder filling and emptying is also informative by ultrasound. This information can be made more accurate by giving furosemide to the mother (19). However, bladder filling can be misleading when significant vesico-ureteral reflux is present (17). Various studies, both in animals and humans, and clinical experience with prenatal intervention, indicate that severe urinary tract obstruction that occurs in the early stages of embryogenesis usually results in irreversible dysplasia (20). Currently, no reliable test exists to assess accurately renal function in utero or the potential for recovery of fetal kidneys with obstructive uropathy. Thus, renal function can be only estimated by the volume of amniotic fluid, a normal amniotic fluid volume indicating that at least one of the kidneys is more or less functioning. In summary, the presence of oligohydramnios, although multifactorial, is a relatively accurate reflection of decreased urinary output and is probably the most important indicator of renal dysfunction.

Several techniques for fetal intervention have been utilized and these include: 1) Needle aspiration of urine from the bladder or from the renal pelvis (transient effect); 2) Diversion of urine into the amniotic sac by internal shunt; 3) Open surgical diversion; and 4) Premature delivery. However, there are significant risks involved with all these procedures. Hemorrhage, sepsis, abortion and premature labor are all possible (17). In addition, post-obstructive diuresis in utero is a theoretical risk leading to shock and eventual fetal death.

Therefore, fetuses with dilated upper urinary tracts should be carefully studied to determine which ones might benefit from in utero intervention. In general, fetuses with unilateral hydronephrosis should be observed. If the hydronephrosis is bilateral and the renal function is preserved (assessed by amount of amniotic fluid and bladder filling), follow-up is indicated with sequential ultrasound studies. If the hydronephrosis is bilateral but with poor renal function, some would recommend intervention. In this situation, there is a higher risk for severe renal-pulmonary hypoplasia. Finally, if bilateral hydronephrosis with equivocal function is present, there is no hard evidence so far to suggest that relief of obstruction in utero will result in improvement in renal or pulmonary function beyond that achieved by surgery in the neonatal period (16, 17). In summary, accumulated experience to date indicates that most fetuses with hydronephrosis should be managed expectantly with serial (even weekly) ultrasound assessments. Only if rapid or sudden deterioration is detected, relief of obstruction should be considered (Figure 4). It seems clear that the natural history of congenital hydronephrosis in the fetus requires more extensive studies before intervention can be widely recommended (16). Nevertheless, prenatal diagnosis is still useful for identification of the high risk pregnancies and early referral to centers where postnatal care can be promptly instituted (21). It is important to repeat the ultrasound studies after delivery to establish an accurate diagnosis and to evaluate the status of the contralateral kidney.

Once the fetus is delivered, there is a new challenge if renal failure develops. Is there an alternative for life if renal damage is severe enough? Certainly, the institution of chronic peritoneal dialysis has modified the natural outcome of patients with these anomalies. There is a growing clinical experience with the use of this still imperfect modality of renal replacement. Many questions remain, including medical, ethical, psycho-social, and financial aspects of this type of life imposed on the family, patient and society.

In summary, great advances have occurred in the past few years in our ability to modify the natural history of congenital anomalies of the kidneys and urinary tract. Still, we are far from understanding which are the mechanisms involved in the development of these malformations and once they have occurred, in their progression to CRF and ESRD. Only with a better understanding of the etiopathogenesis of these disorders, a preventive and more effective therapeutic approach will be developed.

REFERENCES

1. Walker, R.D., Richard, G.A., Bueschen, A.J., et al.: Pathophysiology and recoverability of function and structure in obstructed kidneys. Urol Clin North Am, 7:291, 1980.

2. Mendoza, S.A., Griswold, W.R., Leopold, G.R., et al.: Intrauterine diagnosis of renal anomalies by ultrasonography. Am J Dis Child, 133:1042, 1979.

3. Bezjian, A.A.: Prenatal diagnosis of fetal urinary tract abnormalities. In Strauss J, (ed.) Neonatal Kidney and Fluid-Electrolytes. Boston: Martinus Nijhoff, 1983, p. 23-30.

4. Mayor, G., Genton, N., Torrado, A., et al.: Renal function in obstructive nephropathy: Long-term effect of reconstructive surgery. Pediatrics 56:740, 1975.

5. Fine, R.N., Malekzadeh, M.H., Pennisi, A.J., et al.: Long-term results of renal transplantation in children. Pediatrics 61:641, 1978.

6. Zilleruelo, G., Andia, J., Gorman, H.M., et al.: Chronic renal failure in children: analysis of main causes and deterioration rate in 81 children. Int J Pediatr Nephrology 1:30, 1980.

7. Warshaw, B.L., Edelbrock, H.H., Ettenger, R.B., et al.: Progression to end-stage renal disease in children with obstructive uropathy. J Pediatr 100:183, 1982.

8. Habib, R., Broyer, M. and Benmaiz, M.: Chronic renal failure in children. Nephron 11:209, 1973.

9. Shimamura, T. and Morrison, A.B.: A progressive glomerulosclerosis occurring in partial five-sixth nephrectomized rats. Am J Pathol 79:95, 1975.

10. Hostetter, T.H., Olson, J.L., Rennke, H.G., et al.: Increased glomerular pressure and flow: A potentially adverse adaptation to reduced renal mass. Clin Res 27:498, 1979.

11. Brenner, B.M., Meyer, T.W. and Hostetter, T.H.: Dietary protein intake and the progressive nature of kidney disease: the role of hemodynamically mediated glomerular injury in the pathogenesis of progressive glomerular sclerosis in aging, renal ablation, and intrinsic renal disease. New Engl J Med 307:652, 1982.

12. Torres, V.E., Velosa, J.A., Holley, K.E., et al.: The progression of vesicoureteral reflux nephropathy. Ann Intern Med 92:776, 1980.

13. Pascal, R.R., Sian, C.S., Brensilver, J.M., et al.: Demonstration of an antibody to tubular epithelium in glomerulonephritis associated with obstructive uropathy. Amer J Med 69:944, 1980.

14. Ibels, L.S., Alfrey, A.C., Haut, L., et al.: Preservation of function in experimental renal disease by dietary restriction of phosphate. New Engl J Med 298:122, 1978.

15. Moorhead, J.F., Chan, M.K., El-Nahas, M., et al.: Lipid nephrotoxicity in chronic progressive glomerular and tubulo-interstitial disease. Lancet 2:1309, 1982.

16. Kramer, S.A.: Current status of fetal intervention for congenital hydronephrosis. J Urol 130:641, 1983.

17. Diament, M.J., Fine, R.N., Ehrlich, R., et al.: Fetal hydronephrosis: Problems in diagnosis and management. J Pediatr 103:435, 1983.

18. Harrison, M.R., Filly, R.A., Parer, J.T., et al.: Management of the fetus with a urinary tract malformation. JAMA 246:635, 1981.

19. Wladimiroff, J.W.: Effect of furosemide on fetal urine production. Br J Obstet Gynaecol 82:221, 1975.

20. Beck, A.D.: The effect of intra-uterine urinary obstruction upon the development of the fetal kidney. J Urol 105:784, 1971.

21. Mandell, J., Kinard, H.W., Mittelstaedt, C.A., et al.: Prenatal diagnosis of unilateral hydronephrosis with early postnatal reconstruction. J Urol 132:303, 1984.

RENAL TUBULAR ACIDOSIS

James C. M. Chan, M.D. and Uri Alon, M.D.

Introduction

The fascination of hydrogen ion metabolism for those of us working in the field of renal tubular disorders was eloquently expressed by the words of Hastings (1) in an address to the New York Academy of Sciences in 1966.

"To Faraday we are indebted for naming the products of dissociation - ions - and thus we came by 'hydrogen ions,' a term now synonymous with protons. Tiny though it is, I suppose no constituent of living matter has so much power to influence biological behavior...

It has become widely accepted since the 1966 international meeting sponsored by the New York Academy of Sciences, that an acid is a substance which donates "hydrogen ions" and a base is one that accepts "hydrogen ions." A strong acid is one whose hydrogen ion is easily and completely dissociated from its conjugate base.

Defense against acid-base disturbance

When hydrogen ions are introduced, as in the form of acidifying salts, the body utilizes three systems in defense of the acid-base disturbances (2). The blood buffers are the first line of defense, resulting in the lowering of the blood pH as well as serum bicarbonate concentrations. The respiratory system is then summoned as the second line of defense by hyperventilation in order to lower the partial pressure of CO_2 and to bring the ratio of metabolic/respiratory components of the acid-base equation closer to that of normal. The third and final line of defense which the body calls forth in defense of acid-base disturbances resides with the kidney. The renal response to an acid-load is to lower the urinary pH and to increase the net acid excretion. Let us examine what we know of the renal acidification mechanisms.

Renal bicarbonate reabsorption and acid excretion

In a normal adult, a daily load of 4,500 mmol of bicarbonate is presented to the glomerulus, 90% of which is reabsorbed in the proximal tubule and 10% in the distal tubule (3). In the smaller child, the total load of bicarbonate has been estimated to be 2,500 mmol/day, with 60% of it reabsorbed in the proximal tubule and 40% in the distal tubule (4). The reabsorption of bicarbonate is linked to the reabsorption of sodium in the proximal tubule. Sodium reabsorption, however, is operational linked to hydrogen ion secretion; whether the hydrogen ion-sodium exchange mechanism is carrier-mediated or not is still under study (5).

Hydrogen ions are buffered in the tubule by filtered phosphate to form titratable acid (6). In addition, through the action of glutaminase on glutamine, ammonia is produced, which combines with hydrogen ions in the renal tubule to form ammonium (7). The sum of titratable acid plus ammonium minus any trace amounts of bicarbonate constitutes the net acid excretion (8).

Net acid excretion is usually presented in uEq/min/1.73 sq.m. With spontaneous or induced metabolic acidosis (9), the net acid excretion increases in excess of 65 uEq/min/1.73 sq.m. once acidosis, as represented by plasma bicarbonate of less than 17 mEq/L, is reached. The urinary pH also decreases in response to metabolic acidosis to values of less than 6.5 and in most cases less than 5.5.

Recent studies by Loney and associates (10) demonstrated that patients with renal tubular acidosis were unable to bring the urinary pH to less than 5.5 in comparison to those who had recovered from acute glomerulonephritis (Figure 1).

Renal tubular acidosis

Type 1 renal tubular acidosis is associated with growth retardation and hyperchloremic metabolic acidosis. Such patients fail to achieve urinary pH of less than 5.5 and a net acid excretion of more than 65 uEq/min/1.73 sq.m, despite spontaneous or induced acidosis as represented by plasma bicarbonate content of less than 17 mEq/L (Figure 2).

Type 2 renal tubular acidosis is associated with a proximal bicarbonate reabsorption defect. On normalization of serum bicarbonate content with alkaline loading, bicarbonaturia becomes more than 15%.

Type 3 renal tubular acidosis is associated with bicarbonate leakage of between 5 to 15% on normalization of serum bicarbonate with alkaline loading. This small bicarbonate leak may be specifically related to a maturational factor. It has been suggested by McSherry and associates (11) that this likely is a sub-type of type 1 renal tubular acidosis.

Type 4 renal tubular acidosis is the result of resistance to or deficiency of aldosterone (12-15). Retention of hydrogen ions and potassium ions obtains. The presence of hyperkalemia readily distinguishes type 4 renal tubular acidosis from the other three types which are more often associated with hypokalemia.

Complications of renal tubular acidosis

In addition to the growth failure and hypokalemic muscle weakness, which are features associated with the first three types of renal tubular acidosis, nephrocalcinosis secondary to hypercalciuria and low citrate excretion is a frequent complication in the untreated type 1 renal tubular acidosis (16-17). In contrast, nephrocalcinosis is rare in type 2 as well as type 4 renal tubular acidosis (18-19).

Fig 1 Urinary pH in children with renal tubular acidosis (closed diamonds) compared to those one to 62 months after recovery from acute glomerulonephritis (closed circles). All subjects received intravenous infusion of 150 mEq/sq.m. of arginine hydrochloride. From Loney LC, Norling LL, Robson AM: The use of arginine hydrochloride infusion to assess urinary acidification. J Pediatr 100:95-98, 1982. By permission.

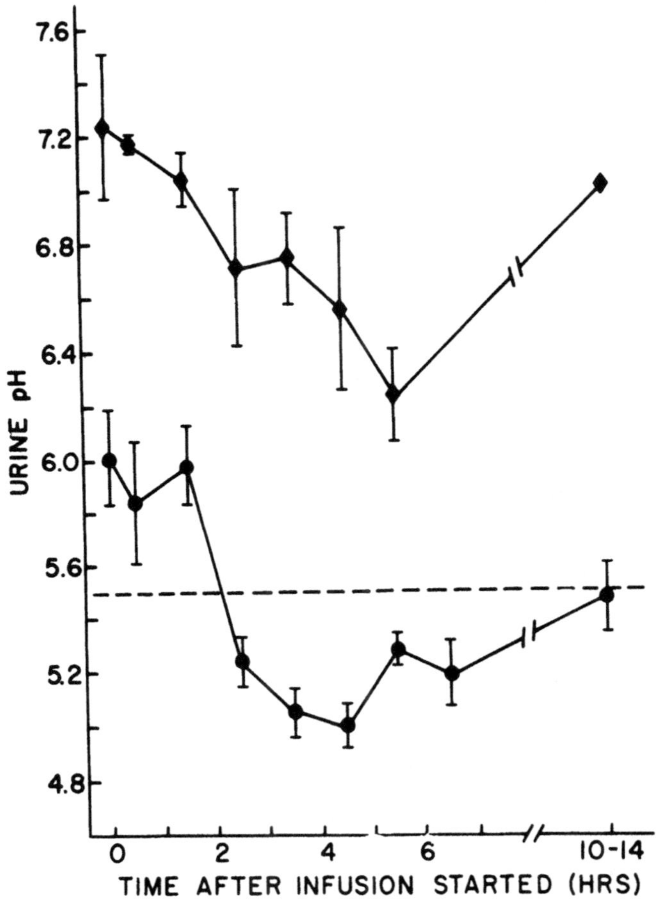

FIG. 2. The relationship between pCO2 and plasma bicarbonate (upper panel); metabolic acidosis and urinary pH (middle panel); and urine net acid excretion (lower panel). From Chan JCM: Nutrition and acid-base metabolism. FASEB 40:2423-2428, 1981. By permission.

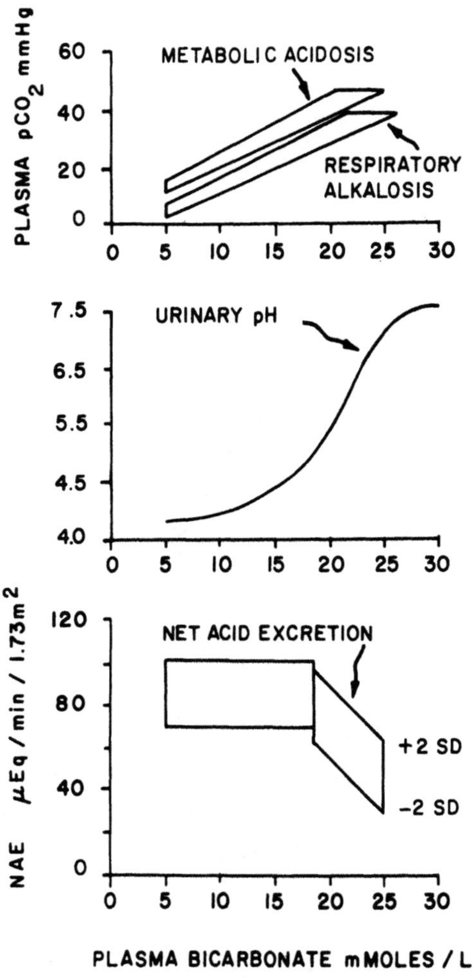

Table 1 Oral Preparations for Alkali Therapy

Name of Drug	How Supplied	Dosage Equivalent
Bicitra	Solution: 5 ml = 500 mg sodium citrate 300 mg citric acid	1 ml = 1 mEq base
Calcium carbonate	Tablet: 420, 650 mg Powder: 1000 mg per 1/2 teaspoon	1000 mg = 22.3 mEq base
Polycitra	Solution: 5 ml = 550 mg potassium citrate, 500 mg sodium citrate, 334 mg citric acid	1 ml = 2 mEq base
Polycitra-K	Solution: 5 ml = 100 mg potassium citrate, 334 mg citric acid	1 ml = 2 mEq base
Sodium bicarbonate	Tablet: 325, 650 mg Solution: 1 ml = 1 mEq base	325 mg = 4 mEq base 650 mg = 8 mEq base
Shohl's solution	Solution: 1000 ml = 140 gm citric acid 90 gram hydrated crystaline sodium citrate	1 ml = 1 mEq base

Glycosuria and aminoaciduria are occasionally found in type 2 renal tubular acidosis.

Treatment with alkali solutions (Table 1) at dosages varying between 2 to 14 mEq/kg/day is associated with a decrease in daily potassium requirements in type 1 renal tubular acidosis. However, with type 2 renal tubular acidosis, correction of acidosis with alkaline treatment aggravates the potassium wasting (20, 21). Thus, in type 2 renal tubular acidosis, the daily potassium requirements are increased with correction of the acidosis.

Undetermined anion gap

The undetermined anion gap in serum is determined by subtracting the sum of chloride and bicarbonate from that of sodium and potassium. The normal anion (UA) gap is less than 12 mEq/L. The UA gap is normal in renal tubular acidosis, diarrhea acidosis, ureteral ileostomy, loss of small intestinal and pancreatic secretions, dilutional acidosis, fluid overload, and in the use of total parenteral nutrition, acidifying salts and cholestyramine resins (22).

The undetermined anion gap is increased (23) under the following conditions: acute and chronic renal failure, ingestion of ethylene glycol, the use of paraldehyde, methyl alcohol and salicylate. The UA gap is also increased by virtue of accumulation of organic acids as in diabetic ketoacidosis, lactate acidosis, phenformin acidosis, inborn errors of metabolism and non-ketotic hyperosmolar coma.

Summary

The advances in our understanding of bicarbonate reabsorption and acid excretion as well as the action of aldosterone on the renal tubules have resulted in the inclusion of several disorders under the general diagnosis of renal tubular acidosis. Early recognition and treatment will result in reversal of the consequential complications. The quotation by Homer W. Smith from Titus Lucretius Carus (95-52 B.C.) poetically anticipated some of our feelings concerning this disorder:

"No single thing abides but all things flow, fragment to fragment clings and the things thus grow, until we know and name them. By degrees...they melt and are no more the things we know...."

Acknowledgements Mrs. Marilyn Reilly provided secretarial assistance; Ms. Martha D. Wellons, B.A., provided research assistance.

References

1. Hastings AB: Introductory remarks. Ann N.Y. Acad Sci 133:16, 1966.

2. Winters RW, Engel K, Dell RB: Acid-Base Physiology in Medicine. A Self-Instruction Program. The Loudon Company, Westlake, Ohio, 1967. 290 pp.

3. Albert MS: Acid-base disorders in pediatrics. Ped Clin North Am 23:639, 1976.

4. Kildeberg P: Clinical Acid-Base Physiology. William & Wilkins Co., Baltimore, 1968. 232 pp.

5. Rector FC, Jr.: Acidification of the urine. Chapter 14; in Orloff J, Berliner RW, Renal Physiology. Am Soc Physiol, Washington, DC, 1973. 23 pp.

6. Rodriguez-Soriano J: Renal tubular acidosis; in Gruskin AB, Norman ME, Pediatric Nephrology. Martinus Nijhoff Publ., Hague, 1981. p. 34

7. Donckerwolcke RA, Van Stekelenburg GJ, Tiddens HA: Therapy of bicarbonate-losing renal tubular acidosis. Arch Dis Child 45:774, 1970.

8. Nash MA, Torrado AD, Greifer I, et al: Renal tubular acidosis in infants and children. J Pediatr 80:738, 1972.

9. Chan JCM: Renal tubular acidosis. J Pediatr 102:327, 1983.

10. Loney LC, Norling LL, Robson AM: The use of arginine hydrochloride infusion to assess urinary acidification. J Pediatr 100:95, 1982.

11. McSherry E: Renal tubular acidosis in childhood. Kidney Int 20:799, 1981.

12. Batlle DC: Hyperkalemic hyperchloremic metabolic acidosis associated with selective aldosterone deficiency and distal renal tubular acidosis. Seminar Nephr 1:260, 1981.

13. Alon U, Kodroff ME, Broecker BH, et al: Renal tubular acidosis type 4 in neonatal unilateral kidney diseases. J Pediatr 104:855, 1984.

14. McSherry E, Portale A, Gates J: Non-azotemic, non-hyporeninemic type 4 renal tubular acidosis (RTA) observed in early childhood. Kidney Int 14:769, 1978. (abstract)

15. McSherry E: Current issues in hydrogen ion transport in Gruskin AB, Norman ME, Pediatric Nephrology. Proceedings of the Fifth International Pediatric Nephrology Symposium 1980. 12 pp.

16. Norman ME, Feldman NI, Cohn RM, et al: Urinary citrate excretion in the diagnosis of distal renal tubular acidosis. J Pediatr 92:394, 1978.

17. Morrissey JF, Ochoa M, Jr., Lotspeich WD, et al: Citrate excretion in renal tubular acidosis. Ann Intern Med 58:159, 1968.

18. Brenner RJ, Spring DB, Sebastian A, et al: Incidence of radiographically evident bone disease, nephrocalcinosis, and nephrolithiasis in various types of renal tubular acidosis. N Engl J Med 307:217, 1982.

19. Morris RC, Jr., Sebastian, A: Renal tubular acidosis and Fanconi syndrome; in Stanbury JB, Wyngaarden JB, Frederickson DS, et al. The Metabolic Basis of Inherited Diseases, 5th ed., McGraw-Hill Book Co., New York, 1983. pp. 1808-1843

20. Sebastian A, McSherry E, Morris RC, Jr: On the mechanism of renal potassium wasting in renal tubular acidosis associated with the Fanconi syndrome (type 2 RTA). J Clin Invest 50:231, 1971.

21. Morris RC, Jr: Renal tubular acidosis. N Engl J Med 304:418, 1981.

22. Kleinmann PK: Cholestyramine and metabolic acidosis. N Engl J Med 290:861, 1974.

23. Narins RG, Goldberg M: Renal tubular acidosis: Pathophysiology, diagnosis and treatment. Disease-a-Month 23:1, 1977.

NEWER DIAGNOSTIC IMAGING PROCEDURES IN NEONATAL RENAL DISEASE

G. N. Sfakianakis, M.D.

INTRODUCTION

At present radioisotope scintigraphy(RS) and ultrasonography(U) are the imaging modalities of choice for the investigation of the kidneys in the neonate. They are relatively(RS) or totally(U) noninvasive and they may be performed in the nursery with portable and relatively inexpensive equipment. Whereas both RS and U provide diagnostic structural information, RS gives functional information, identifies the level of obstruction and detects easily ectopic units, whereas U has a better anatomical resolution independent of function and identifies cystic structures promptly. The two modalities are complimentary, RS is easier to perform and interpret, U requires expertise and dedication, being operator dependent. Our current protocol calls for an IV injection of lmCi of Tc-99m-Glucoheptonate followed by a flow phase, sequential imaging for 20 min and delayed scintigrams 4-6 hours post injection(1). A retrospective analysis concluded in our Institution showed that RS of the kidneys in neonates agreed with the final diagnosis in 96% of the cases, U in 82% and excretory urography(IVP) in only 55% of the cases studies(2).

NEW PROCEDURES

Ultrasonography and Radioisotope Scintigraphy have been applied in the investigation of neonatal renal diseases for a decade. Real-time Ultrasonography is becoming more popular because of its versatility and examiner participation; in experienced hands it is more effective in finding ectopic kidneys and in outlining dilated systems(3). Radioisotope Tomography (Single Photon Emission Computed Tomography or SPECT) has a limited resolution in its current state of the art and with the presently available radiopharmaceuticals it is not expected to affect the application of scintigraphy in the neonatal renal disease(4). A new Tc-99m labeled radiopharmaceutical known with the acromym DADS is a promising tubular agent because it combines the low-dose/high efficiency properties of Tc-99m with the effectiveness of the PAH. It is under clinical investigation(5).

Digital subtraction angiography (DSA) is a recently developed radiographic technique for producing images that accentuate vascular structures and vascular images with the help of powerful computers. Because of the advance in image technology, it has beome possible to perform many angiographic procedures using only intravenous injections of constrast agents (intravenous angiography). The term "subtraction" refers to accentuating the differences between structures filled with radiographic contrast, and the same structures as seen on scout films prior to the injection of contrast. DSA images demonstrate the aorta, renal arteries, and vessels down to the third order. Arterial, capillary, and venous phases can be imaged (6). An estimate of parenchymal renal function can be obtained. Technical problems with renal DSA studies are caused by vessel overlap and patient motion. Indications of DSA for the investigation of neonatal renal disease are very limited. Ultrasonography and Scintigraphy can provide the anatomical and functional information needed for the diagnosis without the dangers of contrast enhancement and with less radiation exposure in the vas majority of neonatal problems. For those cases where a vascular problem is contemplated, DSA may replace or precede traditional angiography.

Nuclear Magnetic Resonance(NMR), the newest diagnostic tomographic imaging modality has stimulated the medical community. The major factor for this is the capability of NMR to generate , without ionizing radiation, high resolution, diagnostic quality tomographic images at any angle and projection of the human body. Based upon magnetic properties of atomic nuclei differentiating not only atoms of different elements but also atoms of the same element according to their location within a molecular structure, NMR may revolutionize medical diagnostic imaging by providing, with no risk, in-vivo data of human biochemistry and pathophysiology (7). The physical basis for NMR imaging involves the interaction of the nuclei of a selected atom within the body, at the present time nearly exclusively hydrogen (protons), a) with an external magnetic field and b) with an external oscillating electromagnetic field that is changing as a function of time at a particular frequency. Energy, absorbed and then released by the particular body nucei (protons), it is detected, characterized and used to produce space distribution images (tomograms) which represent body spaces, organs and tissues. Different physical characteristics of the signal enable more than one kind of NMR images. Normal organs exhibit predictable patterns, and changes in size or location can be identified. Abnormal tissues have different proton content and proton magnetic parameters (relaxation times T_1, T_2) as compared to normal tissues on the tomograms. Paramagnetic agents can be used IV, orally, etc. to enhance the NMR images.

It appears that NMR imaging is able to diagnose many, if not all, of the anatomical changes that are seen with x-ray CT or Ultrasonography. Some kind of functional information can also be provided.

Reports to NMR studies of the kidneys showed that this modality can differentiate cystic from solid lesions and both from normal renal parenchyma in adults (8,9). A piperidinyl nitroxide stable free radical derivative, TES, is rapidly excreted in the urine with a clearance equal to GFR and it has strong paramagnetic properties. TES was used in experimental animals with renal artery, renal vein, or ureteral ligation and NMR images were taken at 0, 15, 30 and 60 minutes after injection. Renal ischemia, vascular congestion and hydronephrosis could be demonstrated on TES-enhanced spin echo (one type of NMR images) renal tomograms, whereas the nonenhanced NMR studies could not depict the abnormalities (10). Chromium or Gadolinium EDTA (another paramagnetic contrast enhancement agent) was also studied in animals and showed the possibility of quantitating renal function on NMR imaging.

By far NMR for the renal studies has not been proven superior to ultrasonography and scintigraphy combined. The NMR contrast enhancement agents have to be proven safe for human use. The cost of NMR is prohibitory for widespread use, unless definite clinical advantage is proven. The cost of cryogenic units is $1.5-2.0 million. The unit requires more space than x-ray computerized tomography. Security around the unit has to be exacting, particularly when patients are in the magnet, because heavy metallic objects may become hazardous missiles flying into the core. In the light of the great potential for NMR, which combines anatomic, physiologic and chemical information, the above drawbacks are not that serious, and if clinical advantage over CT, Ultrasonography and Scintigraphy is proven, this new modality will prevail.

REFERENCES

1. Sfakianakis GN: Radio-Scintigraphic evaluation of the kidneys in the neonate. In Proceedings of Pediatric Nephrology Seminar IX, Strauss J, Editor Martinus Nijhoff Publishers p 139-151, 1983.

2. Sfakianakis GN, Sfakianakis E, Lopez R, et al: Renal Scintigraphy in neonatal and Infantile Clinical Problems. (Abstracted) J Nucl Med 23: 98, 1983

3. Hricak H, Slovis TL, Callen CW, et al: Neonatal Kidneys: Sonographic Anatomic Correlation. Radiology 147: 699-702, 1983

4. Jaszczak RJ, Whitehead FR, Lim CB, et al: Lesion Detection with Single Photon Emission Computed Tomography (SPECT) compared with Conventional Imaging. J Nucl Med 23: 97-102, 1982

5. Fritzberg AR, Kuni CC, Klingensmith WC III, et al: Synthesis and Biological Evaluation of Tc-99m N, N'-bis-(mercaptoacetyl)-2,3-diaminopropionate: A potential replacement for I-131 hippuran. J Nucl Med 23: 592-598, 1982

6. Hillman BJ, Oritt TW, Nudelman S, et al: Digital Video Subtraction Angiography of Renal Vascular Abnormalities. Radiology 139: 277-280, 1981

7. Pylcett IL: NMR Imaging in Medicine. Scientific American 246 (5): 78-101, 1982

8. Hricak H, Crooks L, Sheldon P, et al: Nuclear Magnetic Resonance Imaging of the Kidney. Radiology 146: 425-432, 1983

9. Hricak H, Williams RD, Moon KL Jr., et al:Nuclear Resonance Imaging of the Kidney: Renal Masses. Radiology 147: 765-772, 1983

10. Brasch RC, London DA, Wesbey GE, et al: Nuclear Magnetic Resonance Study of a Paramagnetic Nitroxide Contrast agent for enhancement of renal structures in experimental animals. Radiology 147: 773-779, 1983

PANEL DISCUSSION

Jose Strauss, M.D., Moderator

QUESTION: What would you consider a normal bladder capacity?

RESPONSE: That is a good question. Usually we calculate the bladder capacity as age in years plus two in ounces. That is more or less the rule that has been established by the Pediatric Urologic Society. When you are talking about bladder capacity, you have to consider the voided urine plus the residual urine together. Also, we can attain a very good estimate with radionuclear procedures.

QUESTION: It has been written that in distal RTA in infants and young children, you always see a proximal leak also. So, the amount of bicarbonate that is needed to correct them is a lots higher than one usually would calculate. I wonder if that has been your experience with this disorder.

RESPONSE: Yes. What was referred to was what some people would classify as Type I, Subtype 3, which is a distal renal tubular acidosis associated with a maturation-related bicarbonate leak. The bicarbonate leak is usually quite small, usually about three to five percent or less. It has been suggested that, instead of saying that there is a Type III renal tubular acidosis, it should be eliminated altogether because it is a maturational process. As the child grows older, the bicarbonate leak disappears. They would rather like everyone to use their classification, eliminating Type III RTA and put it into Type I, Subtype 3. Even though the bicarbonate leak is small, one would be required to supplement more than 2 mEq/kg/day of bicarbonate. The rationale for using 2 mEq/kg/day of bicarbonate is primarily to replace what the endogenous acid production is estimated to be in infants and young children. In an adult, the endogenous acid production has been estimated to be 1 mEq/kg/day. It is simply summarized in the following fashion: net excretion in you and I, adults between 60 and 70 kg body weight, is about 70 mEq/day. Dividing that amount of acid excretion by 70 kg, mean weight of men (and some women), it becomes 1 mEq/kg/day. However, in infants and children we have found that the endogenous acid production is between 2 to 3 mEq/kg/day. So, those were the observations that led some people to suggest that we should use enough bicarbonate to achieve sustained correction of acidosis, starting at 2 mEq/kg/day of bicarbonate, progressively increasing up to 14 mEq/kg/day. I would like to ask somebody here to comment on the continuation story of one of the original works I did on four children with distal RTA. Two of them were brothers; I have written to those who were supposed to have continued care for these children but I did not get replies until just now during the coffee break. This person told me that he happens now to be the physician for the family with very astounding findings. Would you care to comment on that?

COMMENT-QUESTION: There are now three of those brothers with RTA instead of two. The oldest brother is now 17. Growth-wise, one is about 5'4", small but not very small. He is currently undergoing a lot of psychological problems in relation to medicational compliance. In consequence, he has been admitted to the hospital on three occasions with severe muscle weakness due to hypokalemia. On x-ray, he has fine nephrocalcinosis throughout both kidneys, not in big chunks of calcium which were shown earlier here. We are not satisfied with his present status; we are trying to deal with the difficulties he is encountering in accepting his disease and being compliant with his medications.

I wonder now if I could ask a question. Time didn't permit you to say much about the Type IV RTA. It is said that this is the commonest type of RTA. I don't know whether they are talking about adults and children or children alone but this is something we need to be aware of. Would you say something more about the Type IV RTA with the hyperkalemia, in terms of the experience in children and their management?

RESPONSE: Type IV renal tubular acidosis has been thought to be one of the more common types of RTA, especially in adults, after obstructive uropathy such as after prostate hypertrophy in a male. The first report was from the group in Chicago; they reported 13 adult patients several months and up to two years after correction of prostate hypertrophy and release of the obstruction to the urinary tract. Up to then, they continued to have hyperkalemic metabolic acidosis. Also, there is a report by another nephrology group with a radiologist as the first author in the New England Journal of Medicine, concerning radiological complications of renal tubular acidosis. They separate their 80 to 90 patients into the pediatric group which consists of 40 to 50 patients and the adult group. Perhaps 20 odd of them had tubular acidosis; however, that has not been my experience up to this point. We will be reporting cases of Type IV in the Journal of Pediatrics after renal vein thrombosis. Any obstruction can cause a Type IV renal tubular acidosis. It is well worth our while to watch out for the metabolic acidosis, growth failure, the alkaline urine pH and hypercalciuria in any children who may be suspected to have RTA and try to determine whether it is a Type IV or the other types of RTA. The fortunate thing is that it is so simple to treat. You just need to use bicarbonate therapy.

MODERATOR: Since we are on that subject, would you care to clarify for us the disagreements that are current on the various nomenclatures? It is important to know that different people have different interpretations of the sub-sub-sub-classifications. Could you clarify that situation for us?

RESPONSE: I wish I could. I don't think there is any general agreement. Basically, one would have to abide either by the San

Francisco group (even among them, they do not agree with all the sub-types) or by other groups. But, perhaps, those sub-types may not be propounded so thoroughly any more, because of various people's new positions.

MODERATOR: Then, the problem will be solved?

COMMENT: At the American Society of Nephrology meeting in Washington, D. C., a few months ago, a Toronto group has started to propound a new system of classification--that we should not say Types I to IV but that we should use the partial pressure of CO_2, the back leak of bicarbonate and hydrogen ion to differentiate the various types. I think that if we have already accepted Types I and II, we might as well go on to accept Types III and IV. The treatments are simple: bicarbonate solution enough to correct and achieve sustained correction of acidosis. As it was said just now, and to my great sorrow and surprise, the brothers who first introduced me to RTA (because they have RTA) are medically non-compliant and nephrocalcinosis is now present in one or both of them. Those brothers have taught us some valuable lessons in that the mother had to insist that the diagnostic work-up be conducted in a younger brother for lack of growth, for constipation that she saw, and it was at her insistence that the diagnostic work-up was performed. Then, she decided she would not need to follow doctor's recommendation and decided that what was good for the older brother would be good for the younger brother. So, it was the same dose being given to the older and the younger brothers. As a result, in retrospect, the younger brother was receiving between 4 and 6 mEq/kg/day long before the data came out about using much higher amounts of bicarbonate. The mother's control trial has shown that at the higher dose the younger brother's height was on the 25th percentile while the older brother was on the first percentile. We presented that to a visitor and he mentioned those brothers subsequently without giving credit to those who had observed them. We learned many things from those two patients. I just wish that they had continued to comply with their medications.

MODERATOR: Since we have mineral metabolism experts here, could I ask one of you to touch upon the possible mechanisms by which nephrocalcinosis occurs? Why does it occur? Why some treatments prevent it and others don't?

COMMENT-QUESTION: I have a question myself in that same vein, about Type IV renal tubular acidosis. In the adult population it has been described as a distinct type of hyporeninemic hypoaldosteronemic type of hyperkalemia with hyperchloremia and RTA. The vast majority of those patients who have interstitial disease or diabetes are not salt-losers. It has been proposed that the hyperkalemia in metabolic acidosis is due to resistance of the tubules to the action of aldosterone. I was wondering if you have encountered that type of patient in the pediatric population and what your thoughts are about the fact that those patients are not salt-losers, despite having a resistance of the tubules to the action of aldosterone.

RESPONSE: I have seen only one or two such cases; I have not really studied them carefully. With reference to the mechanism of nephrocalcinosis, it can be stated, perhaps in a simplistic fashion, that citrate excretion is decreased in these renal tubular acidotic patients and calcium excretion is increased to a very high level. This calcium is being excreted, instead of the normal soluble calcium citrate form, in an insoluble calcium carbonate form and nephrocalcinosis ensues due to that form of calcium being deposited. With correction of acidosis, citrate excretion will return to normal. So, it is not an intrinsic defect of RTA kidneys to excrete citrate, it is just secondary to the presence of metabolic acidosis. With early recognition, one can reverse the hypercitruria, return citrate excretion to normal so that calcium excretion, which will also decrease after acidosis, will be coming out as soluble citrate.

COMMENT-QUESTION: We have been studying the fractional excretion of bicarbonate in very low birth weight infants. We have found that small prematures are able to lower their urine pH even below 5.0 in situations of severe respiratory or metabolic acidosis. Under those conditions, what is the validity of the delta PCO_2? What does it mean? Is the PCO_2 of urine minus that of blood valid in a small infant? This question is prompted by the statement of some, that impaired concentrating ability may be a limiting factor for the evaluation of those results. Do you have any data in children to help interpret what happens with the delta PCO_2 as a reflection of distal hydrogen ion secretion?

RESPONSE: Unfortunately, I only know of other people's work on that. I have not been involved in determining partial pressure of CO_2 in urine. They have assured me that it is a very easy procedure to do. It just happens that I have the titrator to do the acid excretion easily; however, always we confront this problem of completeness of urine collection in small children and in infants. I was pleased to report the study published in Pediatric Research in 1976, that it is possible to acidify both premies as well as term infants after three weeks of age and expect the responses to be that of a normal adult. So, it would seem that the acidifying capacity is different from the delayed maturation of renal concentration.

QUESTION: Do you have any explanation for the difference in development of rachitic bone changes in proximal versus distal RTA?

RESPONSE: The issue of differences or lack of bone complications in Type II RTA as compared with Type I RTA can be simplistically summarized in the following fashion: in Type I RTA it is the distal tubular inability to excrete hydrogen ions that gives rise to accumulation of acid and therefore metabolic acidosis, whereas in Type II RTA there is no accumulation of hydrogen ions. Type II RTA, if we may be so simplistic--there are certain virtues in being simplistic in a complicated situation like RTA--it is that Type II RTA is secondary to a bicarbonate reabsorption defect, perhaps related to maturation factors. So, the infants with Type II RTA will have been spilling bicarbonate after serum bicarbonate exceeds the Tm bicarbonate, exceeding the threshold up to which bicarbonate is reabsorbed. If we were to plot on an axis the bicarbonate concentration so that at a bicarbonate concentration of 26, we begin spilling bicarbonate, in a premature infant the Tm bicarbonate or tubular threshold for bicarbonate is brought down to about 22. At that stage, bicarbonaturia begins. However, in Type II RTA there is a lowering of that threshold even further down to let's say 16, so that bicarbonaturia begins the moment that serum bicarbonate exceeds 16. However, by the same token, they should not get more severe acidosis than reflected by a bicarbonate of 16. They are only wasting bicarbonate; they are not retaining hydrogen ion. The absence of retention of hydrogen ion, then, gives rise to the absence of all the consequences of hydrogen ion retention. I hope that that explanation is clear. It may seem like a circular explanation but, in fact, if you do not have hydrogen ion retention, you should not have the complications of bone diseases, as would occur in chronic renal failure with its retention of hydrogen ion.

MODERATOR: Could we ask a question about the false diagnosis of congenital uropathies in utero, the evaluation of renal function in utero that has been reported and questioned by different people? Also, for the discussion on the renal scan versus the IVP or the ultrasound: what is the final evaluation when there is disagreement among all those tests?

RESPONSE: I'm afraid I don't have the answers. Personally, I have not been involved in the evaluation of pre-natal problems, so I cannot answer that question. What is the merit of nuclear medicine versus sonography? I would say that it is our experience that nuclear studies are very easy to be performed, even without the involvement of physicians at all. They don't need any particular experience for the technology. All you need is a good injection and immobilization of the child. As far as the interpretation, when a person has six months experience, as we find from our residents, he can handle the cases. Ultrasound requires a lot of personal involvement by the ultrasonographer. It is much more difficult to perform; unless the ultrasonographer has great skill and experience, there will be many mistakes. If you have perfectly performed studies, I think ultrasonography is very helpful for the evaluation of structure. Nuclear medicine is more efficient when the question of function is raised.

MODERATOR: What about the disagreements? It has been said that at times there are disagreements about results with the IVP and other procedures. The question is: "What is really happening?" Can you be sued for not correcting something that the IVP is showing, or not showing but is shown by another method? I guess the answer is: "Well, there is confusion". Then, you just settle down, wait, repeat the test and so on. If you are going to repeat, what are you going to repeat? The IVP or the renal scan?

RESPONSE: There is always some greater degree of invasiveness which one can pursue. If there is a problem with renal vein thrombosis, you can do a venogram which is an invasive test and have a more specific answer. If the question is about renal artery stenosis, you can do an arteriogram. If it is an extreme hydronephrosis versus multicystic kidney (which may be a question), it is our experience that hydronephrosis can easily be distinguished with nuclear medicine studies. In hydronephrosis we see always some residual renal functioning tissue around the collecting system, whereas the multicystic kidney does not show this appearance. The question should be answered on an individual basis; I believe that there is always some specific answer for each situation.

COMMENT: I would agree completely with what was said. All these tests complement each other. Probably, the best agreement with the final clinical diagnosis in the neonatal period is still obtained with the renal scan more than with ultrasound and more than with the IVP. There are technical limitations in interpretation, especially of the IVP, in the first few weeks of life. There is a growing problem I could see especially for pediatric nephrologists, a new specialty which is going to be Prenatal Nephrology to handle those calls we get more and more often about babies with problems detected in utero, regarding anomalies of the kidneys or urinary tract. Again, we need to evaluate very carefully with whose hands these tests have been made, the expertise of the ultrasonographer, before making any decision and, even more, before giving information to the parents. We have created great anxiety in parents who were told that the baby may have severe complications only to find after birth that the baby has normal kidneys and GU tract.

MODERATOR: We work as a team with the people in Pediatric Radiology and Nuclear Medicine and with the urologists. One of the main urologists that currently winds up getting us out of (or into) trouble is the urologist on this Panel. When we bring such a patient to you, what do you usually do?

COMMENT: Let me say that I agree and disagree with one of the things that has been said. First, you have a child in whom you want to do a general evaluation. You have questions if you feel a mass, the child has urinary tract infection and you want to do an initial evaluation in the neonatal period. In that situation, I usually request a nuclear medicine study and an abdominal ultrasound, simultaneously. The problem is that many times when we find that there is hydronephrosis we have to make a decision whether or not to do something, perform some type of operation, usually a diversion-the most common procedure we do in infancy. We want the anatomical confirmation of what we are seeing, so that we can decide what we are going to do. If I have a child in whom I suspect posterior urethral valves, I want to get a plain voiding cystogram with contrast material to establish the diagnosis of the disease. Sometimes I want to see if the bladder anatomically looks like a neurogenic bladder; in that case, I also get a cystogram. Another problem would be when we suspect obstruction of the urinary tract and we are not sure sometimes if it is at the uretero-pelvic junction or if it's a lower ureteral obstruction or something rare at the level of the urethra. I should say that Dr. Sfakianakis is very precise with the diagnoses. So, putting together what has been said, with ultrasound and an experienced ultrasonographer to look at renal masses, and radionuclide procedures to bypass the bowel to get a better visualization of the kidneys, in this manner you can do an initial evaluation. But if you have to make a decision for surgery, I think that the iodinated material should be used in an IVP and voiding cystogram.

MODERATOR: What is your understanding of the current situation for intervention in utero? Have you intervened? Do you have any thoughts on that? It's something that has become quite dramatic; it has even appeared in the newspapers!

COMMENT-RESPONSE: No. Not more than what you know about the fetal ultrasound. It has helped us greatly having the diagnosis as soon as the baby is born so we can do more definitive studies right away and start treatment immediately. I don't know. In California a group has done a lot of work on that. The initial work has not been very encouraging. I don't know if there are new data coming from there. Experimentally, you know that early obstruction is usually associated with dysplasia. We would have to be considering doing something at the not too late part of pregnancy to save some function during intrauterine life. There is one team working on that. I think we need to wait for their results to really make a decision for ourselves.

MODERATOR: We currently are involved with such a patient. Our approach is very conservative: try to save the patient rather than the kidneys which anyhow have been subjected to blood pressure changes and obstruction for several months. Accelerating the delivery, we believe, unless there are very, very good indications that there is something acute, does not seem to be wise. We haven't faced that situation yet; so, when we meet with the parents and "meet the baby" through the mother's belly, we try to reassure them, and convey the message that probably there will not be much difference in the outcome if we wait for a term or near-term delivery.

COMMENT: It also depends upon the type of problem that initiated the study in utero. When the fetus has been found to have an abnormality of the kidneys by an ultrasound performed just to assess fetal maturity, in general there are not severe problems and there usually is a very good outcome. The initial experience that we reported in JAMA, maybe two years ago, was in 13 fetuses born with different congenital anomalies; in most of these patients the mothers had olighydramnios and they all had severe anomalies. Four of them died in spite of procedures performed. I think the wave now is to be conservative until we have more information on the subject.

QUESTION: In newborn infants (full-term and premature babies), often we see metabolic acidosis, hyperbicarbonaturia or lack of ability to excrete hydrogen ion. What percent of these patients do you think are reversible and to what extent do you suggest work-up of these patients and follow-up? My question is based on the fact that the work-up of a patient with metabolic acidosis and renal tubular acidosis is expensive and difficult.

RESPONSE: I wish I had the answer. I don't think the answer is truly available. We have been waiting for our results to accumulate to the degree that we would be able to make a statement. To answer your question, to share our experience about what we do, we would be called by our colleagues to see infants and children who have acidosis and some suggestion of alkaline urine. I like to treat them with Shohl's solution because I would like to correct the acidosis to prevent hypercalciuria. I would measure urine calcium divided by urine creatinine on spot tests to assure myself and the patient and the parents that hypercalciuria, if present, is reversed by the alkali treatment. Then, every several months on follow-up of these children, I ask them to stop the bicarbonate treatment a week or two before they come to the clinic visit so that I can follow the natural history of what seems like RTA but it could be primarily a maturational process, or some condition induced by diarrhea, sepsis, or undetected sub-clinical insults to the kidneys. In time, I hope to accumulate enough data to see what we are really dealing with. I am following them with assessment of their acid-base status every second time. That is, I would have them off bicarbonate every second clinic visit so that I know whether or not there is spontaneous resolution of the initial acidosis. I would also follow the urine calcium and creatinine. Perhaps in another few years I will be able to summarize these results. At this point, I can share with you that I am following 30 or more patients who have documented alkaline urine pH's associated with metabolic acidosis. About half of them have hyperkalemia but I am not 100% sure that these are not associated with hemolyzed blood. I would ask my neonatology colleagues to obtain free flowing blood samples and they would document that they are free-flowing and yet we are seeing hyperkalemia. About half of those infants seem to have a Type IV RTA. But as far as the natural history, really the question you want answered and the percentage of involvement, we need a few more years before we have the answers. I hope that that is a satisfactory way of sharing with you what we do.

COMMENT-QUESTION: First a statement; with any "funny looking kid", it is the obligation of the pediatrician to look for secondary congenital anomalies and not to wait for abnormal urines to show since we may not see abnormal urines until later on. My question is: when do you do surgery in the children with myelomeningocele with high pressure bladders?

RESPONSE: Not always do I do surgery in children with high pressure bladders. If they don't have upper tract problems, I try to control the high pressure in the bladder with medication. If the bladder empties well, I do not add intermittent catheterization. If the child has residual urines, then I add intermittent catheterization. That would be the basis of my treatment. We need to know if the child has a high pressure bladder in order to continue following the child, and I should say almost forever or at least until adulthood, because if we let them go to the age of puberty and tell them that everything is ok, then abnormalities like this will appear. What will happen in the future is very hard to say. I do not know. But certainly, the point is that the high pressure bladder group is at risk and if they can handle the problem with intermittent catheterization, we leave them with the problem without surgery as much as possible. If they cannot, then we have to consider different types of surgical procedures. If the bladder capacity is satisfactory, we might do a vesicostomy; if the bladder capacity is not satisfactory or if they have small fibrotic contracted bladders with vesicoureteral reflux and megaureters, then we favor bladder replacement. It is interesting that you brought up that question because now a lot of people are using artificial sphincters for urinary incontinence in these children. What was reported in a very reliable report is that in 71% of these children with high pressure bladders, there is a possibility that if you obstruct the bladder outlet, the intravesical pressure might get worse with time. We have two cases of artifical sphincters placed elsewhere with dilated and tortuous ureters. So, that is something else to consider when debating the possibility of implanting an artificial sphincter. Definitely, that is a group that is at risk.

MODERATOR: What about the other point? That's what we teach, that's what we try to do. Whenever there is a congenital anomaly any place in the body, we try to look at least with ultrasound but ideally, with something more informative, for renal anomalies. Does the panel agree with that position? The heads are nodding in agreement.

QUESTION: Regarding patients with neurogenic bladder and reflux; we know that most times these children have bacteria in their urine. With the problem in differentiating between upper and lower urinary tract infection, how would you follow these children? What is the significance of bacteria in the urine of these children?

RESPONSE: I pass the question to my pediatric nephrology colleagues who have done some work on that. Basically, in patients with myelomeningocele we treat the bladder problem because that is the source of the infection. If you decompress the bladder, usually the problem disappears unless the child has an associated upper tract obstruction. Now, in the child who comes to see you with fever or pyelonephritis-like symptoms and you want to know if it is coming from the bladder or from the kidney, you have a more complex problem. I would like to transfer the question to the Moderator.

MODERATOR: Actually, my associate is the one of our group with the greatest experience. Would you like to answer that question?

RESPONSE: I agree with the previous comment. Indeed, when you are dealing with an asymptomatic patient that is doing self-intermittent catheterization, we do not know what is the significance of the growth of bacteria. Let's say 50,000 to 100,000 colonies/ml. I am not sure that we have the data and if we should place them in active treatment or not. In those patients who are asymptomatic, I agree that we probably could do some non-invasive studies and try to document the level of involvement. The question may be just theoretical because if you have reflux and you have bladder infection, you must assume that the bladder urine is reaching the kidneys. But if the patient has fever, a high sedimentation rate or the C-Reactive Protein is positive, I would be inclined to treat it as an acute pyelonephritis.

QUESTION: You mentioned high pressure and low pressure bladders, above 40 and below 40 cm H_2O. What is the normal pressure usually?

RESPONSE: In a normal bladder the pressure is up to 15 cm H_2O.

QUESTION: How often do you see unilateral reflux in neurogenic bladders and would you approach them differently in re-implanting the ureter since the other side is normal? Since these neurogenic bladders would be colonized with bacteria especially if you catheterize the bladder intermittently, what criteria do you use for treatment of these patients when they have urinary tract infection?

RESPONSE: We have been following our patients with chronic suppressive antibiotics, intermittent catheterization and anticholinergics. It is very difficult to talk about a generalized rule for myelomeningoceles because they present similar pathology at different ages, so the treatment might be different. In these children who are within the post-pubertal age, who are reliable and follow instructions to empty their bladder, by getting urine cultures on a sequential basis and getting assessments of their renal functions periodically, we have not observed deterioration of the upper tract, including renal functions. We have observed, using anticholinergics, that the bladder which is small and retracted, improves; the capacity of the bladder improves. We have observed that the vesico-ureteral reflux sometimes disappears and sometimes diminishes. So, my initial approach to these children is like I said several times, conservative. Now, if they start having uncontrollable infections, if they have problems performing the intermittent catheterizations or if we see any kind of deterioration in the renal functions, then we have to decompress or treat the bladder problem by other means. The other means would be, depending on the capacity of the bladder, a vesicostomy or just a reimplantation if it is a low pressure bladder, or doing a bladder substitution if it is a small retracted bladder. In between, you have all the problems that you can find on a daily clinical basis; you have to adjust your treatment depending on the patient.

COMMENT-QUESTION: I have an answer for a previous question. If by clinical signs or symptoms we cannot localize an infection, we always have radiological studies. There is the galium approach, the labelled leucocyte imaging, or if this has been performed, the ultrasound may give an idea of the localization. I have my own question. We see referrals with myelomeningocele for evaluation of the condition of the kidneys and there are problems with compliance. We see patients who come after being lost to follow-up for two years and they have severe deterioration of their renal functions. We see hydronephrosis with double the size from the previous evaluation. How common is this problem in your practice? Do you have any approach to solve this problem?

COMMENT-RESPONSE: Probably, it is a matter of waiting long enough and you will see those disasters, coming to end-stage renal disease later on in life but of course that affects the nephrologists and not the urologists. We are dealing with a referral population. I would say that, of the large number of patients who come to us referred for any other type of congenital anomaly of the urinary tract (in children, minor degrees of reflux), fortunately, there is a small percent that goes to chronic renal failure and end-stage renal disease.

COMMENT-RESPONSE: I think that the main question for the surgeon who is dealing with these patients on a daily basis, in the deteriorating child in whom you see that the ureter is becoming more dilated, that the kidneys are not growing, that he is developing infections, is when to operate and when to follow the child conservatively. When I was in training, all the children with dilated ureters were operated. Now it has been found that all those ureters that were operated on had problems anyway. So, our general orientation now is to be conservative with these children; plus, we have better antibiotics and we have better methods for following the patients. I really think that conservative methods should be emphasized, but, obviously, with adequate follow-up.

QUESTION: For the record, yes or no, is there ever a place for diversion above the bladder in 1984?

RESPONSE: Very rarely.

MODERATOR: With that briefest of question and answer, we shall adjourn. Thank you.

EDITOR'S COMMENTS

This Panel Discussion attempted to clarify questions on subjects as important as renal tubular acidosis, urinary tract infections in patients with myelomeningocele, bladder capacity, nephrocalcinosis, rachitism, and anomalies of the genito-urinary tract diagnosed in utero with conflicting results from various diagnostic modalities.

Of general interest were the comments on the role played by personalities in creating the complex RTA nomenclatures proposed or actively (passionately?) defended. In contrast, a simple recommendation made during this Panel merits emphasis: that the follow-up of patients with RTA include frequent determinations of urinary calcium/creatinine ratios. This should simplify identification of those patients who are prone to, or in the process of developing nephrocalcinosis.

IV

MINERAL METABOLISM

EARLY NEONATAL HYPOCALCEMIA

Billy S. Arant, Jr., M.D.

Serum calcium concentrations in newborn infants at 24 hours of age vary directly with gestational age, but serum calcium concentrations in the fetus actually exceed the range of normal values and decrease abruptly during the first day of life (1). In premature infants, the decrease in serum calcium concentration following birth is more pronounced than in those born at term. The smallest, least mature neonate at 72 hours of age may have a serum calcium concentration of 6.5-7 mg/dl without symptoms of hypocalcemic tetany (2). In healthy infants fed early, serum calcium concentrations increase spontaneously to within the range of normal values by the end of the first week of life. This pattern of change in serum calcium concentration in the newborn infant is referred to as early neonatal hypocalcemia and is considered normal even though the understanding of this physiologic event in fetal adaptation to postnatal life is incomplete.

Serum calcium concentration in the fetus is approximately 2 mg/dl greater than its mother (1). This observation has been attributed to the relative hyperparathyroidism of pregnancy since serum magnesium concentrations are similar, serum phosphorus concentrations are higher in the fetus than the mother, and 25-hydroxy-vitamin D levels are not different (3). On the other hand, serum 1,25-dihydroxyvitamin D concentration in the mother is more than twice that of the fetus (4).

It has been said that compared to fullterm infants total body calcium in preterm infants is decreased; therefore, serum calcium concentrations decrease rapidly because of inadequate calcium stores. When body calcium is related to fetal weight, however, the accretion rate of calcium is directly related to the gain in body weight (5). At any given weight or maturity, fetuses or newborn infants at birth have relatively similar calcium stores.

Calcium is distributed in the body in a rapidly exchangeable pool; namely, in the serum, the interstitial fluid, and cytesol of surface bone. In addition, there is a slowly exchangeable calcium pool in subcellular organelles and dystrophic calcification, while a nonexchangeable pool exists in the deeper layers of bone. Normally, about 40% of calcium is nondiffusible and bound to protein, and 60% occurs in the diffusible fraction, either in the ionized form or bound to other radicals. Factors which appear to protect the neonate against developing hypocalcemic tetany include normal serum ionized calcium concentrations (6) due, in part, to lower serum albumin concentrations. Moreover, the relative metabolic acidosis of prematurity may predispose to increased serum ionized calcium.

A decrease in serum ionized calcium stimulates parathyroid hormone (PTH) secretion which, in turn, activates renal hydroxylase activity to form 1,25-dihydroxy-vitamin D. This activated form of vitamin D promotes intestinal absorption of calcium and phosphorus. When serum calcium concentration is restored to normal, this stimulus to PTH release ceases. Any phosphorus excess is excreted in the urine by the action of PTH on renal tubules. Moreover, PTH and vitamin D together promote bone resorption to augment the restoration of serum calcium concentration to normal. Early neonatal hypocalcemia, therefore, could be due to decreased PTH activity, to decreased hydroxylase activity, to decreased gastrointestinal absorption of calcium or to decreased responsiveness of bone or renal tubular epithelia to 1,25 dihydroxy-vitamin D or PTH. When serum calcium concentrations were measured during the first week of life and compared to simultaneously measured serum PTH levels, an inverse relationship was found, suggesting that the neonatal parathyroid glands do respond to changes in total serum calcium concentration (7). When neonates were treated with different doses of vitamin D metabolites, early neonatal hypocalcemia was not prevented (8). Since liver metabolism is limited in newborn infants, and since hyperbilirubinemia occurs during the same period of time as early neonatal hypocalcemia, it could be that 25-hydroxy-vitamin D formation is inadequate or that renal hydroxylase activity is deficient for adequate synthesis of 1,25-dihydroxy-vitamin D. However, 25-hydroxy-vitamin D, shown to be normal when compared to maternal values, is directly correlated with the serum concentrations of 1,25-dihydroxy-vitamin D in fullterm infants (9), suggesting no deficiency of vitamin D activation by the neonatal kidney. Therefore, early neonatal hypocalcemia cannot be explained fully by inappropriate or immature hormonal mechanisms.

Serum phosphate concentrations are increased in newborn and growing infants above that of adults. It has been reported previously that the tubular reabsorption of phosphate is inappropriately high for the elevated serum phosphate concentrations in these infants--an observation interpreted as a feature of functional immaturity of the newborn kidney. However, when tubular reabsorption of phosphate in infants at birth was measured prior to phosphate intake, values were unrelated to the maturity of the infants. When formula was introduced, serum phosphate concentrations increased further and tubular phosphate reabsorption decreased, suggesting that changes in the renal handling of phosphate is appropriate to increases in plasma phosphate concentration in the neonate.

Although it had been assumed previously that urinary losses of calcium did not contribute to the development of early neonatal hypocalcemia, serum calcium concentrations in preterm infants were found to be related inversely to the urinary excretion of both calcium and sodium (10). Moreover, urinary excretion of calcium and sodium increased as sodium intake of the infants increased. When the urinary calcium to creatinine ratio, a means of detecting hypercalciuria in children and adults with hematuria and urolithiasis was measured, it was noted that normal, healthy full-term and premature infants excreted very little calcium in their urines; urine calcium:creatinine ratios were <0.15 (11). However, sick newborn infants with or without lung disease excreted 5 to 30-fold more calcium; calcium: creatinine ratios were as high as three. Moreover, intravenous calcium or furosemide increased urinary calcium excretion further. More recently, the urinary excretion of calcium, phosphorus and sodium in infants was studied during the first week of life (12). The data obtained in infants studied on the first day of life were compared with those studied on the second to the seventh days of life. A similar pattern of calcium and sodium excretion with gestational age was observed regardless of postnatal age, i.e., calcium and sodium excretions were highest in the most premature infants and least in infants born at term. Phosphorus excretion on the first day of life also varied inversely with gestational age; however, phosphorus excretion after the first day increased in infants of every gestational age. Fractional urine flow rate, which reflects the percent of glomerular filtrate excreted as urine, decreased with gestational age, both in infants studied at birth or subsequently during the first week of life. When calcium excretion in these infants was related either to phosphate or sodium excretion and to fractional urine flow rate, a direct correlation was noted for each on the first day of life. Between two and seven days of life, similar but less significant correlations were observed. Moreover, fractional urine flow rate varied directly with urinary excretion of calcium, phosphorus and sodium, regardless of postnatal age. Infants studied at birth and subsequently during the first week of life exhibited changes in urinary calcium excretion which varied directly with changes in fractional urine flow rate, but not to changes in urinary phosphate or sodium excretion.

Which factors increase the risk of early neonatal hypocalcemia becoming a clinical problem? One factor could be aggressive fluid therapy. Any factor which increases urine flow rate could be associated with increased urinary losses of calcium and sodium. Excessive sodium intake, provided either as a supplement to formula or in parenteral fluids, will promote urinary sodium and calcium excretion. The recommended treatment for hypercalcemia in adults is aggressive fluid therapy and furosemide to increase urinary calcium excretion. The effect of furosemide, known to inhibit sodium chloride reabsorption and thereby increase urine output, also increases the urinary excretion of potassium and calcium in newborn infants (13). Such treatments are often part of the routine management of high risk neonates, and, therefore, may predispose them to developing symptomatic hypocalcemia. Bicarbonate therapy to treat metabolic acidosis decreases the ionized fraction of serum calcium by increasing calcium binding to serum proteins. Moreover, albumin administration to increase blood volume and raise blood pressure may increase calcium binding and reduce serum ionized calcium concentration below a critical level; symptomatic hypocalcemia may occur after alkali or albumin administration even when total serum calcium concentration is unchanged. Another factor which may affect serum ionized calcium concentration is transfusion with citrated blood. Serum ionized calcium concentration decreases during exchange transfusion with citrated blood. It is only after exchange transfusion that serum ionized calcium returns to near pre-treatment values (1). Magnesium deficiency reported in infants of diabetic mothers places the newborn infant at risk of developing symptomatic hypocalcemia.

How can early neonatal hypocalcemia be avoided or at least minimized? Efforts to increase calcium intake immediately after birth either as intravenous calcium infusion or as increased oral calcium intake have had variable results. When calcium was infused intravenously, the fall in serum calcium concentration was prevented in preterm infants older than 34 weeks gestation (14). Moreover, serum ionized calcium concentrations measured in infants during the first 24 hours of calcium supplementation showed significant improvement when large calcium supplements were provided. Although serum ionized calcium concentrations were lower in untreated infants, each value remained ≥ 2.5 mg/dl, and no infant developed symptomatic hypocalcemia. When supplementation from birth with 1 μg of 1,25-dihydroxy-vitamin D was compared to a lower dose of vitamin D or to a vitamin D_2 preparation, total serum calcium concentrations were increased only in those given the highest doses of activated from of vitamin D; however, serum calcium concentrations did not fall below 8.5 mg/dl in infants given either a smaller dose of activated vitamin D or vitamin D_2 (8). Of interest is the observation that serum PTH concentrations were not suppressed by any of these treatments, and serum ionized calcium concentrations were increased above controls only in those given the higher dose of activated vitamin D.

In conclusion, the approach to minimizing the risks associated with early neonatal hypocalcemia should include the avoidance of aggressive fluid therapy to achieve unnecessary water diuresis in preterm infants and the reduction of augmented urinary sodium excretion produced by aggressive fluid therapy, by diuretics or by increased sodium chloride intake. The casual administration of loop diuretics, especially for the sole purpose of increasing urine flow rate to an arbitrary, value or to "prevent" respiratory distress should not be a supported practice in neonates. The use of colloid does not increase blood pressure in preterm infants, but it is possible to reduce serum ionized calcium by this treatment. Parenteral calcium should be provided infants subjected to exchange transfusion, and magnesium deficiency in infants of diabetic mothers should be anticipated and corrected. Finally, the indiscriminate use of sodium bicarbonate therapy for infants without significant metabolic acidosis should be abandoned.

REFERENCES

1. Tsang, R.C., Chen, I-W., Friedman, M.A. et al.: Neonatal parathyroid function: role of gestational age and postnatal age. J. Pediatr. 83: 728, 1973.

2. Tsang, R.C. and Oh, W.: Neonatal hypocalcemia in low birth weight infants. Pediatrics 45: 773, 1970.

3. Hillman, L.S. and Haddad, J.G.: Human perinatal vitamin D metabolism I: 25-hydroxyvitamin D in maternal and cord blood. J. Pediatr. 84: 742, 1974.

4. Fleischman, A.R., Rosen, J.F., Cole, J., et al.: Maternal and fetal serum 1,25-dihydroxyvitamin D levels at term. J. Pediatr. 97: 640, 1980.

5. Forbes, G.B.: Calcium accumulation by the human fetus. Pediatrics 57: 976, 1976.

6. Brown, D.M., Boen, J. and Bernstein, A.: Serum ionized calcium in newborn infants. Pediatrics 49: 841, 1972.

7. Salle, B.L., David, L., Glorieux, F.H. et al.: Early oral administration of vitamin D and its metabolites in premature neonates. Effect on mineral homeostasis. Pediatr. Res. 16: 75, 1982.

8. Chan, G.M., Tsang, R.C., Chen, I-W. et al.: The effect of 1,25$(OH)_2$vitamin D_3 supplementation in premature infants. J. Pediatr. 93: 91, 1978.

9. Glorieux, F.H., Salle, B.L., Delvin, E.E. et al.: Vitamin D metabolism in preterm infants: serum calcitriol values during the first five days of life. J. Pediatr. 99: 640, 1981.

10. Brown, D.R. and Steranka, B.H.: Renal cation excretion in the hypocalcemic premature human neonate. Pediatr. Res. 15: 1100, 1981.

11. Goldsmith, M.A., Bhatia, S.S., Kanto, W.P., Jr. et al.: Gluconate calcium therapy and neonatal hypercalciuria. Am. J. Dis. Child. 135: 538, 1981.

12. Arant, B.S., Jr.: Renal handling of calcium and phosphorus in normal human neonates. Sem. Nephrol. 3: 94, 1983.

13. Sulyok, E., Varga, F., Nemeth, M. et al.: Furosemide-induced alterations in the electrolyte status, the function of renin-angiotensin-aldosterone system and the urinary excretion of prostaglandins in newborn infants. Pediatr. Res. 14: 765, 1980.

14. Salle, B.L., David, L., Chopard, J.P. et al.: Prevention of early neonatal hypocalcemia in low birth weight infants with continuous calcium infusion: effect on serum calcium, phosphorus, magnesium, and circulating immunoreactive parathyroid hormone and calcitonin. Pediatr. Res. 11: 1180, 1977.

LATE NEONATAL HYPOCALCEMIA

Michael Freundlich, M.D., Gaston Zilleruelo, M.D., Carolyn Abitbol, M.D. and Jose Strauss, M.D.

Hypocalcemia, defined as a serum calcium (Ca) concentration $\leq$ 7.5 mg/dl, constitutes a frequent development during the neonatal period. Since Ca is transferred across the placenta into the fetus at daily rates of up to 150 mg/kg of fetal weight during the last trimester of pregnancy, it is not surprising that upon delivery, the sudden interruption of such a rich supply of calcium should result in hypocalcemia. The latter has two main peaks of occurrence: during the first 48 hours following delivery (early hypocalcemia), or after the second part of the initial week of life (late hypocalcemia or classical neonatal tetany) (1). Early hypocalcemia is dealt with in detail in another chapter of this volume; however, since several mechanisms seem to be operative in both early and late hypocalcemia, some degree of overlap is unavoidable. This chapter attempts to summarize the available information related to the pathogenetic mechanisms involved in late neonatal hypocalcemia (Table 1).

TABLE 1

LATE NEONATAL HYPOCALCEMIA

PATHOGENETIC MECHANISMS

Hyperphosphatemia
Hypomagnesemia
Hypercalcitoninemia
Hypoparathyroidism
Vitamin D Deficiency-Immaturity
Acid-Base Disturbances
Hypercalciuria
Miscellaneous

HYPERPHOSPHATEMIA

Neonatal tetany has been recognized since the early part of this century (2). Hyperphosphatemia, as a result of the increased phosphate load contained in cow's milk, has been identified as an important pathogenetic mechanism (3). Elevated serum phosphorus (P) concentration may lead to hypocalcemia by favoring bone Ca deposition, augmenting calcitonin action at the bone site and by blunting the calcemic action of parathyroid hormone (PTH). In one study (3), serum Ca concentration was lower and that of P higher in infants fed cow's milk as compared to those fed breast milk. The Ca/P ratio of 1.3 of cow's milk is much lower than that of human milk, 2.2. Furthermore, cow's milk contains a much higher phosphorus concentration in absolute terms. Thus, the P load of cow's milk is several fold higher than that of breast milk. In another study on a large number of infants (4), plasma Ca and P were determined at the sixth day of life following the administration of different formulas with various modifications in the Ca/P content ratios. The authors were able to demonstrate a positive linear relationship between plasma Ca concentration and the Ca/P of the formula, as well as a similar but negative correlation for plasma P. They were able to abolish the hypocalcemic effect of cow's milk by increasing the dietary Ca content. Current recommendations for milk formulas, as pertains to the total P content and the CA/P ratio, include those which more closely approximate breast milk.

Since the kidney is the main excretory route for P, and since glomerular filtration rate (GFR) is lower in early infancy than at later ages, it would seem logical to attribute the elevated serum P so characteristic of infants to limitations in renal excretion. Although several studies have addressed this issue, the role of the diminished GFR in the maintenance of a high serum P concentration early in life, remains uncertain (5). Studies in rats (6) have revealed significantly lower maximal tubular reabsorption of P (TRP) in mature as compared to young animals, even after thyroparathyroidectomy. Those differences could not be accounted for by changes in GFR or urinary cyclic AMP, suggesting that the decrease in TRP that occurs with maturation is independent of PTH. Studies in guinea pigs have revealed similar observations, namely, a significantly higher absolute reabsorption rate of P/unit of kidney weight in the young animals as compared to their older counterparts (5). The authors concluded that the renal transport mechanism for P is more efficient in the newborn, and accounts for the maintenance of the positive external balance for this ion in the growing subject. Finally, decreased phosphaturic and urinary cyclic AMP responses have been reported in infants suggesting decreased end organ responsiveness to PTH (7), with its consequent hyperphosphatemia.

HYPOMAGNESEMIA

Calcium and magnesium (Mg), the major divalent cations in the body, share many physiologic characteristics, and their homeostatic regulation is closely interrelated. A detailed review of those interrelationships is beyond the scope of this chapter; suffice it to say, though, that any disturbance in homeostasis of one of these ions is commonly associated with a corresponding disturbance in the other. Hypomagnesemia leads to hypocalcemia through several mechanisms: decreased production of PTH, target organ resistance to PTH, decreased intestinal absorption of calcium, and decreased exchange of Ca for Mg at the bone surface, with reduction of calcium release from bone (8). Several isolated cases of neonatal hypocalcemia associated with hypomagnesemia have been described in the literature. Some selected cases of neonatal hypomagnesemia seem to be hereditary with recessive genetic characteristics (9). Detailed studies in a large group of neonates (10) demonstrated that after 24 hours of age, the mean plasma Mg concentration was consistently and significantly lower in hypocalcemic infants than in normals and than in non-hypocalcemic sick infants.

Other studies (11) in infants with hypocalcemic tetany during the first two weeks of life, found a significant correlation between serum Ca and Mg concentrations. However, hypomagnesemia has not been a consistent finding during the first week of life (12), nor has a significant correlation with serum Ca always been noted (13). Usually the hypomagnesemia is transient and resolves spontaneously. Hypomagnesemia is more frequently encountered in small for gestational age infants of toxemic mothers, asphyxiated babies with metabolic acidosis, and infants of diabetic mothers (13). The hypomagnesemia in the latter seems to be related to functional hypoparathyroidism and maternal hypomagnesemia (14). Other factors associated with hypomagnesemia include: intestinal malabsorption, total parenteral nutrition, use of diuretics, and therapy with aminoglycosides. Shortening of the small intestine by surgery can lead to Mg malabsorption with the consequent hypomagnesemia. Finally, as noted above, hypomagnesemia leads to a decrease in the secretion rate of PTH; this may constitute another mechanism by which hypomagnesemia contributes to the genesis of hypocalcemia.

HYPERCALCITONINEMIA

Calcitonin is a hormone produced by the C-cells of the thyroid gland and acts at the bone site antagonizing the effect of PTH by decreasing the amount of Ca and P released from bone into the blood. Calcitonin has been found to be increased during the first 24 hours of life in full-term (12) as well as premature infants (15). However, few data are available pertaining calcitonin levels after the first couple of days of life. In one study, calcitonin concentration was elevated above the normal adult levels in both premature and term infants at birth, 48 hours and seven days of life (12). The levels at seven days were still above those seen at birth, and slightly higher in the premature infants. These data suggest that calcitonin may be another contributory factor in the pathogenesis of late neonatal hypocalcemia.

VITAMIN D DEFICIENCY

Significant progress has been achieved in understanding the metabolic pathway and mechanisms of action of Vitamin D. In brief, either ingested in the diet or generated by ultraviolet radiation of the skin, Vitamin D reaches the blood circulation and undergoes its first conversion to 25 hydroxycholecalciferol (25 Vitamin D) in the liver. The second and final conversion to 1,25 dihydroxycholecalciferol (1,25 Vitamin D) takes place in the proximal tubular cells of the kidney. This final product, actually a hormone, is the most active and potent of the

Vitamin D metabolites, and is considered the main mediator of its final actions at the bone site and intestinal mucosa (16). In the adult human and animal, Vitamin D clearly plays an important role in intestinal absorption of Ca; however, in the early postnatal period this may not be applicable.

Following birth, the intestinal tract becomes the major organ of calcium acquisition. Although as noted, 1,25 Vitamin D plays a prominent role in this intestinal absorption in adult life, studies of Vitamin D deficient and newborn rats have demonstrated that intestinal Ca transport during the first two weeks of life is not mediated by 1,25 Vitamin D (17). When 1,25 Vitamin D was administered to newborn rats, its effect was noted only after day 25, that is after weaning. Before 1,25 Vitamin D can exert its action at the intestinal level, it requires binding by specific receptors in the cytoplasm of the intestinal cell; the concentration of these receptors was found to be very low in the intestine of suckling rats at 7 and 14 days of life, but substantially increased upon weaning (18). In the adult, the binding of 1,25 Vitamin D to its receptors, stimulates the intestinal synthesis of a Ca binding protein. However, both the concentration and the activity of the Ca binding protein were found to be relatively low in the suckling rat (19).

Intestinal absorption of calcium involves two mechanisms: 1) active, carrier mediated 1,25 Vitamin D dependent, and 2) passive diffusion independent of Vitamin D. During the former, Ca is absorbed from the luminal gut against the existing concentration gradient between intestinal lumen and plasma. In adults, the duodenum and jejunum are mainly involved in carrier mediated Ca transport, whereas the ileum and colon are the sites of passive transport. However, in premature infants, (20, 21) Ca absorption is linear with regards to Ca intake, suggesting a lack of carrier mediated transport. Thus, it could be speculated that 1,25 Vitamin D plays no role in the early postnatal intestinal absorption of Ca and that, consequently, hypocalcemia of prematurity may not respond to the administration of Vitamin D or its metabolites. Studies in the fetal lamb preparation (22) have demonstrated similar results, namely, no difference in the intestinal uptake of Ca nor Ca ATPase activity in the intestinal mucosa of either nephrectomized or normal fetuses. This again suggests that intestinal Ca transport is not Vitamin D dependent, since the nephrectomized fetuses (presumably devoid of circulating 1,25 Vitamin D) showed similar trends as the intact animal (22).

In the infant, cord blood concentration of 25 Vitamin D correlates with maternal levels regardless of gestational age (12). The postnatal changes in 25 Vitamin D were similar in term or premature infants, although the latter had significantly lower serum calcium concentrations at 48 hours of age, suggesting that Vitamin D deficiency played no role, at least in the early hypocalcemia. Vitamin D deficient mothers gave birth to neonates with low 25 Vitamin D levels. Several studies have casted doubt about the inability of premature infants to synthesize Vitamin D. In one study of infants during the first five days of life, with and without Vitamin D administration, the authors concluded that after 32 weeks of gestational age the liver is able to hydroxylate Vitamin D, to maintain and restore normal concentration of 25 Vitamin D, and that the gut can absorb calcium and the kidneys are able to hydroxylate Vitamin D (23). This clearly demonstrates that after 32 weeks of gestation, there is no defect in Vitamin D activation. Furthermore, the authors found normal blood 1,25 vitamin D levels, contrary to low levels reported by others (24).

On the other hand, data from Europe suggest that maternal Vitamin D status may be related to late neonatal hypocalcemia. In one study (25), significantly lower mean Ca concentrations were noted on the 6th day of life in infants of Asian immigrants as compared to other ethnic groups. When those mothers were supplemented with Vitamin D, the incidence of neonatal hypocalcemia decreased substantially. In the same study (25), a significant correlation between maternal alkaline phosphatase concentration at 36 weeks gestation and neonatal hypocalcemia was noted, indicating that maternal Vitamin D deficiency affects Ca homeostasis in the offsprings. Maternal Vitamin D supplementation also resulted in lower alkaline phosphatase levels during pregnancy. The association of late hypocalcemia with eventual teeth enamel hypoplasia (26) supports the contention that both are due to antenatal factors, namely maternal Vitamin D and/or Ca dietary deficiencies.

Few clinical circumstances are clearly associated with a truly decreased synthesis of Vitamin D: neonatal liver disease may lead to decreased synthesis of 25 Vitamin D, while Vitamin D dependent rickets is associated with diminished synthesis of 1,25 Vitamin D. Both may lead to hypocalcemia and rickets (27).

HYPOPARATHYROIDISM

Although low or undetectable at birth, most infants have a noticeable increase in serum PTH concentration by two and seven days (8). However, functional hypoparathyroidism, that is, the inability of the parathyroid gland to respond to hypocalcemia, has been noted in sick infants and in infants of diabetic mothers (14). Maternal hyperparathyroidism leads to maternal and, consequently, fetal hypercalcemia. The latter results in fetal parathyroid gland suppression and eventual postnatal hypocalcemia (28). Transient congenital hypoparathyroidism has also been noted in some infants (29). A more detailed description of hypoparathyroid states in the neonatal period can be found in another chapter of this book (28).

ACID BASE DISTURBANCES

Metabolic acidosis increases the flux of Ca from bone to the extracellular fluid, whereas alkalosis has an opposite effect (30). Alkalosis induced by hyperventilation with mechanical respiration in infants with respiratory disease, may lead to hypocalcemia. This has been prevented by the constant infusion of Ca at the rate of 1 mg/kg/hr in infants requiring the concomitant administration of sodium bicarbonate (31). Alkalosis leads to a decrease in the ionized Ca, due to increased binding of Ca by plasma proteins. In fact, post-acidotic tetany, namely the development of tetany following correction of metabolic acidosis accompanying diarrhea, was described almost four decades ago (32). The same has been described in neonates treated with sodium bicarbonate for the correction of metabolic acidosis (33).

HYPERCALCIURIA

This is another possible contributing factor to the development of neonatal hypocalcemia and is dealt with in detail in another chapter of this book. Suffice it to say that the widespread use of loop diuretics in nurseries, with its consequent hypercalciuric effect, might aggravate the hypercalciuria of neonates (34).

The use of alternative diuretics, like thiazides, which exert a hypocalciuric effect, should be explored in a controlled fashion.

MISCELLANEOUS

Neonates who develop acute renal failure are prone to develop pronounced hypocalcemia. These infants exhibit a substantial daily rise in the blood concentration of inorganic P with the expected fall in plasma Ca (35). The alterations of mineral metabolism in acute renal failure have been recently reviewed (36).

Hypocalcemia has been noted in association with persistence of the ductus arteriosus and with congestive heart failure (37, 38), and seems to play a role in the decreased contractility of the heart muscle. The parenteral administration of Ca had a salutory effect on several hemodynamic parameters (38).

In summary, a multitude of factors seems to determine the genesis and perpetuation of hypocalcemia during the latter part of the first week of life. An attempt has been made here to review the most relevant aspects.

REFERENCES

1. Wald, M.K.: Problems in chemical adaptation: Glucose, calcium and magnesium. In Klauss, M.H. and Fanaroff, A.A. (eds.) Care of the High Risk Neonates. Philadelphia: W. B. Saunders Publishing Co., 1978, p. 224.

2. Pincus, J.B. and Gittleman, J.F.: Infantile tetany: Metabolic study. Am J Dis Child 51:816, 1936.

3. Gardner, L.I., MacLachlan, E.A., Pick, W., et al.: Etiologic factors in tetany of newly born infants. Pediatrics 5:228, 1950.

4. Barltrop, D. and Oppe T.E: Dietary factors in neonatal calcium homeostasis. Lancet 2:1333, 1970.

5. Spitzer, A., Kaskel F.J., Feld, L.G., et al.: Renal regulation of phosphate homeostasis during growth. Semin Nephrol 3:87, 1983.

6. Caversazio, J., Bonjour, J.P. and Fleish, H.: Tubular handling of Pi in young growing and adult rats. Am J Physiol 242:F705, 1982.

7. Linarelli, L. G., Bobik, J. and Bobik, C: Newborn urinary cyclic AMP and developmental responsiveness to parathyroid hormone. Pediatrics 50:14, 1972.

8. Tsang, R.C., Donovan, E.F. and Steichen, J.J.: Calcium physiology and pathology in the neonate. Pediat Clin N Amer 23:611, 1976.

9. Friedman, M., Hatcher G. and Watson, L.: Primary hypomagnesemia with secondary hypocalcemia in an infant. Lancet 1:703, 1967.

10. David L and Anast C.S.: Calcium metabolism in newborn infants. The interrelationship of parathyroid function and calcium, magnesium, and phosphorous metabolism in normal, "sick", and hypocalcemic newborn. J Clin Invest 54:287, 1974.

11. Chiswick, M.L.: Association of oedema and hypomagnesaemia with hypocalcemic tetany of the newborn. Br Med J 3:15, 1971.

12. Hillman, L.S., Rojanasathit, S., Slatopolsky, E., et al.: Serial measurements of serum calcium, magnesium, parathyroid hormone, calcitonin, and 25-hydroxy-vitamin D in premature and term infants during the first week of life. Pediat Res 11:739, 1977.

13. Tsang, R. C. and Oh, W.: Serum magnesium levels in low birth weight infants. Amer J Dis Child 120:44, 1970.

14. Tsang, R.C. and Steichen, J.J.: Disorders of calcium and magnesium metabolism. In Fanaroff, A.A., and Martin, R.J., (eds.): Behreman's Neonatal-Perinatal Medicine. St. Louis: C. V. Mosby, 1983, p. 870.

15. David, L., Salle, B., Putet, G., et al.: Serum immunoreactive calcitonin in low birth weight infants. Description of early changes. Pediat Res 15:803, 1981.

16. Freundlich, M. and Strauss, J.: Calcium, vitamin D and parathyroid hormone related aspects in the neonatal period. In Strauss, J. (ed.): Neonatal Kidney and Fluid-Electrolytes. Boston: Martinus Nijhoff, 1983, p. 127.

17. Halloran, B.P. and DeLuca, H.F.: Calcium transport in small intestine during early development: Role of vitamin D. Am J Physiol (Gastro Intest Liver Physiol) 2:G473, 1980.

18. Halloran, B.P. and DeLuca, H.F.: Appearance of the intestinal cytosolic receptor for 1,25-dihydroxyvitamin D_3 during neonatal development in the rat. J Biol Chem 256:7338, 1981.

19. Gleason, W.A. and Lankford, G.L.: Intestinal calcium-binding protein in the developing rat duodenum. Pediat Res 16:403, 1982.

20. Barltrop, D., Mole, R.H. and Sutton, A.: Absorption and endogenous faecal excretion of calcium by low birthweight infants on foods with varying contents of calcium and phosphate. Arch Dis Chil 52:41, 1977.

21. Shaw, J.C.L.: Evidence for defective mineralization in low birth weight infants: The absorption of calcium and fat. Pediatrics 57:16, 1976.

22. Moore, E.S., Langman, C.B., Loghman, A.M., et al.: Intestinal calcium transport in utero. Clinical implications for the newborn infant. In Strauss, J. (ed.): Neonatal Kidney and Fluid-Electrolytes. Boston: Martinus Nijhoff, 1983, p.3.

23. Glorieux, F.H., Salle, B.L., Delvin, E.B., et al.: Vitamin D metabolism in preterm infants: Serum calcitriol values during the first five days of life. J Pediatr 99:640, 1981.

24. Steichen, J.J., Tsang, R. C. and Gratton, T.L.: Vitamin D homeostasis in the perinatal period. N Engl J Med 302:315, 1980.

25. Watney, P.J.M., Chance, G.W., Scott, P., et al.: Maternal factors in neonatal hypocalcemia: A study in three ehnic groups. Br Med J 2:432, 1971.

26. Purvis, R.J., Mackay, G.S., Cockburn, F., et al.: Enamel hypoplasia of the teeth assocated with neonatal tetany: A manifestation of maternal vitamin-D deficiency. Lancet 2:811, 1983.

27. Chan, J.C.M.: Phosphate losing nephropathies. Semin Nephrol 3:126, 1983.

28. Alon, U. and Chan, J.C.M.: Parathyroid hormone insufficiency and resistance. In this volume.

29. Rosenbloom, A.L.: Transient congenital idiopathic hypoparathyroidism. South Med J 66:666, 1973.

30. Parfitt, A.M. and Kleerekoper, M.: Clinical disorders of calcium, phosphorus, and magnesium metabolism. In Maxwell, M.H., and Kleeman, C.R. (eds.): Clinical Disorders of Fluid and Electrolyte Metabolism. New York: McGraw Hill, 1980, p. 947.

31. Nervez, C.T., Shott, R.J., and Bergstrom, W.H.: Prophylaxis against hypocalcemia in low-birth-weight infants requiring bicarbonate infusion. J Pediatr 87:439, 1975.

32. Rapaport, S., Dodd, K., Clark, M., et al.: Post-acidotic state of infantile diarrhea. Am J Dis Child 73:391, 1947.

33. Tsang, R.C. and Oh, W.: Neonatal hypocalcemia in low-brith weight infants. Pediatrics 45:773, 1970.

34. Arant, B.S.: Renal handling of calcium and phosphorus in normal human neonates. Semin Nephrol 3:94, 1983.

35. Williams, G.S., Klenk, E.L. and Winters, R.W.: Acute renal failure in pediatrics, In Winters, R.W. (ed.): The Body Fluids in Pediatrics. Boston: Little, Brown, 1973, p. 523.

36. Freundlich, M., Zilleruelo, G. and Strauss, J.: Mineral metabolism in acute renal failure. In Strauss, J. (ed.): Acute Renal Disorders and Renal Emergencies. Boston: Martinus Nijhoff, 1984, p. 197.

37. Hammerman, C., Eidelman, A.I. and Gartner, L.M.: Hypocalcemia and the patent ductus arteriosus. J Pediatr 94:961, 1979.

38. Mirro, R. and Brown, D.R.: Parenteral calcium treatment shortens the left ventricular systolic time intervals of hypocalcemic neonates. Pediatr Res 18:71, 1984.

PHARMACOLOGIC AGENTS TO REVERSE HYPERCALCEMIC AND HYPOCALCEMIC STATES

Robert J. Geller, M.D. and James C. M. Chan, M.D.

Introduction

Calcium concentration in the extracellular fluids is precisely maintained within very narrow limits. Substantial deviations from the norm usually result in symptoms, such as tetany from hypocalcemia or anorexia, nausea, polydipsia, polyuria, constipation, depression, fatigue, muscle weakness and failure to thrive from hypercalcemia.

Corvisart, a French physician of the 19th century, was credited as the first to use the word tetany to describe the involuntary muscular contraction of the extremities in adults (1). In 1887, Walter Butler Cheadle, the noted English pediatrician, underscored the muscular spasms, seizures and laryngeal stridor of infantile tetany (2). The French physician, Armand Trousseau, was the first in the 19th century to describe spasm of muscle, induced by pressure on the innervating nerve, seen in hypocalcemic tetany - a physical sign which bears his name.′ The Austrian surgeon, Franz Chvostek in the late 19th century, described the spasmodic contraction of the facial muscle provoked by tapping the facial nerve in the parotid region of the face and seen in tetany associated with hypocalcemia. In contrast, the initial descriptions of hypercalcemic symptoms cannot be traced to any one person.

Supported by Public Health Service, National Institutes of Health
Research Grants AM HD 31370.

Hypercalcemia

Even the exact definition of hypercalcemia provokes controversy. Probably the most commonly used criterion is a serum concentration of total calcium exceeding 11.0 mg/dl (2.75 mmol/l) in the absence of serum protein abnormalities, although many laboratories use serum calcium concentrations of 10.5 mg/dl as their upper limit of normal. Common symptoms of hypercalcemia include listlessness, irritability, and anorexia. Signs commonly associated with hypercalcemia include hypotonia, weakness, headaches, weight loss, constipation, vomiting, polyuria and polydipsia. Prolonged or marked hypercalcemia can result in nephrocalcinosis, hypertension, and renal failure.

Incidence. The incidence of hypercalcemia exceeds 500 new cases per million adults per year, extrapolating from Mundy and Martin's experience (3). Of these hypercalcemic individuals, 50% were caused by primary hyperparathyroidism and another 30% had an underlying malignancy causing the hypercalcemic state (3). Table 1 lists the more common causes of hypercalcemia seen in clinical practice.

Hyperparathyroidism. Hypercalcemia secondary to hyperparathyroidism is most commonly detected in asymptomatic outpatients (during screening procedures or laboratory tests ordered for other reasons). However, although common in adults, hyperparathyroidism appears to be relatively rare in adolescents and even more uncommon in young children (4, 5). Boys are affected more commonly than girls (6). The underlying pathophysiology in infants is usually parathyroid hyperplasia and may result in severe hypercalcemia. However, infants of hypoparathyroid mothers may also be afflicted with transient hyperparathyroidism and symptomatic hypercalcemia (6). Older children more commonly develop hyperparathyroidism as a result of parathyroid tumors.

Malignancies. Malignancy-related hypercalcemia is usually mediated through increased osteoclastic activity. The relative increase in osteoclastic activity may, on occasion, result from the secretion of a PTH-like substance, the secretion of a poorly characterized substance called osteoclast activating factor, or by direct tumor metastasis to bone (7). Under normal circumstances, the increased mobilization of calcium resulting from this osteoclastic activity might be adequately compensated for by the usual mechanisms of increased osteoblastic activity and skeletal deposition of calcium, and by increased renal excretion. However, in malignancy-related hypercalcemia, osteoblastic activity is usually decreased (8), and renal clearance of calcium is also frequently subnormal.

The most frequently associated hematologic lesions include multiple myelomas and, less commonly, leukemias. Renal and breast tumors are the adenocarcinomas most commonly associated with hypercalcemia. Squamous cell carcinoma of the lung is also commonly associated. Although the tumors themselves are rare, thyroid cancers and cholangiocarcinomas frequently cause hypercalcemia when they do occur.

Table 1. Differential Diagnosis of Hypercalcemia

Diseases	Drug-Related
Hyperparathyroidism	Calcium excess
Malignancies	Thiazide diuretics
hematologic	Hypervitaminosis D
adenocarcinoma	Alkali (antacids)
squamous cell	Phosphate deficiency
Protracted immobilization	Hypervitaminosis A
Dehydration	Estrogens
Sarcoidosis	Androgens
Tuberculosis	Tamoxifen
Dysmorphic syndromes	Progestins
Renal transplantation	Pepto-Bismol tablets
Acute renal failure (recovery)	Prostaglandin E2
Hyperthyroidism	Aluminum toxicity
Hypothyroidism	Lithium
Paget's disease	
Subcutaneous fat necrosis	
Metabolic alkalosis	
Adrenal insufficiency	

Immobilization. Hypercalcemia secondary to protracted immobilization occurs most commonly following major injuries where loss of weight-bearing occurs for extended periods. It is most commonly seen in adolescents who have sustained spinal cord injuries, and is attributed to an imbalance between osteoblastic and osteoclastic activity (although this remains an unproven hypothesis). It typically begins about 10 days post injury, is maximal at 10 weeks post injury, and lasts at least six months (9).

Dehydration. Dehydration is almost universally present in states of severe hypercalcemia, but because hypercalcemia itself may produce dehydration, it is frequently unclear which entity preceded which.

Dysmorphic syndromes of infancy. Hypercalcemia in infancy may be associated with a malformation syndrome. Lightwood's Syndrome (comprised of supravalvular aortic stenosis, mild to moderate mental retardation and "elfin" facies) has been associated with hypercalcemia in early infancy, sometimes resolving by the age of two years (10). Hypercalcemia has also been reported to sometimes be associated with Williams' Syndrome (moderate short stature, prominent lips, and moderate mental retardation) (11).

Renal transplantation. Renal transplantation following chronic renal failure associated with secondary hyperparathyroidism has been reported to cause elevation of calcium, lasting up to two years or longer post-transplant (12). In one study of 95 patients (13) evaluated six months to 12 years following surgery, 47 (51%) had an elevated serum ionized calcium. However, total serum calcium was elevated in only 10 of the 95 (12). Immunoreactive PTH concentrations were not related to serum calcium, serum phosphorus, or to time since transplantation. Hypercalcemic patients did have an increased incidence of subperiosteal erosions and arterial calcifications. The degree of osteitis fibrosa on bone biopsy done at the time of transplantation was found to be most predictive of the subsequent development of post-transplantation hypercalcemia. The authors concluded that "hyperparathyroidism may indeed be an important factor in post-transplant hypercalcemia and hypophosphatemia." For a further review of this area, the reader is referred to the article by Conceicao et al (13).

Medication-related. The drugs presented in Table I have been reported to cause hypercalcemia in humans (14-18). Excessive calcium intake may overwhelm the body's compensatory mechanisms, with predictable results. Thiazides decrease the kidney's excretion of calcium, thereby predisposing to hypercalcemia. The milk-alkali syndrome is a well recognized entity consisting of hypercalcemia, alkalosis, and renal impairment. Although the pathophysiology is incompletely understood, the ingestion of large amounts of both calcium and alkali (antacids, etc.), especially as calcium carbonate, appears to cause an impairment in renal calcium and bicarbonate excretion (17).

Other commonly used agents, including theophylline and thyroxine, are suspected to cause hypercalcemia in animals, but have not been documented to do so in humans. A careful drug history should be obtained from a patient with otherwise unexplained hypercalcemia, bearing the possibility of an etiologic relationship in mind.

Hypocalcemia

Hypocalcemia is usually defined as a serum calcium less than 7.5 mg/dl, although some laboratories use different limits. Its clinical presentation usually includes some combination of tetany, carpopedal spasm, muscle cramps and twitching, seizures, paresthesias, and laryngeal stridor. Infants may also demonstrate lethargy, poor feeding, and vomiting (10, 19).

Prematurity. Hypocalcemia may present at any age (Table 2). The neonate, especially the stressed premature neonate and the infant of a diabetic mother, may present in the first few days of life with significant hypocalcemia. The 5 to 7 day old infant may develop hypocalcemia related to a diet high in phosphate relative to its calcium content. Older children may develop hypocalcemia due to dietary deficiencies of calcium or vitamin D, defective metabolism of vitamin D, renal disease or any other cause of chronic hyperphosphatemia, or syndromes involving parathyroid dysfunction.

Early infantile hypocalcemia is thought to be related to the premature infant's decreased ability to respond to hypocalcemic stimuli by releasing PTH. The risk of hypocalcemia is increased in infants who receive citrate or bicarbonate containing fluids (20). Hypocalcemia in the first few days of life may also be caused by maternal hyperparathyroidism or by primary hypomagnesemia (by decreasing both the quantitative release of PTH and the end-organ responsiveness to PTH). Although the hypocalcemia related to these problems usually resolves promptly after correction of the underlying abnormality, the hypoparathyroid state has been reported to last up to one year in rare cases (21).

Parathyroid and other disorders. Hypocalcemia in older children may result from DiGeorge syndrome, from the hyperphosphatemia of chronic renal failure, or from hyposecretion by multiple endocrine organs (parathyroids, adrenals, pancreatic beta cells, thyroids, ovaries). Hypocalcemia may also result from pseudohypoparathyroidism, despite adequate or even increased production of PTH, in the presence of end-organ unresponsiveness to the hormone. The specific type of pseudohypoparathyroidism may be classified on the degree of involvement of skeletal muscle, bone, or the kidney individually or in combination. PTH receptors may also fail to respond adequately to endogenous hormone but respond to exogenous PTH, qualitatively implicating the hormone itself.

Vitamin D-dependent rickets, presenting in the first year of life with hypocalcemia, hypophosphatemia, elevation of alkaline phosphatase and aminoaciduria, is associated with high 25-hydroxyvitamin-D and low 1,25-dihydroxyvitamin-D secondary to deficiency of renal 25-hydroxyvitamin-D 1 alpha-hydroxylase. Hypocalcemia also occurs secondary to hypoproteinuria of nephrotic syndrome, metabolic alkalosis, congenital malformation syndromes and hemorrhagic pancreatitis (Table 2).

Table 2. Differential Diagnosis of Hypocalcemia

Diseases	Drug-Related
Prematurity	Excess phosphate
Infant of a diabetic mother	Hypovitaminosis D
Hypoparathyroidism	Magnesium deficiency
Pseudohypoparathyroidism	Radiologic Contrast
Vitamin D-dependent rickets	Anticonvulsants
Chronic renal failure	Citrated transfusions
Hypoproteinemia	Fluorides
Alkalosis	Acetazolamide
Malformation syndromes	Colchicine
Hemorrhagic pancreatitis	Ethylene glycol
	Sodium EDTA

Glucocorticoids and other medications. Hypocalcemia may result, less commonly from a poor dietary intake of calcium, or from decreased calcium absorption from the gut. Glucocorticoids, in particular, may decrease calcium absorption if used chronically (22, 23). Indeed, glucocorticoids have been shown to produce osteomalacia with chronic use, and to result in a higher rate of rib and vertebral fractures in recipients (24). Chronic renal disease or hepatic disease may interfere with the production of the active compound calcitriol (1,25-dihydroxycholecalciferol) from its precursors, thereby decreasing calcium absorption (25, 26).

Drug-related disorders. Drugs may also alter calcium homeostasis. Inadequate vitamin D intake is one common exacerbating factor; low sunlight exposure only compounds this. The use of phenytoin or phenobarbital have been shown to produce a relative vitamin D deficient state (27-29), and other anticonvulsants and sedative-hypnotics may also do so to a lesser extent (29). Decreased absorption of vitamin D itself, increased consumption, and altered metabolism of the 25-OH-cholecalciferol moiety have all been implicated in the pathogenesis of this phenomenon, but the relative contribution of each remains unclear. Increased intake of vitamin D has been shown to offset the imbalance produced by the anticonvulsants (29-31).

Citrate-containing products have also been shown to produce hypocalcemia, probably by the chelating action of the citrate. Radiologic contrast agents containing diatrizoate have been shown to produce a drop in serum calcium and a corresponding increase in serum immunoreactive PTH. However, products containing citrate and diatrizoate (e.g., Renografin, Reno-M-DIP) have been shown to cause a significantly greater drop in serum calcium and greater increase in PTH than diatrizoate-containing agents without citrate or edetate (e.g. Hypaque) (32-33).

Other drugs, such as acetazolamide, have also been shown to interfere with the hypercalcemic response to vitamin D in rats but, thus far, this has not yet been reported in man (34).

Treatment of Hypercalcemia

Multiple therapeutic modalities are available for the treatment of severe hypercalcemia. The lack of consensus regarding the indications for each approach probably indicates the suboptimal effectiveness of any available therapy. Furthermore, little if any information is available dealing specifically with the treatment of the pediatric patient with hypercalcemia. However, depending on an analysis of all the circumstances, the clinician faced with this problem must choose from amongst the commonly available treatment modalities; we hope the information summarized here will provide a basis for an informed choice.

A primary consideration in selecting a therapeutic approach is the urgency of the situation. As defined by Mundy and Martin (3), total serum calcium exceeding 13 mg/dl after correction for plasma protein abnormalities is severe hypercalcemia and requires a treatment regimen with rapid onset of action. Similarly, the patient with symptoms directly attributed to hypercalcemia requires intervention with rapid therapeutic effect. The patient with mildly elevated serum calcium whose disease is indolent, will not require such rapidity of effect but will be best served by the simplest and safest therapeutic strategy, such as fluids and diuretics.

The underlying disease state causing the hypercalcemia also serves to govern the selection of therapy, as different conditions give rise to hypercalcemia by different pathophysiologic mechanisms. If the underlying problem can itself be easily remedied, this is certainly the best approach, as in the case of substitution for or elimination of thiazide diuretics.

Rehydration. Most patients with hypercalcemia are significantly dehydrated. The vomiting and polyuria associated with hypercalcemia, compounded by the renal effects of hypercalcemia (reduction in glomerular filtration rate, and impairment in renal concentrating ability and sodium-reabsorbing ability) all contribute to depletion of body water. This reduction in total body water perpetuates a "vicious cycle" of further exacerbation of the hypercalcemia. The kidney attempts to compensate for the intravascular volume depletion by increasing proximal tubular reabsorption of water and sodium, thereby increasing calcium reabsorption as well, as calcium and sodium reabsorption in the proximal tubule are thought to be coupled (35).

The first treatment for seriously hypercalcemic patients should be aimed at rapid restoration of intravascular volume, although in certain patients, this may be difficult to achieve due to their underlying cardiopulmonary disorder. Other relative contraindications include preexisting renal failure or inappropriate antidiuretic hormone secretion. Treatment must first be aimed at volume repletion with 0.9% saline. The sodium chloride administration reduces proximal renal tubular reabsorption of sodium and concurrently reduces reabsorption of calcium (36). The rate of administration should be adjusted to produce a brisk diuresis at 3-5 liters/day for the adult, supplemented by potassium 20-40 mEq/l and magnesium 10-20 mEq/l (14), augmented if necessary by the additional administration of loop diuretics. Once the circulating intravascular volume has been restored, dextrose containing fluids with lower sodium content may be used.

Table 3. Treatment of Hypercalcemia

Agent	Administration	Dosage	Onset	Comments
Fluids	IV, PO	maximum tolerated	<6-12 hr	Normal Saline preferred Monitor for electrolyte imbalances
Calcitonin	SC, IM	2-8 MRC Units/kg/day divided at least every 6 hours	<4 hr	Escape phenomenon occurs within days Use with glucocorticoids may delay escape Hypersensitivity reactions may occur - ?skin test before first dose Use with mithramycin may cause hypocalcemia
Mithramycin	slow IV over 3-6 hrs	25 mcg/kg ?reduce in renal or hepatic disease	12-24 hr	Monitoring of hepatic, renal, and coagulation status necessary Toxicity probably cumulative Use with calcitonin may cause hypocalcemia
Phosphates	PO	0.25-0.5 mmol/kg/day, in 3 divided doses; may increase as tolerated to max. 90 mmol/day if hypophosphatemia persists	?12 hr	Monitor for hyperphosphatemia Use with extreme caution in preexisting hyperphosphatemic states 32 mmol phosphorus = 1 gm phosphorus
	slow IV over 6-8 hr	0.25-0.5 mmol/kg; max. 4 doses	?1 hr	Possible seizures, cardiotoxicity
Prednisone	IV, PO	1-2 mg/kg/dose, every 6-24 hrs	12-24 hr	Most effective in sarcoidosis and vitamin D excess

Although volume repletion is widely cited as efficacious, there is little data extant regarding this. The available data suggest that 70% of patients treated with aggressive fluid repletion will have at least a 50% reduction in the elevation of the serum calcium concentration (35). If fluid repletion is effective, the decrease in serum calcium will begin in several hours and probably continue over 48 hours to a total decline of 2-3 mg/dl.

Diuretics. Forced diuresis, involving administration of fluids (as discussed above) at rates up to 500 ml/hr plus up to 80-100 mg of furosemide or 20-40 mg of ethacrynic acid every 1-2 hours for the adult, has been widely used for the treatment of severe hypercalcemia. Diuretics should not be administered during the first one to two hours of this regimen, to avoid exacerbating the already depleted intravascular volume which usually coexists with the hypercalcemia. After the first two hours, diuretic therapy should be initiated at the smallest dose producing a satisfactory diuresis.

When effective, the decrease in serum calcium concentration secondary to this therapy should be seen within a few hours. Toxicities associated with this regimen include ototoxicity and nephrotoxicity from high doses of diuretics, as well as problems related to excessive fluid administration and electrolyte imbalance.

Calcitonin. As presently in use, calcitonin (Calcimar) is the synthetic form of salmon calcitonin, the most potent form of the hormone recognized. It is an inhibitor of osteoclastic activity (probably by blocking the stimulatory effects of PTH on the osteoclast), and also causes increased calcium loss from the kidney (36, 37).

The major advantage of calcitonin is its rapid onset of action: the maximal hypocalcemic effect is usually achieved by 4 to 6 hours after the first dose, but the effect lasts only about 24 hours. It is, therefore, recommended that calcitonin be given either in divided doses every 6 to 12 hours or by continuous infusion. (There does not seem to be adequate data showing any significant difference between these two methods of administration.) (38) About 80% of patients will respond to calcitonin therapy initially (38, 39), but most will show an "escape" phenomenon (probably mediated by the development of antibodies against the calcitonin) after several days of therapy. The concomitant use of glucocorticosteroids seems to block the escape phenomenon and to prolong the effectiveness of therapy (40), although the exact duration for which this therapeutic combination remains effective is controversial (36, 38, 40).

The "standard" dose of calcitonin in use is 2-4 MRC units/kg/day, although it remains unclear whether this is indeed the optimum dose. Recommendations vary between 2-4 MRC units/kg/day to 8 MRC units/kg/dose to be repeated every 12 hours (14, 38, 41). The only significant side effects of calcitonin noted are nausea, vomiting, and flushing, although these may occur in up to 25% of drug recipients.

Mithramycin. Derived as a cytotoxic agent, mithramycin is included in several antineoplastic chemotherapeutic regimens (42). Its main use, however, is in the treatment of severe hypercalcemia, when used in a fraction of its antineoplastic dose. Its advantages as an anti-hypercalcemic agent are its high rate of efficacy while the complication of hypocalcemia is rarely encountered. The other advantage of mithramycin is long duration of its action of 3 to 15 days (36, 39).

However, disadvantages include its long latency before onset of response (24-48 hours), and its propensity to cause quantitative and qualitative platelet dysfunction, hepatotoxicity (manifest as elevated transaminases), and nephrotoxicity. Less common side effects include nausea, vomiting, diarrhea, fever, stomatitis, lethargy, acneiform dermatitis, toxic epidermal necrolysis, and phlebitis (14, 36).

The usual therapeutic dose is 25 mcg/kg/dose, given by slow intravenous infusion over six hours. Toxicity is most common with doses exceeding 30 mcg/kg/dose, or when more than 150 mcg/kg/week or 250 mcg/kg total dose are given (3, 16, 36, 39).

The use of mithramycin has been recommended by some authorities for the chronic treatment of hypercalcemia of malignancy, by administration of weekly doses (14). Others note, however, that sudden elevation of serum calcium, sufficient to prove lethal, may occur before the onset of the mithramycin effect (36, 39).

Glucocorticosteroids. These agents have been shown to retard bone resorption due to causes other than PTH (3, 43), and to reduce absorption of calcium from the gut, especially in hypercalcemia secondary to hypervitaminosis D and sarcoidosis (3, 36). Hyperparathyroid-induced hypercalcemia does not respond to therapy with glucocorticoids, and in fact this lack of response forms the basis for the diagnostic test differentiating hyperparathyroidism from other causes of hypercalcemia (3, 36).

Glucocorticosteroids are effective in 30% to 50% of patients with hypercalcemia not related to primary hyperparathyroidism, although some of these patients respond only incompletely (3, 39). Furthermore, the response to glucocorticoids is variable and unpredictable. If effective, the onset of action is noted within 24 to 48 hours after the onset of therapy. The recommended dosage is approximately 1-2 mg/kg/day of prednisone (36).

Phosphates. Phosphates act by precipitating calcium, both in the gut and in total body water. Given intravenously, phosphates have the ability to rapidly and predictably remove calcium, which is the primary advantage of this method of therapy. However, complications include hyperphosphatemia (especially in those patients with pre-existing renal compromise) and extraskeletal calcifications, and when given intravenously, seizures and cardiotoxicity. These potential risks have made intravenous phosphate treatment less than desirable in most cases (39, 44).

The use of oral phosphate supplements is an attractive therapy for mild cases of chronic hypercalcemia. Oral phosphates are not as rapidly, nor as predictably effective, but only infrequently result in extraskeletal calcifications. Oral phosphate therapy is, however, poorly tolerated by some patients. Gastrointestinal side effects, primarily nausea, vomiting, and diarrhea, occur in 20% to 30% of adults receiving oral phosphates in doses of 0.5 gm twice daily to 1 gm three times a day (39, 44).

Diphosphonates. This new class of agents has recently become available for the therapy of Paget's disease. The only agent available commercially in the United States at this time is etidronate, for oral use. The use of etidronate for hypercalcemia other than that of Paget's disease has largely been disappointing (39). Other agents, such as aminohydroxypropane diphosphonate (APD) and dichloromethylene diphosphonate Cl_2MDP) available abroad and for investigational use, have proven promising in the hands of some investigators although not all (3, 36, 39).

Prostaglandin Synthetase Inhibitors. Prostaglandins have been implicated in bone resorption caused by bone tumors (45). Therapeutic trials with indomethacin and aspirin, however, have largely proven disappointing (36, 39).

Dialysis. Dialysis may be beneficial for the patient with acute renal impairment and hypercalcemia. However, this will only temporize for a period of days, until other therapy can be undertaken to directly address the causes of hypercalcemia.

Surgery. Parathyroidectomy has served as a time-honored cure for severe hypercalcemia due to primary hyperparathyroidism. Although some authorities continue to advocate emergent parathyroidectomy for this problem, others advocate medical therapy with vigorous fluid repletion followed by parathyroidectomy on a less emergent basis (46).

Other Agents. Other agents previously utilized in the management of hypercalcemia include EDTA and sodium sulfate. These agents, because of their high toxicity compared to their efficacy, are no longer recommended for the treatment of hypercalcemia.

Precis of Therapeutic Approach to Hypercalcemia

The treatment of hypercalcemia remains an area of little agreement. Therapeutic options are summarized in Table 3. A rational approach probably includes vigorous fluid repletion with normal saline as a first line of therapy, followed by either calcitonin (with or without prednisone) or mithramycin. Treatment of the underlying etiology should be undertaken wherever possible. Diphosphonates seem promising, but the currently available agent does not appear to be a significant addition to the therapeutic armamentarium for the urgent treatment of severe hypercalcemia.

Treatment of Hypocalcemia

The treatment of symptomatic hypocalcemia falls into two broad categories:

(a) non-specific replacement of calcium, usually as an emergency procedure by intravenous calcium infusion and

(b) specific therapeutic measures based on the underlying causes of the hypocalcemia.

Neonatal tetany. The often severe hypocalcemia of neonatal hypoparathyroidism and the consequent risk of mental retardation from convulsions, demands prompt intervention with calcium gluconate or calcium gluceptate infusions. (Table 4) The recommended rate of infusion of calcium gluconate is 500 to 1,000 mg/sq.m./day. Tissue necrosis and sloughing results from extravasation of such infusate and must be avoided by the use of a well-placed intravenous catheter.

Table 4. Calcium Preparations for Treatment of Hypocalcemia

Name	How Supplied	Dosage	Comments
Calcium gluceptate injection	23% solution = 18 mg or 0.9 mEq Ca^{++}/ml 5 ml ampules	0.1-0.5 ml/kg up to 10 ml per dose	transient tingling (IV) sense of oppression or "heat waves"; mild local reaction (IM)
Calcium gluconate injection	10% solution = 9 mg or 0.45 mEq Ca^{++}/ml	0.25-1.0 ml/kg up to 20 ml per dose	transient tingling (IV); abscess formation precludes IM injection
Calcium gluconate tablets	325, 500, 650 or 1000 mg tablet = 1.5, 2.3, 3.0 or 4.6 mEq Ca^{++}, respectively	(not settled)	non-irritating to gastric mucosa
Calcium chloride injection	5-10% solution = 0.68 to 1.36 mEq Ca^{++}/ml	0.1-0.2 ml/kg of 10% solution up to 10 ml	Inject slowly to avoid syncope, irritating to vein, peripheral vasodilation, hypotension, cutaneous burning sensation, metabolic acidosis
Calcium chloride powder	27%	use with milk to avoid gastric upset	gastric irritation, intestinal necrosis precludes use in infants
Calcium glubionate (Neo Calglucon)	345 mg elemental calcium/15 ml	1-2 tablespoons, t.i.d.	administer before meals to enhance absorption, hypercalcemia, hypercalciuria rare

Table 4. **Calcium Preparations for Treatment of Hypocalcemia (continued)**

Name	How Supplied	Dosage	Comments
Calcium carbonate	40% calcium powder or 650 mg calcium carbonate tablets	1-3 tablets, t.i.d.	converted to stable salts in intestine before absorption; unable to solubilize this preparation. Used as antacid
Calcium phosphate	dibasic and tribasic insoluble; used as antacids		
Calcium levulinate	13% calcium powder or 10% solution = 0.69 mEq Ca^{++}/ml		bitter, saline taste

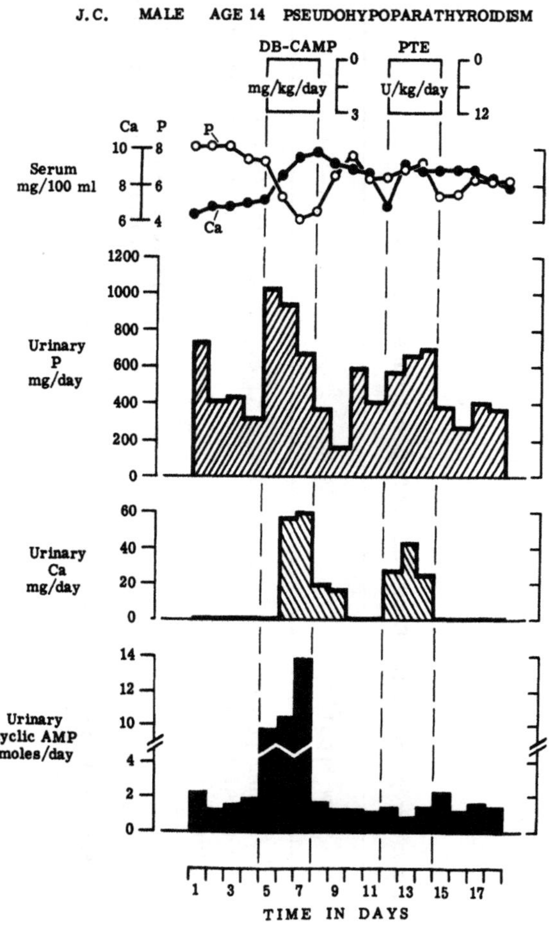

Fig. 1. The reversal of severe hypocalcemia (initial serum calcium concentration of 6 mg/100 ml) after dibutyryl cyclic adenosine mono-phosphate (DB-CAMP) and normalization of serum calcium (Ca) concentration is maintained with acute parathyroid extract (PTE) excretion. The phosphaturia induced by DB-CAMP is associated with decrease in serum phosphorus (P) concentration and the reciprocal elevation in serum calcium concentration.

From Bell, NH, Avery S, Sinoish OT, et al: The effects of dibutyryl cyclic adenosine 3,5-monophosphate and parathyroid extract on calcium and phosphorus metabolism in hypoparathyroidism and pseudohypoparathyroidism. J Clin Invest 51:816-823, 1972. Reprinted by permission.

Calcium chloride should not be used except into large veins during dire emergencies because tissue damage at the site of injection may be particularly severe with this agent. For the same reason, no calcium salts should be given intramuscularly.

Care must be exercised in not mixing bicarbonate solutions with the calcium solutions because of the well-known occurrence of calcium precipitation in an alkaline medium. After neonatal tetany and convulsions are controlled by the above measure, the infant should receive calcium supplementation daily of 500 to 1,000 mg of elemental calcium and regular vitamin D of 10,000 units or 1,25-dihydroxyvitamin-D 20-40 ng/kg/day. The dosage of vitamin-D or its metabolites should be monitored by repeated calcium determinations to maintain serum calcium between 8 to 10 mg/dl and urine calcium/urine creatinine ratio of less than 0.25.

The possible association of hypothyroidism and hypomagnesemia also needs to be evaluated, especially in refractory cases. Correction of these defects facilitates correction of hypocalcemia.

The utilization of low phosphate milk formulae or the use of human milk with lower phosphorus content compared to cow's milk are also important adjunct measures.

Neonatal hypocalcemia may also be associated with acute infection and associated with hypernatremia. Reversal of hypocalcemia occurs secondary to successful treatment of these underlying causes.

Hypoparathyroidism. Tetany a few days following thyroidectomy arises due to severe damage to the parathyroid glands. Mild parathyroid insufficiency from tissue scarring occurring without overt symptoms of hypocalcemia post-thyroidectomy may give rise to cataracts. Parathyroid function tests should be carried out routinely within six months post-thyroidectomy. The specific treatment of tetany is the intravenous infusion of calcium gluconate (Table 4). Oral supplementation of calcium and restriction of dietary phosphate content constitute general measures. If hypocalcemia persists for a few days despite these measures, vitamin D or its metabolites will be needed and should be continued for three to four months; after which, the vitamin-D preparation can be discontinued to test whether the parathyroid function has returned (48). In rare cases, post-operative osteitis fibrosis - the "hungry bone" syndrome - may require the most vigorous pursuit of all the above measures.

Idiopathic hypoparathyroidism and the various types of pseudohypoparathyroidism, presenting with severe hypocalcemia, will require the emergency treatment outlined above. Long-term maintenance doses of calcium, up to 2 to 4 grams daily of elemental calcium, are often administered orally (49). The use of calcium chloride administered orally has been advocated because of its mild acidifying action to augment the ionized calcium content in the extracellular fluids. Severe hypocalcemia is also reversed after dibutyryl cyclic adenosine monophosphate and parathyroid hormone infusion (Fig. 1), but these substances are not available commercially. The use of vitamin D or its active metabolite 1,25 dihydroxyvitamin D is needed to promote intestinal calcium absorption (50, 51) and in the case of pseudohypoparathyroidism for the additional reason of compensating for the defective 1 -hydroxylation of 25-hydroxyvitamin-D (52, 53).

Table 5. Vitamin-D Preparations and Metabolites

Pharmacologic Agent	Trade Name (Pharmaceutical Co.)	Preparation
Vitamin D	Calciferol (Kremers-Urban)	50,000 units (1.25 mg) per tablet (bottle of 100 tablets)
Dihydrotachysterol	Dihydrotachysterol or DHT (Philips-Roxane)	0.125, 0.2, 0.4 mg tablet (bottle of 50 or 100)
	Hytakerol (Winthrop)	0.25 mg/ml in oil (bottle of 15 ml) 0.125 mg/capsule (bottle of 50)
25-hydroxyvitamin D	Calderol (Upjohn)	20 ug/capsule 50 ug/capsule (bottle of 50)
1,25-dihydroxyvitamin D	Rocaltrol (Hoffman-LaRoche)	0.25 ug/capsule 0.50 ug/capsule (bottle of 50)
1-hydroxyvitamin D	One-alpha (Leo)	0.25 ug/capsule 0.50 ug/capsule (bottle of 50)

Table 6. Calcium metabolism before and with treatment by $1,25(OH)_2D_3$ in a child with steroid-resistant minimal-change nephrotic syndrome. From Alon U and Chan JCM: Int. J. Pediatr. Nephr. 4:115–118, 1983.

Period	Total Protein gm/dl	Albumin gm/dl	Total Calcium mg/dl	Ionized Calcium mg/dl	PTH µlEq/l	Urine Calcium mg/kg/24h
Control	3.2	1.1	7.2	4.1	1.6	0.8
Calcitriol 0.5 mcg/day and	3.0	1.1	9.2	6.0	0.8	0.60
Calcitriol 0.25 mcg/day	3.2	1.2	8.5	5.0	0.9	0.21
Normal values	5.0-8.0	3.0-5.0	9.0-10.6	4.4-5.1	0.7-1.3	< 4.0

The use of vitamin D or its metabolites must be closely monitored to detect hypercalcemia which may occur months or even years after stable maintenance doses of the vitamin D therapy (25). Due to the absence of the effect of parathyroid hormone on normal tubular reabsorption of calcium in hypoparathyroid and pseudoparathyroid patients, the hypercalciuric tendency of vitamin D and its metabolites becomes magnified with increasing risks of nephrocalcinosis and nephrolithiasis after prolonged use of vitamin D therapy. Careful monitoring to maintain a urinary calcium to creatinine ratio of less than 0.25 must be part of the follow-up of such vitamin D therapy. A useful criteria to follow is to use enough vitamin D and calcium supplements to maintain serum calcium in the low normal ranges.

Alternatively, it has been advocated that thiazides be used to reduce the rate of urinary calcium excretion (53). However, the benefits must be balanced by the risk of hypercalcemia induced by the diuretic. The use of a low-salt diet to augment tubular reabsorption of calcium and the hypocalciuric effect of thiazide can also be considered.

Magnesium deficiency is a well-known complication of hypoparathyroidism (54). The repletion of this deficiency restores sensitivity to vitamin D.

Magnesium deficiency. In refractory hypocalcemic tetany, concomitant hypomagnesemia must be considered. Symptomatic hypomagnesemia is treated with magnesium replacement: 10% solution of magnesium sulfate over one hour at a dose of 600-1000 mg/sq.m.

Hypovitaminosis D. Hypocalcemia and rickets in nutritional deficiency may develop in severe and prolonged malnutrition. The vitamin D storage of a newborn is depleted by six months if breast-fed infants are not supplemented with vitamin D because of the low vitamin D content in human milk. However, an infant born of a vitamin D deficient mother is without such storage and develops hypocalcemic episodes within a week. Intravenous infusion of 1 ml/kg up to 20 ml per dose of 10% calcium gluconate (Table 4) with the usual precautions (vide supra) meets the initial emergency. This is followed by vitamin D at 600,000 units given as a single dose or in divided doses over 24 to 48 hours (55). Alternatively, vitamin D at 10,000 units/day for three weeks is sufficient. Careful monitoring for hypervitaminosis as discussed before must be followed. Drisdol or other vitamin D preparations in propylene glycol are to be avoided because of the systemic depressant side effects of propylene glycol in neonates.

In vitamin D deficiency due to the intestinal malabsorption of intestinal bypass surgery, biliary and hepatic diseases, or celiac syndrome, the use of large, pharmacologic doses of vitamin D is needed, or the more specific vitamin D metabolites may be preferred. In anticonvulsant-induced hypovitaminosis D, the use of Calcidiol (25-hydroxyvitamin D), 20 to 50 mcg/day, is the treatment of choice. In nephrotic syndrome during relapse, serum vitamin D metabolites are significantly reduced due to urinary loss of these metabolites bound to vitamin D-binding globulin (56). Controversy exists regarding the use of vitamin D metabolites in nephrotic patients. The majority of nephrotic syndrome patients do not need vitamin D supplements because of prompt arrest of proteinuria in response to prednisone therapy. However, in a few rare cases with prolonged and massive proteinuria from steroid-resistance (57), symptomatic hypocalcemia and hypovitaminosis D require the use of 1,25-dihydroxyvitamin D. However, the risk of vitamin D-induced hypercalcemia must be carefully monitored even in the face of normal or low total serum calcium concentration and and low calculated ionized calcium fraction (56), as the actual measurement by selective ion electrode method may reveal hypercalcemia which is not detectable by conventional estimations (Table 6).

In vitamin D-dependent-rickets, the use of 25-hydroxyvitamin D (Table 5) is preferred because the use of 1,25-dihydroxyvitamin D bypasses the feedback regulation mechanism.

Precis of Therapeutic Approach to Hypocalcemia

The emergency treatment of hypocalcemic tetany consists of intravenous administration of 10% calcium gluconate (Table 4) with the usual precautions for differences in body weight. The specific treatment of hypocalcemia is dependent on the underlying cause and may require the administration of vitamin D or its metabolites (Table 5) as well as maintenance of oral calcium supplementation (Table 4). The risks of hypercalcemia and hypercalciuria must be carefully monitored. The recognition of concurrent hypomagnesemia in refractory cases must also be recognized.

Acknowledgements. The authors thank Mrs. Betty W. Timozek and Mrs. Marilyn Reilly for secretarial assistance; Martha D. Wellons, B.A. and Martha D. Massie, B.A., R.D. for research assistance.

References

1. Corvisart, L.: These de Paris: De la contracture des extremites on tetamie chez l'adulte, 1852.

2. Cheadle, W. B.: Pathology and treatment of laryngismus tetany and convulsions, illustrated by cases of these disorders in childhood, and also by a case of the tetany of adult life. Lancet 1:919, 1887.

3. Mundy, G. R. and Martin T. J.: The hypercalcemia of malignancy: pathogenesis and management. Metabolism 31:1247, 1982.

4. Mannix, H.: Primary hyperparathyroidism in children. Am. J. Surg. 129:528, 1975.

5. Bjernulf, A., Hall, K., Sjogren I. et al: Primary hyperparathyroidism in children. Acta. Ped. Scand. 59:249, 1970.

6. Landing, B. H. and Kamoshita, S.: Congenital hyperparathyroidism secondary to maternal hypoparathyroidism. J. Pediatr. 77:842, 1970.

7. Ibbotson, K. J., D'Souza, S. M., Kanis, J. A. et al: Physiological and pharmacological regulation of bone resorption. Metab. Bone Dis. Rel. Res 2:177, 1980.

8. Stewart, A. F., Vignery, A., Silverglate, A., et al.: Quantitative bone histomorphometry in humoral hypercalcemia of malignancy: uncoupling of bone cell activity. J. Clin. Endocr. Metab. 55:219, 1982.

9. Maynard, F. M. and Imai, K.: Immobilization hypercalcemia in spinal cord injury. Arch. Phys. Med. Rehabil. 58:16, 1977.

10. Hung, W., August, G. P., and Glasgow, A. M.: Parathyroids, calcium, and vitamin D. In Pediatric Endocrinology. New York: Medical Examination Publishing Company, 1978, p. 193.

11. Smith, D. W. and Jones, K. L.: Williams Syndrome. In Recognizable Patterns of Human Malformation. Philadelphia, W. B. Saunders, 1982, p. 100.

12. David, D. S., Sakai, S., Brennan, L. et al.: Hypercalcemia after renal transplantation: Long-term follow-up data. New Engl. J. Med. 289:398, 1973.

13. Conceicao, S. C., Wilkinson, R., Feest, T. G. et al.: Hypercalcemia following renal transplantation: causes and consequences. Clin. Nephrol. 16:235, 1981.

14. Elliott, G. T. and McKenzie, M. W.: Treatment of hypercalcemia. Drug Intell. Clin. Pharm. 17:12, 1983.

15. Ragavan, V. V., Smith, J. E. and Bilezikian, J. P.: Vitamin A toxicity and hypercalcemia. Am. J. Med. Sci. 283:161, 1982.

16. Levine, R. A.: Risk of hypercalcemia from prophylaxis of Travelers' Diarrhea. JAMA 249:1151, 1983.

17. Orwoll, E. S.: The milk-alkali syndrome: current concepts. Ann. Int. Med. 97: 242, 1982.

18. Boyce, B. F., Fell, G. S., Elder, H. Y. et al.: Hypercalcemic osteomalacia due to aluminum toxicity. Lancet 2:1009, 1982.

19. Tsang, R. C., Noguchi, A. and Steichen, J. J.: Pediatric parathyroid disorders. Ped. Clin. N. Am. 26:223, 1979.

20. Tsang, R. C., Chen, I., Friedman, M. A. et al.: Neonatal parathyroid function: Role of gestational age and postnatal age. J. Pediatr. 83:728, 1973.

21. Rosenbloom, A. L.: Transient congenital idiopathic hypoparathyroidism. South. Med. J. 66:666, 1973.

22. Hahn, T. J., Halstead, L. R. and Haddad, J. G.: Serum 25-hydroxyvitamin D concentrations in patients receiving chronic corticosteroid treatment. J. Lab. Clin. Med. 90:399, 1977.

23. Boyle, I. T. and Fogelman, I.: Glucocorticoids and estrogens in management of hypercalcemia. Metab. Bone Dis. Rel. Res. 2:203, 1980.

24. Adinoff, A. D. and Hollister, J. R.: Steroid-induced fractures and bone loss in patients with asthma. N. Engl. J. Med. 309:265, 1983.

25. Chan, J. C. M., Young, R. B., Alon, U. et al.: Hypercalcemia in children with disorders of calcium and phosphate during long-term treatment with 1,25-dihydroxyvitamin D3. Pediatr. 72:225, 1983.

26. Long, R. G., Wills, M.R. and Skinner, R. K.: Serum 25-hydroxyvitamin-D in untreated parenchymal and cholestatic liver disease. Lancet 2:650, 1976.

27. Hunter, J., Maxwell, J. D., Stewart, D. A. et al.: Altered calcium metabolism in epileptic children on anticonvulsants. Br. Med. J. 4:202, 1971.

28. Tolman, K. G., Jubiz, W., Sanella, J. J. et al.: Osteomalacia associated with anti-convulsant drug therapy in mentally retarded children. Pediatr. 56:45, 1975

29. Hahn, T. J. and Avioli, L. V.: Anticonvulsant osteomalacia. Arch. Int. Med. 135: 997, 1975.

30. Jubiz, W., Haussen, M. R., McCain, T. A. et al.: Plasma 1,25-dihydroxyvitamin D levels in patients receiving anticonvulsant drugs. J. Clin. Endocr. Metab. 44:617, 1977.

31. Peterson, P., Gray, P. and Tolman, K. G.: Calcium balance in a drug induced osteomalacia: response to vitamin D. Clin. Pharm. Ther. 19:63, 1976.

32. Berger, R. E., Gomez, L. S. and Mallette, L. E.: Acute hypocalcemic effects of clinical contrast media injections. AJR 138:283, 1982.

33. Mallette, L. E. and Gomez, L. S.: Systemic hypocalcemia after clinical injections of radiographic contrast media: amelioration by omission of calcium chelating agents. Radiol. 147:677, 1983.

34. Pierce, W. M., Lineberry, M. D. and Waite, L. C.: Effect of sulfonamides on the hypercalcemic response to vitamin D. Horm. Metab. Res. 14:670, 1982.

35. Sleeboom, H. P. and Bijvoet, O. L. M.: Hypercalcemia due to malignancy: role of the kidney and treatment. Contr. Nephrol. 33:178, 1982.

36. Stewart, A. F.: Therapy of malignancy associated hypercalcemia. Am. J. Med. 74:475, 1983.

37. Hosking, D. J.: Treatment of severe hypercalcemia with calcitonin. Metab. Bone Dis. and Rel. Res. 2:207, 1980.

38. Avioli, L. R.: Calcitonin therapy for bone disease and hypercalcemia. Arch. Int. Med 142:2076, 1982.

39. Mundy, G. R., Wilkinson, R. and Health, D. A.: Comparative study of available medical therapy for hypercalcemia of malignancy. Am. J. Med. 74:421, 1983.

40. Binstock, M. L. and Mundy, G. R.: Effect of calcitonin and glucocorticoids in combination on the hypercalcemia of malignancy. Ann. Int. Med. 93:269, 1980.

41. Wisneski, L. A., Croom, W. P., Silva, O. L. et al.: Salmon calcitonin in hypercalcemia. Clin. Pharm. Ther. 24:219, 1978.

42. Coombes, R. C., Dady, P., Parsons, C. et al.: Mithramycin therapy: an adjunct to conventional treatment of hypercalcemia and bone metastases in breast cancer. Metab. Bone Dis. and Rel. Res. 2:199, 1980.

43. Strumpf, M., Kowalski, M. A. and Mundy, G. R.: Effects of glucocorticoids on osteoclast activating factor. J. Lab. Clin. Med. 92:272, 1978.

44. Heath, D. A.: The use of inorganic phosphate in the management of hypercalcemia. Metab. Bone Dis. and Rel. Res. 2:213, 1980.

45. Martin, T. J. and Partridge, N. C.: Prostaglandins, cancer and bone: pharmacological considerations. Metab. Bone Dis. and Rel. Res. 2:167, 1980.

46. Baker, J. R. and Wray, H. L.: Early management of hypercalcemic crisis: case report and literature review. Milit. Med. 147:756, 1982.

47. Wills, M. R., Bruns, D. E. and Savory, J.: Disorders of calcium homeostasis in the fetus and neonate. Ann. Clin. Lab. Sci 12:79, 1982.

48. Parfitt, A. M.: Surgical, idiopathic and other varieties of parathyroid hormone deficient hypoparathyroidism. In DeGroot LJ, LaHill GF Jr, Odell WD, Martini L, Potts JT Jr, Nelson DH, Steinberger E, Winegred AI (eds): Endocrinology. New York: Grune & Stratton, Inc., 1979.

49. Beale, M. G., Chan, J. C. M., Oldham, S. B. et al: Vitamin D: The discovery of its metabolites and their therapeutic applications. Pediatr. 57:729, 1976.

50. Mazzuoli, G. F., Coen, C. and Antonozzi, I.: Study on calcium metabolism, thyro-calcitonin assay and effect of thyroidectomy in pseudohypoparathyroidism. Int. J. Med. Sci. 3:627, 1967.

51. Drezner, M. K., Neelon, F. A., Haussler, M. et al: 1,25-dihydroxycholecalciferol deficiency: The probable cause of hypocalcemia and metabolic bone disease in pseudohypoparathyroidism. J. Clin. Endocrinol. Metab. 42:621, 1976.

52. Kooh, W. W., Fraser, D., DeLuca, H. F. et al: Treatment of hypoparathyroidism and pseudohypoparathyroidism with metabolites of vitamin D. Evidence for impaired conversion of 25-hydroxyvitamin D to 1,25-dihydroxyvitamin D. N. Engl. J. Med. 293:840, 1973.

53. Alon, U., Wellons, M. D. and Chan, J. C. M.: Reversal of vitamin-D-induced hypercalciuria by chlorothiazide. Pediatr. Res. 17:117, 1983.

54. Suh, S. M., Tashjian, A. H. and Mutuso, N.: Pathogenesis of hypocalcemia in primary hypomagnesemia: Normal end-organ responsiveness to parathyroid hormone, impaired parathyroid gland function. J. Clin. Invest. 52:153, 1973.

55. Harrison, H. E. and Harrison, H. C.: In Disorders of Calcium and Phosphate Metabolism in Childhood and Adolescence. Philadelphia: W. B. Saunders Co., 1979, p. 314.

56. Alon, U. and Chan, J. C. M.: Calcium and Vitamin-D homeostasis in the nephrotic syndrome. Nephron 36:1, 1984.

57. Alon, U. and Chan, J. C. M.: Calcium and vitamin-D metabolism in nephrotic syndrome. Int. J. Pediatr. Nephrol. 4:115, 1983.

RENAL HYPOPHOSPHATEMIC RICKETS

James C. M. Chan, M.D. and Uri Alon, M.D.

Introduction

Renal hypophosphatemic rickets is a renal tubular disorder which has fascinated workers in the field for a long time (1-7). The condition is concurrently known as sex-linked dominant hypophosphatemic rickets, vitamin D resistant rickets and familial hypophosphatemia. Recent advances in phosphate metabolism, pathophysiology, and treatment will be reviewed here.

Tubular reabsorption of phosphate

Fifty percent of filtered phosphate is reabsorbed in the proximal tubule and 40% in the distal tubule. Thus 90% of filtered phosphate is reabsorbed. However, the tubular reabsorption of phosphate is influenced by a large number of factors. Reabsorption is increased in the presence of dietary insufficiency of phosphate, low dietary calcium intake, after parathyroidectomy, and in the presence of contracted extracellular fluids such as after dehydration (8,9). The tubular reabsorption of phosphate is decreased secondary to dietary excess, infusion of parathyroid hormone or cyclic AMP, or in the presence of metabolic acidosis and hypercalcemia or after the use of carbonic anhydrase inhibitors. In view of the fact that tubular reabsorption of phosphate is influenced by all these variables, estimation of the TRP and its interpretation requires adequate knowledge of these influencing factors. Thus, through the work of several investigators, the tubular threshold for phosphate fractionated by glomerular filtration rate (TmP/GFR) has been utilized in place of the tubular reabsorption of phosphate in evaluation of renal phosphate handling (10,11).

Metabolic aspects of renal hypophosphatemic rickets

Glorieux and Scriver (12) have proposed over the last decade that there is a selective disorder of parathyroid hormone, resulting in exaggerated phosphaturic response to parathyroid hormone in patients with renal hypophosphatemic rickets.

Renal hypophosphatemic rickets is characterized by persistent hypophosphatemia secondary to phosphate wasting as suggested by a reduction in the tubular reabsorption of phosphate from 90% to 30% or lower. Renal hypophosphatemic rickets is also characterized by metabolic bone diseases (13,14), which manifests as rickets in a child and osteomalacia in an adult.

Another feature of renal hypophosphatemic rickets is the resistance to even superpharmacological dosages of vitamin D2 (15). There is no associated acidification defect. Thus renal hypophosphatemic rickets can be differentiated from Fanconi syndrome - one of the other phosphate-wasting disorders. Finally, moderate renal glycosuria may occur especially in the younger child.

Clinical features of renal hypophosphatemic rickets

Renal hypophosphatemic rickets is manifested by growth failure, rachitic bone diseases, most particularly coarse trabeculation and thickened cortices of the long bones. As noted earlier, the serum phosphate concentration is below the 5th percentile. It is important to note that the serum phosphate concentration is high in the younger age group (Figure 1).

The serum calcium concentrations are usually normal, but occasionally may be depressed. The serum parathyroid hormone concentrations may be elevated or depressed and, as we shall discuss in greater detail later in this presentation, have important physiologic implications. The alkaline phosphatase concentrations are usually normal, but occasionally may be elevated.

The best characterized form of renal hypophosphatemic rickets is the sex-linked dominant type. Thus, as can be expected from the Lyon hypothesis, males are more severely affected (14,16).

The clinical features of rickets, bone deformities and short stature, as noted earlier, are well recognized. Less familiar to most physicians is the presence of dental abscesses due to the hypophosphatemia (Figure 2).

Other aspects of renal hypophosphatemic rickets include decreased intestinal absorption of calcium and phosphate. The plasma 25-hydroxyvitamin D concentrations are usually normal. Plasma 1,25-dihydroxyvitamin D concentrations may be normal or low (17,18). Several lines of evidence have pointed to inadequacy in 1,25-dihydroxyvitamin D production especially in relation to the hypophosphatemia (19,20).

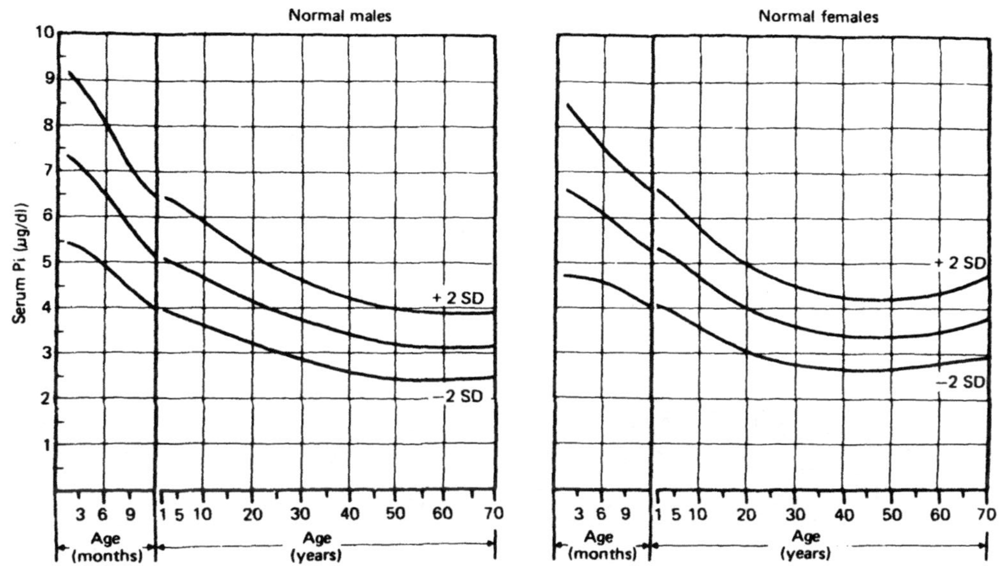

FIG. 1. Ninety-fifth percentile confidence limits of serum phosphate concentrations correlated with age. From Scriver CR, Fraser D, Kooh SW: Hereditary rickets. Chapter 1 in Heath DA and Marx SJ (eds.): Calcium Disorders. Butterworth Scientific, London, 1982. pp. 1-46. By permission.

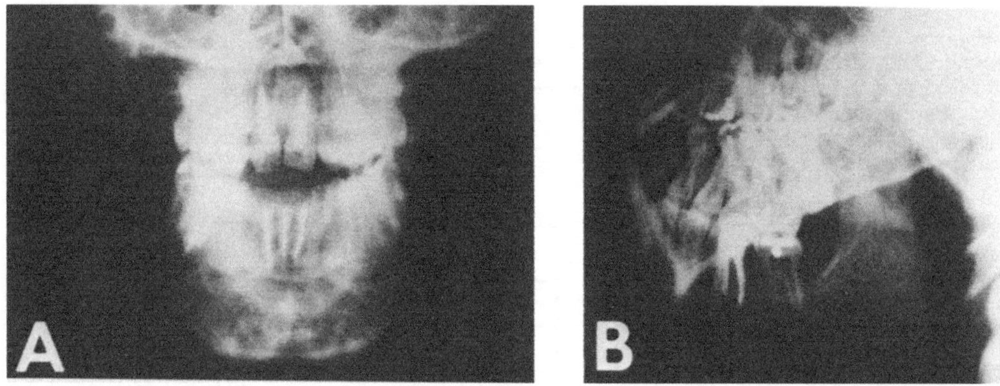

FIG. 2. Radiographs of the maxillofacial region at age 17 years. (A) Poor subperiosteal mineralization, root-canal and other fillings which obtained from spontaneous tooth abscesses over the preceding ten years. (B) Lamina dura is not well seen. Generalized demineralization is present. From Chan JCM, Bartter FC: Hypophosphatemic rickets: Effect of 1α,25-dihydroxyvitamin-D on growth and mineral metabolism. Pediatrics 64:488-495, 1979. By permission.

Pathophysiology and treatment consideration

Administration of 1,25-dihydroxyvitamin D to children with hypophosphatemic rickets has resulted in dramatic growth responses (21-28). Before the availability of 1,25-dihydroxyvitamin D, healing of bone in X-linked hypophosphatemic rickets required large amounts of vitamin D and phosphate (29). The margin between therapeutic benefit and toxicity was quite narrow. In addition, hypophosphatemia may persist even with treatment consisting of 80,000 units of vitamin D2 and 3,000 units of buffered phosphate supplements.

As illustrated by Figure 3, the use of vitamin D2 and phosphate in certain difficult cases did not reverse the rachitic changes, until 1,25-dihydroxyvitamin D was used in place of conventional vitamin D2 therapy. It has also been found that fairly large doses of 1,25-dihydroxyvitamin D need to be utilized (23), giving rise to the question of whether there is a 1-hydroxylase defect in these patients.

Data from Drezner and associates (30) as well as Chesney and associates (17) showed that in untreated patients with hypophosphatemic rickets, the serum 1,25-dihydroxyvitamin D concentration is indeed depressed compared to that of normal controls. Recent data by Tenenhouse (20) further demonstrated that in hypophosphatemic mice, the set point for 1-hydroxylase activity is lowered compared to that of normal control mice. These lines of evidence would, therefore, point to a defective renal 1-hydroxylase in this disorder.

Summarizing these recent lines of evidence, the following pathophysiology of this disorder can be considered. The X-linked dominant defects give rise to increased renal tubular threshold for phosphate, which is modulated by parathyroid hormone and perhaps other, as yet unidentified, humoral factors. This gives rise to hypophosphatemia. In addition, defective renal 1-hydroxylase activity results in inadequate serum 1,25-dihydroxyvitamin D production relative to the hypophosphatemia. It is likely that there is partial end-organ resistance to 1,25-dihydroxyvitamin D as well as parathyroid hormone. The net effect of these disorders is the decrease in intestinal absorption of calcium and phosphate, further aggravating the hypophosphatemia. All these defects then give rise to the clinical features of rickets, bone deformities, short stature, dental abscesses and osteomalacia.

Recent advances in treatment of renal hypophosphatemic rickets

Hirschman, DeLuca and Chan (21) in 1978 documented the beneficial effects of 1,25-dihydroxyvitamin D in the child with hypophosphatemic rickets. It was found later that large doses of 1,25-dihydroxyvitamin D are needed occasionally to attain normalization of serum phosphorus and healing of rickets (23,26). The recent data of Drezner and associates (30) as well as Chesney and associates (17,26) and Tenenhouse (20), referred to above, provide the rationale for the requirement of larger doses of 1,25-dihydroxyvitamin D, because their data suggest a defect in the 1-hydroxylase system.

FIG. 3. X-ray of the wrist in a patient with X-linked dominant hypophosphatemic rickets. Upper panel: at age 14 years, after seven years of treatment with vitamin D2 at 40,000 to 60,000 units per day, plus phosphate supplementation of 2,000 to 4,000 mg per day, severe rickets persisted. Middle panel: 6 months of 1,25-dihydroxyvitamin D at 20-80 ng/kg per day in place of vitamin-D2 and continued phosphate supplement, dramatic reconstitution of provisory zone of calcification, narrowing of epiphyseal plate and disappearance of the irregular metaphysis. Lower panel: continued improvement at 12 months. From Chan JCM, Lovinger RD, Mamunes P: Renal hypophosphatemic rickets: growth acceleration after long-term treatment with 1,25-dihydroxyvitamin-D3. Pediatrics 66:445-454, 1980. By permission.

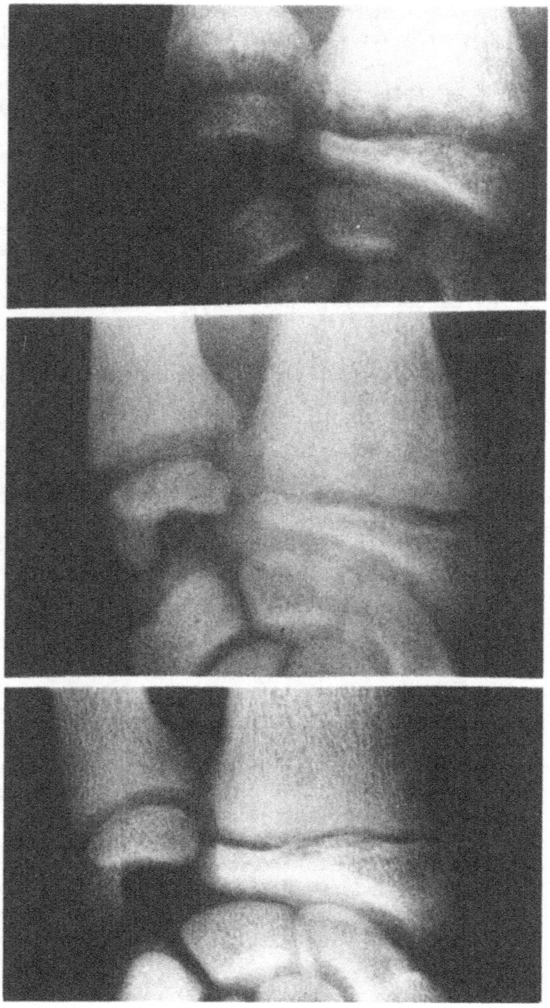

FIG. 4. The height velocity of children with X-linked dominant hypophosphatemic rickets. Arrows indicate initiation of treatment of 1,25-dihydroxyvitamin D. Interrupted line indicates periods without 1,25-dihydroxyvitamin D, but with vitamin D2. Phosphate supplementation is maintained throughout the study. Markedly accelerated growth velocity is demonstrated. From Chan JCM, Lovinger RD, Mamunes P: Renal hypophosphatemic rickets: growth acceleration after long-term treatment with 1,25-dihydroxyvitamin-D3. Pediatrics 66:445-454, 1980. By permission.

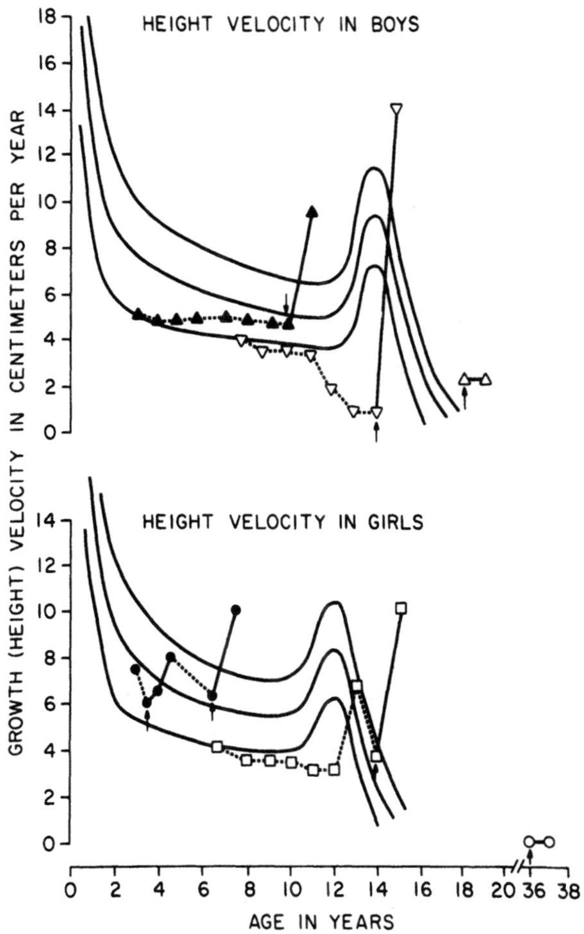

Data by Kristiansen et al (27) and Rasmussen et al (24) have also demonstrated the beneficial effects of 1-alpha-hydroxyvitamin D, an analog of 1,25-dihydroxyvitamin D.

Administration of 1,25-dihydroxyvitamin D to children with X-linked hypophosphatemic rickets has resulted in dramatic growth responses (Figure 4), but the higher doses of 1,25-dihydroxyvitamin D often required to maintain normalization of serum phosphate are complicated by the occurrence of hypercalciuria.

Reversal of hypercalciuria with hydrochlorothiazide and amiloride

In order to reverse the hypercalciuria and the risk of hypercalcemia induced by the introduction of high doses of 1,25-dihydroxyvitamin D, a three-year study on five patients with renal hypophosphatemic rickets was conducted to evaluate the effect of thiazide to reverse hypercalciuria (31). Their usual dose of 1,25-dihydroxyvitamin D (0.5 to 1 mcg/day) as well as Neutra-Phos (1 to 3 gm/day) was continued. In addition, hydrochlorothiazide, at a dosage of 1.5 to 2.2 mg/kg/day, in conjunction with amiloride, at a dosage of 1 mg to every 5 mg of hydrochlorothiazide, was introduced.

The serum phosphate concentration demonstrated (31) mean values of 3.1 mg/dl before this combined therapy and improved to 3.7 mg/dl after therapy ($P < 0.01$). In addition, the TmP/GFR was 1.31 mg/dl before and improved to 1.74 mg/dl after the combined therapy ($P < 0.01$).

In addition, when comparing hydrochlorothiazide alone to hydrochlorothiazide plus amiloride in these 1,25-dihydroxyvitamin D and phosphate treated patients, it was shown that the drop in potassium concentration was as much as 1 mEq/L with the hydrochlorothiazide alone and showed a mean change of only 0.1 mEq/L with the hydrochlorothiazide and amiloride treated group ($P < 0.02$). Metabolic alkalosis, secondary to the hypokalemia, which was prevalent in the hydrochlorothiazide treated group did not appear in the hydrochlorothiazide and amiloride treated group (32).

Follow-up study of 38 months showed that the mean alkaline phosphatase level which was previously 447 IU/1 improved by returning to mean values of 287 IU/1. In addition, the growth velocity which previously was 5.5 ± 1.6 cm/yr before therapy increased to 7.7 ± 3.4 cm/yr after therapy. By examining the height for age, we were able to demonstrate that, whereas, before therapy this variable showed mean values of -2.2 standard deviations below the mean, after treatment this had improved to -1.8 standard deviations below the mean.

Therefore, we conclude that diuretic-induced extracellular fluid contraction results in an increase in TmP/GFR, plasma phosphate and linear growth as well as continued healing of rickets, especially in the more difficult cases of renal hypophosphatemia. The combined use of hydrochlorothiazide and amiloride eliminates the complication of hypokalemic metabolic alkalosis and would appear to be a useful therapeutic adjunct to the 1,25-dihydroxyvitamin D and Neutra-Phos regimen. This is especially so in the more difficult cases in which high doses of 1,25-dihydroxyvitamin D are required to maintain normophosphatemia and continued healing of rickets.

Summary

We hope that this interpretative review of recent advances has provided a background on the diagnosis and treatment of this phosphate disorder.

Acknowledgements Mrs. Marilyn Reilly provided secretarial assistance; Ms. Martha D. Wellons, B.A., and Mrs. Martha D. Massie, B.A., R.D., provided research assistance. Supported in part by N.I.H. grant AM HD 31370.

References

1. McEnery PT, Silverman FN, West CD: Acceleration of growth with combined vitamin D-phosphate therapy of hypophosphatemic resistant rickets. J Pediatr 80:763, 1972.

2. Stickler GB, Jowsey J, Bianco AJ: Possible detrimental effects of large doses of vitamin D in familial hypophosphatemic vitamin D-resistant rickets. J Pediatr 79:68, 1971.

3. Field MH, Reiss E: Vitamin D-resistant rickets: The effect of calcium infusion on phosphate reabsorption. J Clin Invest 39:1807, 1960.

4. Falls WF Jr, Carter NW, Rector FC Jr, et al: Familial vitamin-D-resistant rickets: Study of six cases with evaluation of the pathogenic role of secondary hypoparathyroidism. Ann Int Med 68:553, 1968.

5. Fraser D, Leeming JM, Cerwenka EA, Kenyeres K: Studies of the pathogenesis of the high renal clearance of phosphate in hypophosphatemic vitamin D-refractory rickets of the simple type. Am J Dis Child 98:586, 1959.

6. Blackard WG, Robinson RR, White JE: Familial hypophosphatemic report of a case with observations regarding pathogenesis. N Engl J Med 266:899, 1962.

7. Arnstein AR, Hanson CA: Nature of renal phosphate leak. N Engl J Med 281:1427, 1969.

8. Harrison HE, Harrison HC: Disorders of calcium and phosphate metabolism in childhood and adolescence. Philadelphia, 1979, W. B. Saunders.

9. Scriver CR: Rickets and the pathogenesis of impaired tubular transport of phosphate and other solutes. Am J Med 57:43, 1974.

10. Alon U, Chan JCM: Effects of PTH and $1,25(OH)_2D_3$ on tubular handling of phosphate in hypophosphatemic rickets. J Clin Endocrinol Metabol 58:681, 1984.

11. Kruse K, Kracht U, Gopfert G: Renal threshold phosphate concentration ($TmPO_4$/GFR). Arch Dis child 57:217, 1982.

12. Glorieux FH, Scriver CR: Transport, metabolism and clinical use of inorganic phosphate in X-linked hypophosphatemia. In Frame B, Parfitt AM, Duncan H, editors: The clinical aspects of metabolic bone disease. Amsterdam, 1973, Excerpta Medica ICS, p 421.

13. Rasmussen H, Anast C: Familial hypophosphatemic rickets and vitamin-D dependent rickets. In Stanbury JB, Wyngaarden JB, Frederickson DS, et al, editors: The metabolic basis of inherited disease, ed. 5, New York, 1983, McGraw-Hill, p 1743.

14. Winters RW, Graham JB, Williams TF, McFalls VW, Burnett CH: A genetic study of familial hypophosphatemic and vitamin D-resistant rickets with a review of the literature. Medicine 37:97, 1958.

15. Balsam S, Garabedian M, Gorgniard R, Holick MF, DeLuca HF: 1,25-dihydroxyvitamin-D_3 and 1 alpha-hydroxyvitamin-D_3 in children: biologic and therapeutic effects in nutritional rickets and different types of vitamin D resistance. Pediatr Res 9:586, 1975.

16. Burnett CH, Dent CE, Harper C, Warland BJ: Vitamin D-resistant rickets: Analysis of 24 pedigrees with hereditary and sporadic cases. Am J Med 36:222, 1964.

17. Chesney RW, Mazess RB, Rose P, et al: Supranormal 25-hydroxyvitamin D and subnormal 1,25-dihydroxyvitamin D. Am J Dis Child 134:140, 1980.

18. Mason RS, Rohl PG, Lissner D, Posen S: Vitamin D metabolism in hypophosphatemic rickets. Am J Dis Child 136:909, 1982.

19. Lyles KW, Clark AG, Drezner MK: Serum 1,25-dihydroxyvitamin D levels in subjects with X-linked hypophosphatemic rickets and osteomalacia. Calcif Tissue Int 34:125, 1982.

20. Tenenhouse HS: Abnormal mitochondrial 25-hydroxyvitamin D_3-1-hydroxylase activity in the vitamin D and calcium deficient X-linked Hyp mouse. Endocrinology 113:816, 1983.

21. Hirschman GH, DeLuca HF, Chan JCM: Hypophosphatemic vitamin D-resistant rickets: Metabolic balance studies in a child receiving 1,25-dihydroxyvitamin-D_3, phosphate and ascorbic acid. Pediatrics 61:451, 1978.

22. Chan JCM, Bartter FC: Hypophosphatemic rickets: Effect of 1α, 25-dihydroxyvitamin-D_3 on growth and mineral metabolism. Pediatrics 64:488, 1979.

23. Chan JCM, Lovinger RD, Mamunes P: Renal hypophosphatemic rickets: Growth acceleration after long-term treatment with 1,25-dihydroxyvitamin-D_3. Pediatrics 66:445, 1980.

24. Rasmussen H, Pechet M, Anast C, Mazur A, Gertner J, Broadus AE: Long-term treatment of familial hypophosphatemic rickets with oral phosphate and 1α-hydroxyvitamin-D_3. J Pediatr 99:16, 1981.

25. Glorieux FH, Marie PJ, Pettifor JM, Delvin EE: Bone response to phosphate salts, ergocalciferol, and calcitriol in hypophosphatemic vitamin D-resistant rickets. N Engl J Med 303:1023, 1980.

26. Chesney RW, Mazess RB, DeLuca HF: Long-term influences of calcitriol and supplemental phosphate in X-linked hypophosphatemic rickets. Calcif Tissue Int 33:307, 1981.

27. Kristiansen JH, Pedersen VF: Hypophosphatemic vitamin D-resistant rickets treated with 1α-hydroxyvitamin-D . Int J Ped Nephr 2:245, 1981.

28. Russell RGG, Smith R, Preston C, Walton RJ, Woods CG, Henderson RG, Norman AW: The effect of 1,25-dihydroxycholecalciferol on renal tubular reabsorption of phosphate, intestinal absorption of calcium and bone histology in hypophosphatemic renal tubular rickets. Clin Sci Mol Med 48:177, 1975.

29. West CD, Blanton JC, Silverman FN, et al: Use of phosphate salts as an adjunct to vitamin D in the treatment of hypophosphatemic vitamin D-refractory rickets. J Pediatr 64:469, 1964.

30. Drezner MK, Lyles KW, Haussler MR, Harrelson JM: Evaluation of a role for 1,25-dihydroxyvitamin-D in the pathogenesis and treatment of X-linked hypophosphatemic rickets and osteomalacia. J Clin Invest 66:1020, 1980.

31. Alon U, Chan JCM; Thiazides as adjuvant therapy in X-linked dominant renal hypophosphatemic rickets. 67th annual meeting of the Feder Am Soc Exp Biol (Chicago, April 1983).

32. Alon U, Costanzo LS, Chan JCM: Additive hypocalciuric effects of amiloride and hydrochlorothiazide in patients treated with calcitriol. Min Electrolyte Metabl 10:379, 1984.

CONTINUOUS PERITONEAL DIALYSIS IN INFANCY WITH PARTICULAR EMPHASIS ON THE NEONATAL PERIOD

Michael Freundlich, M.D., Carolyn Abitbol, M.D., Gaston Zilleruelo, M.D., and Jose Strauss, M.D.

Advanced renal failure in infancy represents a difficult therapeutic dilemma, particularly when it rapidly advances to end-stage renal disease (ESRD) during the neonatal period (1-3). Once ESRD is reached (creatinine clearance of around 5 ml/min/1.73m^2), most patients require the institution of some kind of renal replacement therapy. The latter can be offered through either hemodialysis or peritoneal dialysis. Hemodialysis requires the passage of a given extracorporeal blood volume through a filter (dialyzer), and is usually performed during three weekly sessions of two to four hours duration each. Although extensively used in children, adolescents, and adults, its implementation in small infants has been limited (4). This is mainly due to the infant's small vessel size and circulating volume. Thus, the surgical creation of an adequate vascular access, and the presence of a large extracorporeal blood volume during dialysis, turn hemodialyis into a rather cumbersome proposition. In addition, infants are particularly susceptible to rapid transcellular volume and solute shifts (disequilibrium) (4), and the life of vascular accesses is relatively shortened as compared to larger patients. Therefore, very few infants have been maintained on hemodialysis for prolonged periods of time.

Continuous Ambulatory Peritoneal Dialysis (CAPD) was first described as a dialytic modality in 1976 (5) and its widespread use began in 1978 with the introduction of dialysis plastic bags (6). From the technical point of view, CAPD is simple, requiring a permanent intraperitoneal catheter connected to a bag containing dialysis fluid that is changed three to five times per day. The ultimate goals of peritoneal dialysis are the removal of water and solutes across the peritoneal membrane and the achievement of a stable clinical and chemical profile. These can be accomplished successfully by the addition of hypertonic glucose to the dialysate, creating an osmotic gradient favoring the withdrawal of water from the extracellular fluid. Solute transport across the membrane from patient to dialysate occurs primarily by passive diffusion. Large molecular weight substances (500-5,000 daltons, middle molecules) have been incriminated as important toxins causing uremia (7). By operating continuously (24 hours per day, 7 days a week), CAPD achieves clearances of those solutes as much as six times more efficiently than that of 12 hours of hemodialysis (8). Because of its inherent advantages (Table I), CAPD appeared as a promising therapeutic modality in a suitable pediatric population. This led to its application in an increasing number of pediatric patients with ESRD (9-13). However, few infants, particularly in the first six months of life, have been treated with CAPD (11,14).

TABLE 1

CONTINUOUS PERITONEAL DIALYSIS
MAIN ADVANTAGES IN PEDIATRICS

MEDICAL

Technically easy
Avoids blood products and blood losses
Avoids vascular access
Avoids extracorporeal blood volume
Avoids disequilibrium
Excellent control of hypertension
Improves nutrition
Improves mineral metabolism
Improves growth

PSYCHO-SOCIAL

Procedure performed at home
Promotes family unity
Promotes independence (adolescents)
Minimal interference with daily activities
Better school attendance

In the pediatric population in general and in infants in particular, growth can be easily and adversely affected. Several aspects pertaining to an adequate nutritional intake and utilization, metabolic and endocrine disturbances, mineral metabolism and renal osteodystrophy (ROD), are of special relevance and require careful scrutiny in order to fully assess the potential benefits of any dialytic therapy. We have been particularly interested in assessing the impact of CAPD on mineral metabolism (13). Thus, much of the following discussion will be centered around these aspects.

Included in the patients we have studied in detail (15, 16), is a neonate whose clinical course is summarized as follows: A full-term girl was born to a healthy mother. The birth weight was 3,300g and the immediate neonatal course was unremarkable. Blood pressure was 83/63 mm Hg, and the abdominal examination elicited large bilateral masses. Radiologic evaluation revealed a left multicystic and a right hydronephrotic obstructed kidney. The renal scan demonstrated poor function bilaterally. On the second day of life, BUN was 20 mg/dl and serum creatinine 2.1 mg/dl. Because of continuous clinical and biochemical deterioration (creatinine 6.5 mg/dl, calcium 7.8 mg/dl, phosphorus 7.4 mg/dl, CO_2 18 mEq/L), and after extensive discussions with the family, peritoneal dialysis was initiated on the 11th day of life. The biochemical abnormalities were rapidly corrected and after two months of dialysis those were as following: BUN 40 mg/dl, creatinine 4.3 mg/dl, calcium 9.4 mg/dl, phosphorus 3.8 mg/dl, potassium 5.6 mEq/L, and CO_2 17-19 mEq/L. The serum immunoreactive parathyroid hormone (PTH) level was 150 μlEq/ml (normal less than 90). Nutrition consisted of Similac PM 60/40 formula with addition of MCT oil according to tolerance.

Peritoneal dialysis was attained through a single-cuff Tenckhoff catheter. Eight daily, three hour cycles of 100 ml each of the 4.25 g/dl dextrose dialysate were instilled. Peritoneal mass transfer (MT) and flux studies of different substances were performed and calculated by the following formula: MT=(dialysate concentration instilled x dialysate volume instilled)-(dialysate effluent concentration x dialysate effluent volume). A positive net MT represented the amount accrued within the patient and the negative MT the amount removed. These calculations revealed substantial daily phosphorus, protein and sodium losses into the dialysate, as well as variable calcium MT (Table II).

TABLE II

DAILY PERITONEAL LOSSES IN AN INFANT ON CAPD

Calcium (N=11) (mg)	Phosphorus (N=11) (mg)	Sodium (N=10) (mEq)	Protein (N=10) (g)
12±8.0	59±6.0	34±8.0	0.6±0.1

N = number of mass-transfer studies.

Several aspects in the management of this infant are worth emphasizing: because of the small amount of desired instilled dialysate volume, and since such small volume bags are commercially unavailable, the implementation of a Y system was required. This allowed one single daily change of the 1,000 ml dialysate bag.

Peritoneal losses of sodium were substantial and averaged 34 mEq/day; this necessitated the replacement of those losses with supplemental sodium chloride. In order to achieve adequate daily ultrafiltration, the high dextrose containing dialysate (4.25 g/dl) was required. This has been noted by others and seems to be due to the fast rate of dialysate glucose absorption across the peritoneal membrane of the neonate and infant (17). Previous studies in adults (18) and our data in children (13, 15, 16) have revealed efficient daily peritoneal phosphorus removal; most certainly, this contributed to the maintenance of a normal serum phosphorus without the utilization of phosphate binders. Although some have reported phosphate levels just above normal in CAPD patients without the use of aluminum containing binders and on a relatively free phosphate diet (19), most series, particularly in children, have included phosphate binders (9, 20-21). The amount of phosphorus removed per exchange is higher in those exchanges utilizing higher dextrose concentration.

The potential impact of calcium and hormonal losses into the peritoneal dialysate on bone structure of the growing infant remains unknown at the present time. We have reported losses of Vitamin D metabolites and PTH into the dialysate in older children (13); however, similar data in infants are not available. It seems reasonable, though, to assume that in patients on CAPD, the administration of some form of Vitamin D is needed, and should be adjusted according to peritoneal losses. On the other hand, the maintenance of a rather stable serum concentration of immunoreactive PTH noted in our patient, may have been, in part, due to its losses into the peritoneal effluents (16, 20).

Although troubled by medical and ethical considerations, our preliminary results and those of others (10, 11,14), suggest that continuous peritoneal dialysis represents a viable therapeutic modality for infants with end-stage renal disease.

REFERENCES

1) Alexander SR: Chronic peritoneal dialysis in infants less than one year of age. In Fine RN and Gruskin AB (eds): End-Stage Renal Disease in Children. Philadelphia: WB Saunders Co., In Press.

2) Hurley JK: Kidney transplantation in infants (Letter). J Pediatr 93:538, 1978.

3) Dialysis and transplantation in young children (Editorial). Brit Med J 2:1033, 1979.

4) Mauer SM, Lynch RE: Hemodialysis techniques for infants and children. Pediatr Clin North Am 23: 843-856, 1976.

5) Popovich RP, Moncrief JW, Dechard JB et al: The definition of a novel portable/wearable equilibrium peritoneal dialysis technique. Am Soc Artif Inter Organs 5:64, 1976 (abstr).

6) Oreopoulos DG, Robson M, Izatt, S et al: A simple and safe technique for continuous ambulatory peritoneal dialysis (CAPD). Trans Am Soc Artif Intern Organs 24:484-487, 1978.

7) Babb A, Popovich RP, Christopher TG et al: The genesis of the square meter-hour hypothesis. Trans Am Soc Artif Intern Organs 117:81-91, 1971.

8) Nolph KD, Popovich RP, Moncrief JW: Theoretical and practical implications of continuous ambulatory peritoneal dialysis. Nephron 21:117-120, 1978.

9) Balfe JW, Vigneux A, Willumssen J et al: The use of CAPD in the treatment of children with end-stage renal disease. Perit Dial Bull 1:35-38, 1981.

10) Alexander SR, Tseng CH, Maksym KA et al: Clinical parameters in continuous ambulatory peritoneal dialysis for infants and children. In Moncrief JW, Popovich RP (eds): CAPD Update. New York: Masson, 1981, pp 195-207.

11) Kohaut E, in this volume.

12) Salusky JB, Lucullo L, Nelson P, Fine RN: Continuous ambulatory peritoneal dialysis in children. Pediatr Clin N Am 29: 1005-1012, 1982.

13) Freundlich M, Zilleruelo G, Strauss, J: Mineral metabolism in children and adults receiving continuous ambulatory peritoneal dialysis. Semin Nephrol 3:159-165, 1983.

14) Alexander, SR, Lubischer JT: Continuous ambulatory peritoneal dialysis in pediatrics: three years' experience at one center. Nefrologia (Madrid) 11 (Supp 2): 53-62, 1982.

15) Freundlich, M, Zilleruelo G, Abitbol C et al: Peritoneal mass transfer of minerals and bone-modulating hormones in children on continuous ambulatory peritoneal dialysis., Pediatr Res 18:361 A 1984 (abstr).

16) Freundlich M, Zilleruelo G, Abitbol C et al: Minerals and bone modulating hormones in children on continuous ambulatory peritoneal dialysis. Nephron (In Press).

17) Kohaut EC, Alexander SR: Ultrafiltration in the young patient on CAPD. In Moncrief JW, Popovich RP (eds): CAPD Update. New York: Masson, 1981, pp 221-226.

18) Blumenkrantz JK, Kopple JD, Moran JK et al: Metabolic balance studies and dietary protein requirements in patients undergoing continuous ambulatory peritoneal dialysis. Kidney Int 21:849-861, 1982.

19) Gokal R, Ellis HA, Ramos JM et al: Improvement in secondary hyperparathyroidism in patients on continous ambulatory peritoneal dialysis. In Gahl GM, Kessel M, Nolph KD (eds): Advances in Peritoneal Dialysis: Proceedings of the Second International Symposium on Peritoneal Dialysis, Berlin (-West), June 16-19, 1981. Amsterdam, Excerpta Medica, 1981, pp 461-466 (International Congress Series no 567)

20) Delmez JA, Slatopolsky E, Martin K et al: Minerals, vitamin D, and parathyroid hormone in continuous ambulatory peritoneal dialysis. Kidney Int 21:862-867, 1982.

21) Calderaro V, Oreopoulus DG, Meema EH, et al: Renal osteodystrophy in patients on continuous ambulatory peritoneal dialysis: A biochemical and radiological study. In Moncrief JW, Popovich RP (eds) CAPD Update, New York: Masson, 1981, pp 243-247.

22) Baum M. Powell D, Calvin S et al: Continuous ambulatory peritoneal dialysis in children. Comparison with hemodialysis. N Engl J Med 307:1537-1542, 1982.

INSUFFICIENCY AND RESISTANCE TO PARATHYROID HORMONE

Uri Alon, M.D. and James C. M. Chan, M.D.

Introduction

Although the parathyroid glands were discovered in dogs and the rhinocerous earlier on, it remained for the great German pathologist, Rudolph Ludwig Virchow, to describe them in man in the mid-19th century and for the Swedish anatomist, Ivor Victor Sandstrom, to document four parathyroid glands in most men and women. However, controversy persisted for awhile as to whether the parathyroid glands were distinct entities or part of the thyroid gland. By the turn of the century, it was clearly delineated that the parathyroid glands have distinct functions with biological actions at both bone cells and renal tubular cells (1-5).

Parathyroid hormone

The circulating form of parathyroid hormone consists of a single-chain polypeptide with 84 amino acids weighing 9,500 daltons (6-8). The parathyroid hormone initially appeared as pre-pro-parathyroid hormone, a 115 amino acid-chain synthesized in the ribosomes of the parathyroid chief cells (9-11). Subsequently, at the rough endoplasmic reticulum, a 25 amino acid-chain is cleaved from the amino terminal to form pro-parathyroid hormone. However, the pro-parathyroid hormone is still not quite active because the amino terminal is blocked by the addition of a 6 amino acid-chain. The next step occurs in the Golgi apparatus where the pro-parathyroid hormone is proteolyzed into parathyroid hormone which is stored in the secretory granules (12-14).

Regulation of PTH secretion

The principal cellular regulator of the parathyroid hormone secretion is the intracellular concentration of cyclic AMP (15). Ionized calcium has a profound effect on the concentration of cyclic AMP. Even as small a decrease as 0.1 mg/dl of ionized calcium results in stimulation of cyclic AMP and PTH secretion. As is generally known, hypercalcemia inhibits parathyroid hormome secretion (16). On the other hand, hypocalcemia stimulates parathyroid hormone secretion (17). Similarly, the magnesium ion exerts an effect on parathyroid hormone secretion, with hypomagnesemia stimulating and hypermagnesemia inhibiting PTH secretion. However, the effect of magnesium is not as strong as that of calcium, although the two ions have a synergistic action on parathyroid hormone secretion (18). Recent evidence has pointed to binding sites at the parathyroid glands for 1,25-dihydroxyvitamin D. In addition, in the last few years, data have been accummulating to support the contention that 1,25-dihydroxyvitamin D can directly inhibit parathyroid hormone secretion. Finally, serum phosphate concentration exerts an indirect effect on parathyroid hormone secretion via its reciprocal action on the serum calcium concentrations (19).

Circulating parathyroid hormone

About 10% of circulating parathyroid hormone is the I-84 polypeptide chain. The biological half-life of the intact parathyroid hormone is a few minutes (20). Similarly, the other active component of circulating parathyroid hormone is the amino terminal fragment which constitutes about 10% of the total circulating PTH. The biological half-life is also in terms of minutes. The third fraction of circulating parathyroid hormone is the inactive carboxyl terminal fragment (21). This constitutes 80% of circulating PTH and has a biological half-life of hours in normal subjects and up to several days in patients with chronic renal insufficiency.

Biphasic action on bone

The early action of parathyroid hormone on bone is to stimulate osteocytes and osteoclasts, resulting in osteolysis and bone resorption (22). In addition, in the early phase, parathyroid hormone stimulates the conversion of phagocytes to osteoclasts. Furthermore, it has been suggested that parathyroid hormone prolongs the life of osteoclasts. Finally, in the early phase, parathyroid hormone inhibits osteoclasts and bone collagen.

However, in the second phase of action of parathyroid hormone on bone, osteoblasts are stimulated and new collagen synthesis and mineralization are enhanced. These actions together constitute the remodeling process of bone (23).

Metabolic fate of parathyroid hormone

The I-84 parathyroid hormone, (24-26) is likely to be metabolized in the liver into C terminal fragments as well as possibly N terminal fragments. The C terminal fragment is secreted by the parathyroid gland. The N terminal fragment is likely to be secreted also by the parathyroid gland. In addition, the renal tubules may play a role in the conversion of I-84 parathyroid hormone to the C terminal fragment.

About 60% of I-84 parathyroid hormone is catabolized in the liver and 30% either filtered and excreted through the glomeruli or secreted by the renal tubules (27-30). The renal tubules are likely responsible for the elimination of C as well as N terminal fragments of parathyroid hormone. The bone may contribute a small part in the consumption of the N terminal fragments.

Interrelationship between parathyroid hormone and chronic renal insufficiency

The physiological action of parathyroid hormone in promoting intestinal absorption of phosphate is counter-balanced by the normal physiological action of parathyroid hormone in promoting phosphate excretion through the renal tubules. Thus, phosphate homeostasis is maintained and the calcium plus phosphate product remains within the normal range. However, in the face of chronic renal insufficiency, the renal tubule is no longer responsive to the phosphaturic actions of parathyroid hormone and thus with increasing intestinal absorption of phosphate, hyperphosphatemia occurs resulting in elevation in the calcium plus phosphate product to variables in excess of 70, and consequently increasing the risk of metastatic calcification (31-33).

Tubular effects of parathyroid hormone

As alluded to earlier, parathyroid hormone decreases tubular absorption of phosphate. It has a secondary action on reducing the tubular reabsorption of bicarbonate and it has been suggested at one time, that this effect of parathyroid hormone may contribute to the development of metabolic acidosis in chronic renal insufficiency (34-36). However, current evidence would tend to downgrade the importance of secondary hyperparathyroidism on the development and perpetuation of metabolic acidosis in chronic renal insufficiency. In addition, parathyroid hormone has an effect on reducing amino acid reabsorption and aminoaciduria may be encountered in cases of elevated circulating parathyroid hormone. Finally, parathyroid hormone has an important action in stimulating the conversion of 25-hydroxyvitamin D to 1,25-dihydroxyvitamin D. This has important clinical implications which will be brought up later on in this presentation concerning pseudohypoparathyroidism (34-36).

Cellular action of parathyroid hormone

The urinary concentration of cyclic AMP is elevated even before the phosphaturic action of parathyroid hormone can be demonstrated. Parathyroid hormone exerts its effect on bone and kidney cells through the activation of adenylate cyclase and increasing cytosolic secondary messenger concentration (37-39).

Parathyroid hormone has an important action on the entry of calcium into the cells as stated earlier in promoting the conversion of 25-hydroxyvitamin D to 1,25-dihydroxyvitamin D. Because calcium entry into the cells as well as extracellular calcium concentration are affected by 1,25-dihydroxyvitamin D, it would seem that the effect of parathyroid hormone on the end-organ must result from the interactions between the hormone itself, 1,25-dihydroxyvitamin D and calcium in circulation (40-42).

Evaluation of parathyroid hormone function

Serum concentrations of parathyroid hormone, calcium, phosphate, alkaline phosphatase are all important variables in evaluating the functions of parathyroid hormone. In addition, the estimation of tubular reabsorption of phosphate (TRP) may provide some insight into parathyroid hormone function. Although as stated previously, TRP can be interpreted between individuals if the variables such as dietary intake and the status of extracellular fluid compartments are examined under controlled conditions (43). In an attempt to overcome the influence of these variables, Bijvoet and associates (44) have perfected a nomogram which they established initially with phosphate infusions to establish the tubular threshold for phosphate (TmP). Because glomerular filtration rate (GFR) is another variable which needs to be controlled in the interpretation of tubular threshold, they

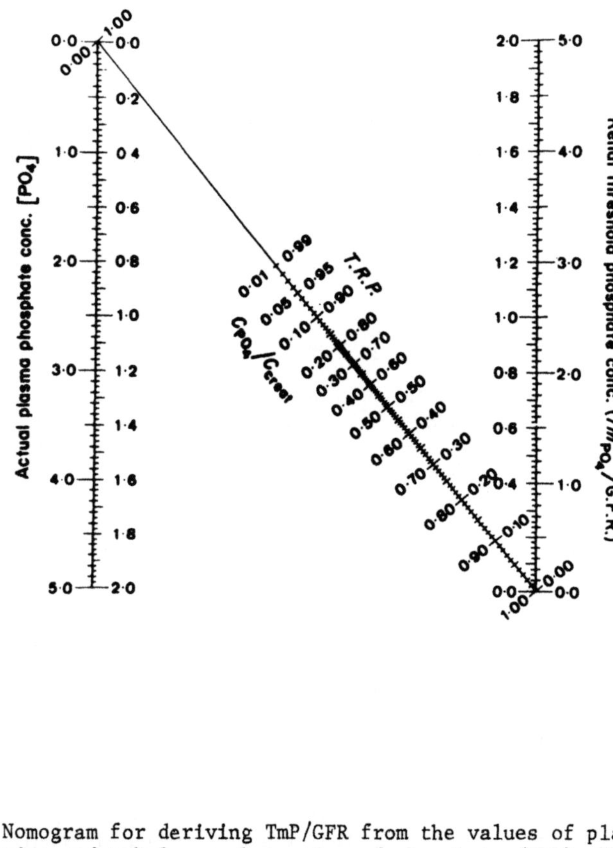

FIG. 1. Nomogram for deriving TmP/GFR from the values of plasma phosphate concentration and tubular reabsorption of phosphate (TRP). The outer scale on each ordinate represents units in mg/dl and the inner scale in mmol/l. The values to the right of the diagnonal line represent TRP. The derivation of TmP/GFR is made by drawing a straight line through the known values of plasma phosphate concentration and TRP. The point of intersection with the right ordinate gives the corresponding TmP/GFR value. The units used (mg/dl or mmol/l) should be the same. From Walton, R.J., Bijvoet, O.L.M.: Nomogram for derivation of renal threshold phosphate concentration. Lancet 2:309, 1975. Reprinted by permission.

fractionated the TmP by the GFR. In addition, they demonstrated that with the simple nomogram (Figure 1), TmP/GFR can be obtained by determining the serum phosphate concentration and plotting it against the tubular reabsorption of phosphate.

Broadus and associates (45) have shown that nephrogenous cyclic AMP is another important variable in estimating parathyroid hormone functions. This is especially true in the case of hypoparathyroid patients in which the nephrogenous cyclic AMP is very low in comparison to the hyperparathyroid patients when the nephrogenous cyclic AMP concentrations are remarkably high (Figure 2).

As stated earlier, parathyroid hormone (46) stimulates the conversion of 25-hydroxyvitamin D to 1,25-dihydroxyvitamin D. Thus, in the absence of parathyroid hormone, or in the cases of parathyroid hormone resistance as occurs in pseudohypoparathyroidism, the serum 1,25-dihydroxyvitamin D concentration can be expected to be low (Figure 3).

Mechanisms of parathyroid hormone resistance

It is well established that hypomagnesemia can lead to symptomatic hypocalcemia even in the presence of normal calcium and vitamin D intakes. Profound hypomagnesemia results in parathyroid hormone resistance due partly to the fact that adenylate cyclase activity in the parathyroid chief cells are dependent on the presence of magnesium (47-49).

In 1942, Albright et al (50) described the association of severe, symptomatic hypocalcemia associated with hyperphosphatemia, skeletal defects (Figure 4), mental retardation, obesity, coarse skin, moon-face, and a thick-set and short body. They also described a preponderance of female:male in a ratio of 2:1. Because of the end-organ resistance to parathyroid hormone, the word pseudohypoparathyroidism has been used to describe the syndrome originally elucidated by Albright and associates. In recent years, two types of pseudohypoparathyroidism have been described.

Type 1 pseudohypoparathyroidism is associated with a decrease in intracellular cyclic AMP concentration. In contrast, type 2 pseudohypoparathyroidism is associated with receptor defects at the end-organ. Thus, hypocalcemia obtains from the parathyroid hormone resistance, prompting the continued secretion of parathyroid hormone (51-53). After a standard parathyroid hormone stimulation test, in both type 1 and type 2 pseudohypoparathyroidism, there is a lack of the normal phosphaturic response. However, the urinary cyclic AMP will be increased in type 2 pseudohypoparathyroidism because the basic disorder resides in the receptor in the renal tubule (53). However, in type 1 pseudohypoparathyroidism, there is no increase in urinary cyclic AMP. It has also been repeatedly documented that the skeletal abnormalities are more marked in pseudohypoparathyroidism type 1. Recent studies (54-56) have demonstrated a sub-type of pseudohypoparathyroidism type 1 and that is related with defective cyclic AMP production in the renal tubule, but the skeletal production of cyclic AMP is intact. Therefore, with the increase in parathyroid hormone secretion, osteitis fibrosa becomes apparent (57-59).

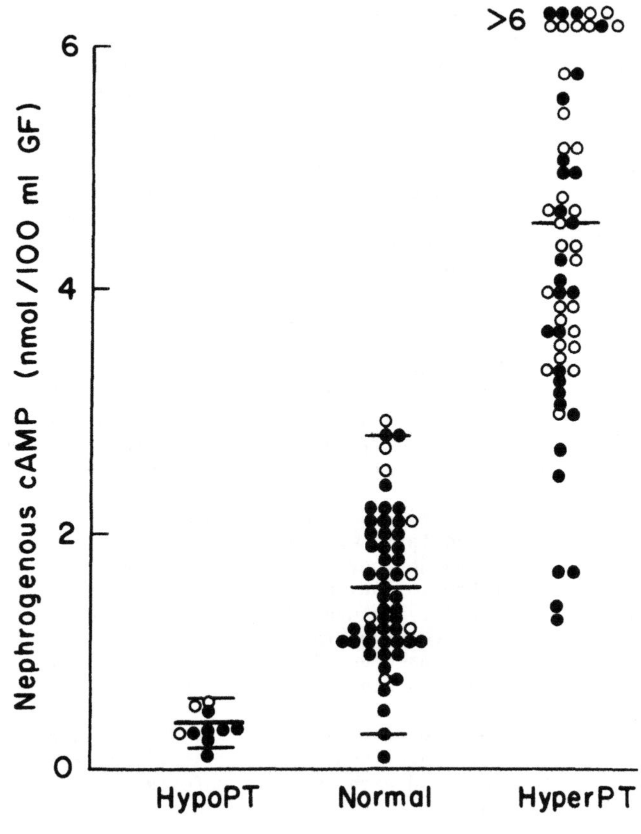

FIG. 2. Nephrogenous cyclic adenosine monophosphate (NcAMP) in patients with hypoparathyroidism (Hypo-PT) and hyperparathyroidism (Hyper-PT) compared to normal controls. From Broadus, A.E., Mahaffey, J.E., Bartter, F.C., Neer, R.M.: Nephrogenous cyclic adenosine monophosphate as a parathyroid function test. J Clin Invest 60:771-783, 1977. Reprinted by permission.

Parathyroid hormone deficiency

Parathyroid hormone deficiency (60-63) may ensue transiently in the neonate or secondary to maternal hyperparathyroidism. In addition, parathyroid deficiency may follow hypomagnesemia, or may result from hypercalcemic suppression.

Transient parathyroid deficiency in the neonate

Infants with low birth weight, birth asphyxia or diabetic mothers incur a 30% to 35% risk of transient hypocalcemia secondary to one or a combination of the following factors: "functional" hypoparathyroidism, hyperphosphatemia from high milk intake of phosphate, hypercalcitonemia, inadequate calcium supply, low tubular absorption of phosphate, vitamin D deficiency or resistance to parathyroid hormone (64-67).

Maternal hyperparathyroidism

Although the elevated parathyroid hormone in the mother with hyperparathyroidism does not cross the placenta, the elevated calcium concentrations on transversing the placenta result in suppression of the fetal parathyroids. Diagnostic work-up for hyperparathyroidism in the asymptomatic mother would, therefore, be important in such a situation. (64-67).

Hypomagnesemia

In adults, hypomagnesemia occurs secondary to chronic alcoholism, presumably from inadequate dietary intake and hepatic insufficiency. It is also possible that anti-convulsants and rhabdomyolysis contribute to the hypomagnesemia. In contrast, hypomagnesemia in infants and children (68-70) is usually associated with malabsorption syndromes, steatorrhea, inadequate magnesium supply in total parenteral nutrition or with the use of diuretic therapy. In addition, it is important to recognize that certain antibiotics such as aminoglycosides are associated with renal magnesium wasting. Associated complications of such renal magnesium wasting include hypocalcemia and hypoparathyroidism.

Suppression by hypercalcemia

As alluded to earlier, hypercalcemia suppresses parathyroid hormone secretion. However, atrophy does not obtain secondary to even prolonged suppression by hypercalcemia. No new parathyroid tissue is generated on normalization of serum calcium concentration (71-72).

Congenital hypoparathyroidism

There are several disorders of congenital hypoparathyroidism, but we will consider here the sporadic hypoparathyroidism; the autoimmune disorder associated with mucocutaneous candidiasis and the DiGeorge syndrome (34,35).

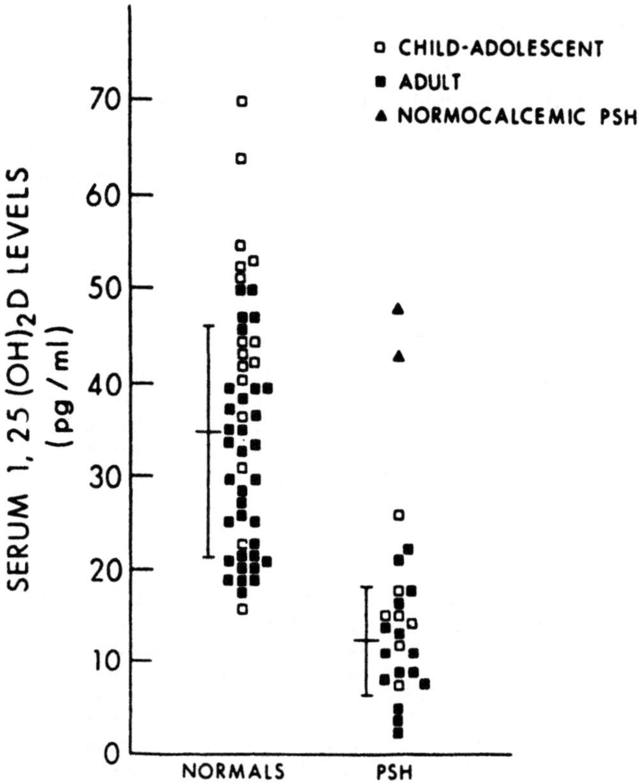

FIG. 3. Serum concentrations of 1,25-dihydroxyvitamin-D, 1,25-$(OH)_2D_3$, in pg/ml in normal subjects, with higher values in children and adolescents, and in untreated, hypocalcemic pseudohypoparathyroidism (PSH) type 1 patients. The serum concentrations of 1,25-$(OH)_2$-D_3 from 3 to 26 pg/ml are substantially lower than the normal subjects. The lack of stimulation on 1-hydroxylase activity obtains from the failure of renal tubules to respond to parathyroid hormone in PSH patients. From Drezner, M.K., Neelon, F,A,: Pseudohypoparathyroidism, Chapter 69 in Stanbury, J.B., Wyngaarden, J.B., Frederickson D.S., Goldstein, J.L., Brown, M.S. (eds): The Metabolic Basis of Inherited Disease. 5th edition, McGraw-Hill Book Co., NY, 1983. pp 1508-1527. Reprinted by permission.

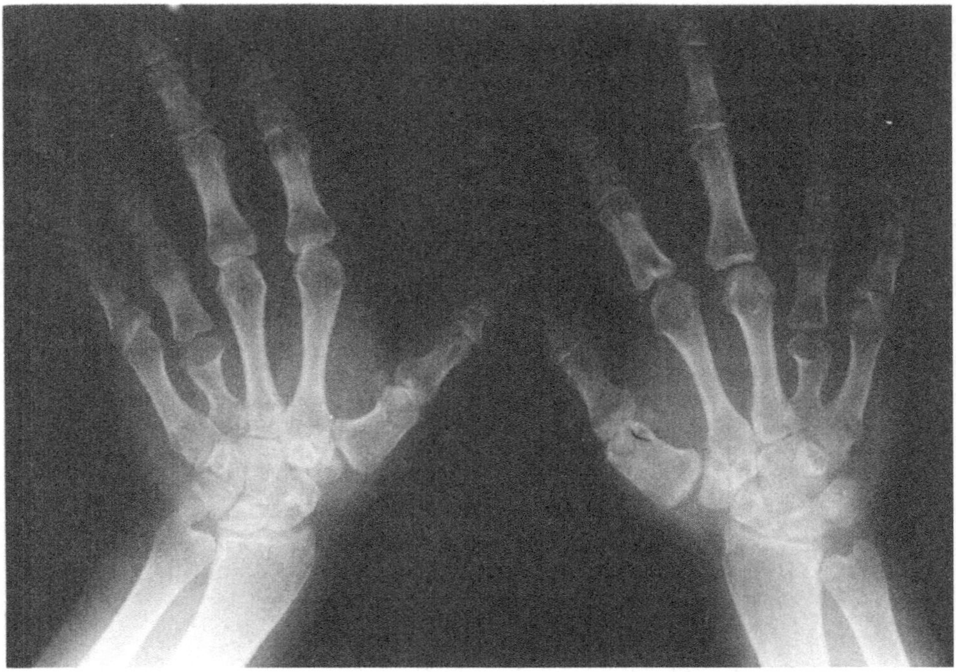

FIG. 4. X-ray of hands and wrists in a 14.3-year-old, white female with pseudohypoparathyroidism. Note the first metacarpal is short and broad. The fourth metacarpal is also short. All epiphyses are fused with irregularity and deformity.

Isolated, congenital hypoparathyroidism

This is a relatively rare condition and usually occurs sporadically although X-linked or autosomal recessive transmission has been described (22).

Autoimmune disorders with mucocutaneous candidiasis

The presence of parathyroid antibodies in conjunction with other autoimmune disorders accentuated by mucocutaneous candidiasis may occur in childhood as well as adulthood. This disorder is usually associated with adrenal insufficiency, lymphocytic thyroiditis, pernicious anemia, chronic hepatitis and premature ovarian insufficiency (47).

DiGeorge syndrome

The aplastic, hypoplastic parathyroid gland associated with thymic immune deficiency has been described by DiGeorge in 1968, secondary to failure of development of the third and fourth pharyngeal pouches. The other associated congenital lesions include cleft-lip, cleft-palate, malformed ears, micrognathia as well as congenital heart diseases. Occasionally, cases have been described in association with hypothyroidism. Experience with transplantation of the fetal thymus is limited and usually unsuccessful due to intractable diarrhea, failure to thrive, hypocalcemic tetany and progressive lymphopenia and intercurrent infections. (34,35).

Acquired hypoparathyroidism

Surgical hypoparathyroidism denotes accidental removal or damage to the parathyroid glands, usually as a complication of thyroidectomy. Infiltration by amyloid tissues, iron, hemosiderin and malignancy give rise to hypoparathyroidism. In addition, hypoparathyroidism may also be acquired secondary to irradiation.

Treatment

The emergency treatment of severe, symptomatic hypocalcemia (69) is the intravenous infusion of 10% calcium gluconate (90 mg of elemental calcium/10 ml) at a rate of 1 ml/min with careful, electronic cardiac monitoring.

Maintenance of normal serum calcium requires the use of oral calcium supplementation at between 500 to 2000 mg/day. In addition, vitamin D or one of the vitamin D metabolites are also needed.

Complications of treatment

The usual complications of calcium and vitamin D supplementation include hypercalcemia, hypercalciuria and nephrocalcinosis (73).

In a five-year study conducted at the Medical College of Virginia to evaluate children with congenital hypoparathyroidism and pseudo-

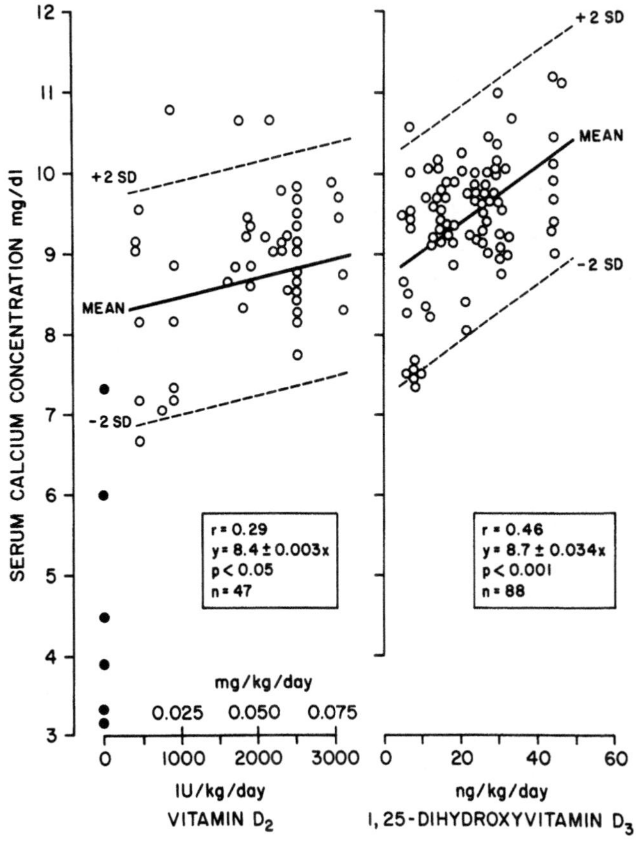

FIG. 5. The linear correlation of serum calcium concentration to the dosage of vitamin D in oral dosages of 2,000 to 4,000 IU/kg/day and 1,25-dihydroxyvitamin D in oral dosages of 10 to 40 ng/kg/day in patients with idiopathic hypoparathyroidism and pseudohypoparathyroidism. The initial serum concentrations of calcium before treatment are shown in black circles and not included in the statistical analysis. The serum calcium concentrations during treatment were presented in open circles. To achieve sustained correction of serum calcium above 8 mg/dl, the dosages of vitamin D need to exceed 2,000 IU/kg/day and 1,25-dihydroxyvitamin D above 10 ng/kg/day. From Chan, J.C.M., Young, R.B., Hartenberg, M.A., Chinchilli, V.M.: Calcium and phosphate metabolism in children with idiopathic hypoparathyroidism or pseudohypoparathyroidism: effects of 1,25-dihydroxyvitamin D3. J Pediatr (in press).

hypoparathyroidism, we found that the incidence of hypercalcemia is very low (Figure 5). The initial dose of 1,25-dihydroxyvitamin D was 0.5 mcg/day which was gradually advanced to 1.5 mcg/day in order to achieve normalization of serum calcium; so far, even at this high dose, hypercalcemia is not common. Regular vitamin D2 at dosages of 1,000 to 3,000 IU/kg/day or 0.024 to 0.075 mg/kg/day, maintains calcium concentrations at 8 to 9 mg/dl. In contrast, the use of 1,25-dihydroxyvitamin D at dosages of 20 to 40 ng/kg/day achieves mean serum calcium concentrations of 9 to 9.6 mg/dl.

Summary

The recent advances in our understanding of parathyroid hormone, its biological characteristics and tubular and skeletal actions are reviewed to provide a basis for understanding syndromes of parathyroid hormone resistance and deficiency. The recent introduction of 1,25-dihydroxyvitamin D to the treatment of these hypocalcemia states has proven to enjoy patient acceptability. In addition, prompt reversal of toxicity in the relatively infrequent episodes of hypercalcemia and hypercalciuria may prove to support the earlier expectations of 1,25-dihydroxyvitamin D as the drug of choice in these conditions.

Acknowledgements Mrs. Marilyn Reilly provided secretarial assistance; Michael A. Hartenburg, M.D. provided the x-rays of the hands and wrists of the patient with pseudohypoparathyroidism. Supported in part by Public Health Service N.I.H. research grants R01-AM HD 31370 and RR 0065.

References

1. MacCallum WG, Voegtlin C: On the relation of tetany to the parathyroid glands and to calcium metabolism. J Expt Med 11:118, 1980.

2. Greenwald I: The effect of parathyroidectomy upon metabolism. Amer J Physiol 28:103, 1911.

3. Greenwald I: Some chemical changes in the blood of dogs after thyroparathyroidectomy. J Biol Chem 61:649, 1924.

4. Thompson DL, Collip JB: The parathyroid glands. Physiol Rev 12:309, 1932.

5. Raisz LG, Kream BE: Regulation of bone formation. N Engl J Med 309:29, 1983.

6. Broadus AE: Mineral metabolism, in Endocrinology and Metabolism eds. P. Felig, J.D. Baxter, et al, 1981, New York (McGraw-Hill).

7. Kemper B, Habener JF, Ernest MD, et al. Pre-proparathyroid hormone: Analysis of radioactive tryptic peptides and amino acid sequence. Biochemistry 15:15, 1976.

8. Habener JF, Potts JT: Biosynthesis of parathyroid hormone. N Engl J Med 299:580, 1978.

9. Habener JF, Potts JT, Rich A: Pre-proparathyroid hormone. J Biol Chem 251:3893, 1976.

10. Hamilton JW, Niall HD, Jacobs HW: The N-terminal amino acid sequence of bovine pro-parathyroid hormone. Proc Natl Acad Sci, USA 71:653, 1974.

11. Aurbach GD, Potts JT: Parathyroid hormone. Amer J Med 42:1, 1967.

12. Aurbach GD, Marx SJ, Spiegel AM: Parathyroid hormone, Calcitonin and the Calciferols, in Textbook of Endocrinology ed. R. H. Williams, 1981, Philadelphia (Saunders).

13. Rasmussen H, DeLuca HF, Arnaud C, et al: The relationship between vitamin D and parathyroid hormone. J Clin Invest 42:1940, 1963.

14. Hanley DA, Takatsuki K, Sultan JM, et al: Direct release of parathyroid hormone fragments from functioning bovine parathyroid glands in vitro. J Clin Invest 62:1247, 1978.

15. Williams GA, Hargis GK, Bowser EN, et al: Evidence for a role of adenosine 3'5'-monophosphate in parathyroid hormone release. Endocrinology 92:687, 1973.

16. Mayer GP, Keaton JA, Hurst JG, et al: Effects of plasma calcium concentration on the relative proportion of hormone and carboxyl fragments in parathyroid venous blood. Endocrinology 104:1778, 1979.

17. Blum JW, Fischer JA, Schworer D, et al: Acute parathyroid hormone response: Sensitivity relationship to hypocalcemia, and rapidity. Endocrinology 95:753, 1974.

18. Anast CA, Mohs JM, Kaplan SL, et al: Evidence for parathyroid failure in magnesium deficiency. Science 177:606, 1972.

19. Sherwood LM, Mayer GP, Rammberg CF Jr, et al: Regulation of parathyroid hormone secretion: Proportional control by calcium, lack of effect of phosphate. Endocrinology 83:1043, 1968.

20. Segre GV, D'Armour F, Rosenblatt M, et al. Heterogeneity and metabolism of parathyroid hormone, in Endocrinology of Calcium Metabolism eds. D. H. Copp, R. V. Talmage, 1978, Amsterdam (Excerpta Medica).

21. Coburn JW, Slatopolsky E: Vitamin D, parathyroid hormone and renal osteodystrophy, in The Kidney eds. B. M. Brenner, F. C. Record, 1981, Philadelphia (Saunders).

22. Harrison HE, Harrison HC: Disorders of calcium and phosphate metabolism in childhood and adolescence, 1979, Philadelphia, (Saunders).

23. Shils ME: Magnesium, calcium, and parathyroid hormone interactions. Ann N.Y. Acad Sci 355:165, 1980.

24. Berson SA, Yalow RS: Immunochemical heterogeneity of parathyroid hormone in plasma. J Clin Endocrinol Metab 28:1037, 1968.

25. Kemper B, Habener JF, Rich A, et al: Parathyroid secretion: Discovery of a major calcium-dependent protein. Science 184:167, 1974.

26. Majzoub JA, Kronenberg HM, Potts JT, et al: Identification and cell-free translation of mRNA coding for a precursor of parathyroid secretory protein. J Biol Chem 254:7445, 1979.

27. Agus ZS, Gardner LB, Beck LH, et al: Effects of parathyroid hormone on renal tubular reabsorption of calcium, sodium and phosphate. Am J Physiol 224:1143, 1973.

28. Ichikawa I, Humes HD, Dousa TP, et al: Influences of parathyroid hormone on glomerular ultrafiltration in the rat. Am J Physiol 394:F393, 1978.

29. Wen SF: Micropuncture studies of phosphate transport in the proximal tubule of the dog. The relationship to sodium reaborption. J Clin invest 53:143, 1974.

30. Sraer J, Sraer JD, Chransel D, et al: Evidence for glomerular receptors for parathyroid hormone. Am J Physiol 4235:F96, 1978.

31. Alon U, Brewer WH, Chan JCM: Nephrocalcinosis: Detection by ultrasonography. Pediatrics 71:970, 1983.

32. Chan JCM, Wellons MD: Hypercalciuria of 1,25-dihydroxyvitamin-D and circadian rhythms of excretion of calcium, phosphate, magnesium and hydrogen ions in sex-linked dominant hypophosphatemic rickets, in Vitamin D Chemical Biochemical and Clinical Endocrinology of Calcium Metabolism eds. A. W. Norman, K. Schaefer, D. V. Herrath, et al, 1982, New York (Walter de Gruyter).

33. Alon U, Wellons MD, Chan JCM: Reversal of vitamin D-induced hypercalciuria and chlorothiazide. Pediatric Res 17:117, 1983.

34. DiGeorge AM: Disorders of the parathyroid glands, in Nelson Textbook of Pediatrics (12th ed.) eds. R. E. Behrman, V. C. Vaughan, 1983, Philadelphia (Saunders).

35. DiGeorge AM: Congenital absence of the thymus and its immunologic consequences: Concurrence with congenital hypoparathyroidism, in Birth Defects, Original Article Series, No. 1, Vol. IV. eds. D. Bergman, R. A. Good, 1968, New York (The National Foundation).

36. Chan JCM: Disorders of water and electrolyte balance, in Pediatrics (Chapter 19) ed. H. M. Maurer, 1983, New York (Churchill-Livingstone).

37. Dennis VW: Actions of parathyroid hormone on isolated renal tubules. Ann N.Y. Acad Sci 372:552, 1981.

38. Garg LC: Effect of parathyroid hormone and adenosine-3',5'-monophosphate on renal carbonic anhydrase. Biochem Pharmacol 24:437, 1975.

39. Chase LR, Aurbach GD: The effect of parathyroid hormone on the concentration of adenosine 3',5'-monophosphate in skeletal tissue in vitro. J. Biol Chem 245:1520, 1970.

40. Chertow BS, Baylink DJ, Wergedal JE, et al: Decrease in serum immunoreactive parathyroid hormone in rats and in parathyroid hormone secretion in vitro by 1,25-dihydroxycholecalciferol. J Clin Invest 56:668, 1975.

41. Canterbury JM, Lerman S, Claflin AJ, et al: Inhibition of parathyroid hormone secretion by 25-hydroxycholecalciferol and 24,25-dihydroxycholecalciferol in the dog. J Clin Invest 61:1375, 1978.

42. Martin KJ, Hruska KA, Freitag JJ, et al: The peripheral metabolism of parathyroid hormone. N Engl J Med 301:1092, 1979.

43. Spiegel AM, Marx SJ, Aurbach GD, et al: The phosphaturic response to parathyroid hormone. N Engl J Med 308:104, 1983.

44. Bijvoet OLM: Kidney function in calcium and phosphate metabolism, in Metabolic Bone Disease eds. L. V. Avioli, S. M. Krane, 1977, New York (Academic Press).

45. Broadus AE, Mahaffey JE, Bartter FC, et al: Nephrogenous cyclic adnosine monophosphate as a parathyroid function test. J Clin Invest 60:771, 1977.

46. Drezner MK, Neelon FA, Haussler M, et al: 1,25-dihydroxycholecalciferol deficiency: The probable cause of hypocalcemia and metabolic bone disease in pseudohypoparathyroidism. J Clin Endocrinol Metab 42:621, 1976.

47. Parfitt AM, Kleerekoper M: Clinical disorders of calcium, phosphorus, and magnesium metabolism, in Clinical Disorders of Fluid and Electrolyte Metabolism (3rd ed.) eds. M. H. Maxwell, C. R. Kleeman, 1980, New York (McGraw-Hill).

48. Shils M: Experimental human magnesium depletion. Medicine 48:61, 1969.

49. Seelig MS: Magnesium deficiency in the pathogenesis of disease, 1980, New York, (Plenum Medical Book Co.).

50. Albright F, Reifenstein EC: The Parathyroid Glands and Metabolic Bone Disease, 1948, Baltimore (Williams and Wilkins).

51. Bell NH, Avery S, Sinha T, et al: Effects of dibutyryl cyclic adenosine 3',5'-monophosphate and parathyroid extract on calcium and phosphorus metabolism in hypoparathyroidism and pseudohypoparathyroidism. J Clin Invest 51:816, 1972.

52. Drezner MK, Burch WM Jr: Altered activity of the nucleotide regulatory site in the parathyroid hormone-sensitive adenylate cyclase from the renal cortex of a patient with pseudohypoparathyroidism. J Clin Invest 62:1222, 1978.

53. Farfel Z, Brickman AS, Kaslow HR, et al: Defect of receptor-cyclase coupling protein in pseudohypoparathyroidism. N Engl J Med 303:237, 1980.

54. Lucas PA, Woodhead JS: The assessment of parathyroid function, in Calcium Disorders eds. D. A. Heath, S. T. Marx, 1982, London (Butterworth).

55. Lambert PW, Hollis BW, Bell NH, et al: Demonstration of a lack of change in serum 1,25-dihydroxyvitamin D in response to parathyroid extract in pseudohypoparathyroidism. J Clin Invest 66:782, 1980.

56. Aksnes L, Aarskog D: Effect of parathyroid hormone on 1,25-dihydroxyvitamin D formation in type 1 pseudohypoparathyroidism. J Clin Endocrinol Metab 51:1223, 1980.

57. Drezner MK, Neelon FA: Pseudohypoparathyroidism, in The Metabolic Basis for Inherited Disease eds. J. B. Stanbury, J. B. Wyngaarden, D. S. Frederickson, et al, 1983, New York (McGraw-Hill).

58. Moses AM, Breslau N, Coulson R: Renal responses to PTH in patients with hormone-resistant (pseudo) hypoparathyroidism. Am J Med 61:184, 1976.

59. Spiegel AM, Levine MA, Marx SJ, et al: Pseudohypoparathyroidism: The molecular basis for hormone resistance - a retrospective. N Engl J Med 307:679, 1982.

60. Tsang RC, Donovan EF, Steichan JJ: Calcium physiology and pathology in the neonate. Pediatr Clin North Am 23:611, 1976.

61. David L, Anast CS: Calcium metabolism in newborn infants: The interrelationship of parathyroid function and calcium, magnesium, and phosphorus metabolism in normal, "sick," and hypocalcemic newborns. J Clin Invest 54:287, 1974.

62. Greer FR, Chesney RW: Disorders of calcium metabolism in the neonate. Seminars Nephr 3:100, 1983.

63. Steichen JJ, Tsang RC, Gratton TL, et al: Vitamin D homeostasis in the perinatal period: 1,25-dihydroxyvitamin D in maternal, cord, and neonatal blood. N Engl J Med 302:315, 1980.

64. Tsang RC, Light IJ, Sutherland JM, et al: Possible pathogenic factors in neonatal hypocalcemia of prematurity. J Pediatr 82:423, 1973.

65. Hillman LS, Rojanasathit S, Slatopolsky E, et al: Serial measurements of serum calcium, magnesium, parathyroid hormone, calcitonin and 25-hydroxyvitamin D in premature and term infants during the first week of life. Pediatr Res 11:739, 1977.

66. Linarelli LG, Bobik J, Bobik C: Newborn urinary cyclic AMP and developmental renal responsiveness to parathyroid hormone. Pediatrics 50:14, 1972.

67. Chan GM, Tsang RC, Chen IW, et al: The effects of $1,25(OH)_2$ vitamin-D_3 supplementation in premature infants. J Pediatr 93:91, 1978.

68. Friedman M, Hatcher G, Watson L: Primary hypomagnesaemia with secondary hypocalcaemia in an infant. Lancet 1:703, 1967.

69. Robson AM: The pathophysiology of body fluids, in Nelson Textbook of Pediatrics (12th ed.) eds. R. E. Behrman, V. C. Vaughan, 1983, Philadelphia (Saunders).

70. Anast CS, Winnacker JL, Forte LR, et al: Impaired release of parathyroid hormone in magnesium deficiency. J Clin Endocrinol Metab 42:707, 1976.

71. Parfitt AM: Surgical idiopathic and other varieties of parathyroid hormone deficient hypoparathyroidism, in Endocrinology ed. L. J. DeGroot, 1979, New York (Grune & Stratton, Inc.).

72. Johnston CC Jr, Schnute RB: A case of primary hyperparathyroidism with spontaneous remission following infarction of the adenoma with development of hypocalcemic tetany. J Clin Endocrinol Metab 21:196, 1961.

73. Chan JCM, Young RB, Alon U, et al: Hypercalcemia in children with disorders of calcium and phosphate metabolism during long-term treatment with 1,25-dihydroxyvitamin-D . Pediatrics. 72:225, 1983.

PANEL DISCUSSION

Jose Strauss, M.D., Moderator

MODERATOR: I would like, first, to ask the nurse of the Panel, about her experience with that baby that was presented. What are the thoughts that you would like to share? Applicability of that procedure--how do you see it from the nursing point of view?

COMMENT: I have a question for the people who have more experience in neonatology because as nurses, we had lots of troubles in achieving some of the goals we had for that baby who was on dialysis. I think the main problem we had was that we weren't able to give her the amount of calories with all the vitamins and minerals required for her treatment. The main problem was to give the feeding. We started several different kinds of formulas. We used one for about three days, and then she started vomiting consistently; so, the baby had to stay 24 hours without feedings. Then, we used PM 60-40 formula. We added kayexalate. We also used breast milk in combination with the PM 60-40. The baby also had difficulties with that. Then, we added supplements of sodium, Polycose, etc., and the baby just didn't tolerate all that. We used first bottle feeding, then we started tube feeding. Finally, the baby stayed with continuous feeding plus hyperalimentation. We had a lot of troubles. Since the panelists have a lot of experience, perhaps they know how to achieve nutrition goals.

COMMENT: This is a tremendous problem that we face and I think other people have faced. We heard about similar problems from some of the other speakers. It is a problem--how to manage those little babies nutritionally, how to provide an adequate nutritional support in order to achieve adequate intake and growth. We are just starting to learn about it. I think that more aggressive nutritional intervention will be the way to go. Once we have decided to commit ourselves to a complex therapy like this, one is in for life. That might entail continuous gavage feedings. There are data from people who have managed those babies from very early in life with continuous tube feeding with quite nice results. However, here we are just starting to learn about those problems. Definitely, it is a tremendous challenge. There is no clear answer to it.

COMMENT: I sympathize with you for all the problems. In fact, I am amazed that that's the only aspect you are questioning. At my institution, not only were they questioning the feeding problems but the kind of "quality of life" that this patient is having or will have, and all the ethical considerations that would go into subjecting somebody to this form of treatment. The way we have dealt with this has been to pass it to the Ethic's Committee and discuss the whole situation with them. We now have a patient who is fairly small, only nine kilograms, and had this problem. She was vomiting every feeding. What we finally did was to put a naso-gastro-jejunal tube so she couldn't vomit everything that went into her stomach.

MODERATOR: May I ask you to enlarge a little bit on the point you just made about the Committee on Ethics? I imagine it is similar to our Committee for the Protection of Human Subjects. Do you have an Ethics Committee that determines not necessarily research but other types of issues related to medical treatment?

RESPONSE: This is an Ethics Committee which is related only to medical treatment, entirely separate from the research aspects. This is composed of an ethicist, a priest, the nurses, the doctors, and eventually, of course, the parents get involved.

MODERATOR: That is very interesting. I don't think we have such a committee. We used to have a committee to decide for transplantation purposes or dialysis purposes who would be allowed to die and who to continue living but that has been discontinued for many years. The point is that when we were studying this baby, it was suggested that we were studying her for research purposes. We thought we were doing it for treatment purposes. Is that research? Where do you draw the line? Like we have said during the Seminar, is ultrafiltration in the neonate an experimental procedure that should go through a research evaluation? Is administration of captopril in the neonate a research project?

RESPONSE: I wish our neonatologist was here. She probably could answer that better than I. I don't really know. As you probably know our University is one of the original places where Institutes for Bioethics were developed. Therefore, we enlisted their help in dealing with this complex issue--what sort of treatment should be given to whom. It's always a difficult situation. Yes, they did ask us also whether what we were doing to this patient was experimental and, therefore, if we should not be going to the Research Committee. If it is indeed experimental, one cannot do anything until after the Research Committee approves the protocol. If it is not experimental, one has to show evidence that it has been successful elsewhere. So, it becomes circuitous. What happened to us, of course, is that everybody got convinced at one time that, yes, it could be experimental. But by the same token, different treatment modalities that we do in pediatrics have not been approved by the FDA either. So, you cannot go running to the Human Research Committee each time. I will give you an example. Propranolol is not approved for treatment of high blood pressure in children and yet everybody is using it. So, eventually it was decided that this sort of discussion would be more appropriately handled in the realm of bioethics.

COMMENT: As far as my approach, in any patient, regardless of size, be it adult or older pediatric or newborn, I consider that experimental because it certainly is not definitive and it's only temporarily therapeutic. It is not the final answer for anyone. As far as whether it is experimental and ethical, a research tool in the newborn, I see it as being no more of a research tool than it is in the adult. But it still is research. Is it ethical? I have wondered greatly about many things being ethical in the newborn and older children. But when you see the pictures and the data that have been put out, you have to say that the results with peritoneal dialysis and tube feedings starting in infants in the first months of life are more impressive than any data from an adult dialysis unit. The numbers look good, the patients look great and they are doing well. You almost wonder if they would do as well if they were transplanted. It's very impressive. I think this is a precedent that this kind of therapy works some of the time—enough of the time that it can be offered as treatment. That does not make the delivery of that care easier. We need to be careful that we don't promise a good result, when we counsel parents of infants. I do everything I can to discourage them from getting involved without telling them "no". I tell them that I will go along with their decision because the modalities are available and other people have used them. They must understand that they are participating in something that is going to be difficult. The hard decision is to say "no", not to do anything for these babies. The easy decision is to say, "Yes, let's do whatever we can to save this baby". That's the easy, cop-out decision. I finally had parents refuse treatment to a newborn this fall. It was a tough decision for them and I would have supported them either way. I am glad for my own personal, selfish nature that they didn't opt to go with treatment because it would have been a tremendous workload that we would have experienced as you have reported to us. It's not only just dialysis and renal failure and feeding. We know with dialysis patients, if we over-dialyze them, over-filtrate them and dry them out, they vomit. And we know that if they are over-hydrated and edematous, they vomit. If their calciums are high, they vomit; if their calciums are low, they vomit. If their sodiums are high, they vomit,; if their sodiums are low, they vomit. It's a tremendous job to keep all these variables in balance. Just one derangement can throw off your whole ability to deliver adequate nutrition. If they don't grow, it's not successful; it's a tough area. Experimental? All dialysis is experimental. Experimental in the newborn? No more experimental in the newborn. Is it ethical? It is as ethical as a lot of other things that we accept and allow to be done in the newborn.

MODERATOR: What about the reverse reasoning? Might you not be breaking a law? For instance, in Florida there is the Child Abuse Law that says, basically, that if the child is sick, he is entitled to treatment, among other things. One form of child abuse is withholding treatment. We had a patient a few years ago before we became aggressive with dialysis and tranplantation. Basically, the parents didn't want to go through hemodialysis. I was talking at the time with the lawyer who sat on the Committee for the Protection of Human Subjects and, passing by, mentioned to him our dilemma in terms of taking a position with those parents and treating the child or not. He said, "You actually are breaking the law because dialysis nowadays is an accepted modality of treatment. You are withholding treatment from that child". Now, without going into questionable laws that are currently being discussed, what are we obligated to do? Can we decide what will be done? Do the parents have the right to decide whether the child will live or die? Do we have that right? Those are tough questions. Does anyone have the answer?

COMMENT: This is a difficult question. We agonize with our kids as well as adults. I had a colleague who in an argument with a surgeon topped off "I don't practice law; I practice medicine". I wish that we could do that but we can't ignore the medico-legal ramifications of what we do. Really, the best we can do is try to be honest with the parents-patients and give them the information as we currently know it. I also tend to try to discourage them but the three patients that I have had, all had parents who wanted aggressive treatments. I think that is the best you can do. There is nothing you can do to protect yourself from a politically over-ambitious district attorney. I don't think you can always be looking over you shoulder to do that. All you can do is the best as far as educating the parents and then go ahead.

One comment about nutrition, if I may go back to that. With adults, it seems that in both acute and chronic renal failure, the more aggressive you get with nutritional support, the better they do, even if more patients require more aggressive dialysis and more aggressive ultrafiltration. I've come full circle with that approach in adults. In children, because of initial technical problems with dialysis, it seemed better to back down on allowed protein intake. Now, I've learned that I need to be more aggressive with nutrition. What I do notice in the three children that we have, a 10 weeks old, a seven months old and one we had on dialysis for a year before she was transplanted, is that the better their nutrition is, the better they feed. That's also true in adults. There has been a long-recognized syndrome--if you go back and look in the literature of the fifties--functional bowel disorders with low albumin which you can correct simply by infusing albumin. We don't infuse albumin into the children or into the adults, not for nutritional support, but clearly by giving them adequate protein and getting the albumin up, they seem to do better.

QUESTION: Would you mind commenting further on the hypercalciuria in patients who are treated with 1,25-D for hypophosphatemic rickets? Does the use of the diuretics make any difference in the calcium excretion? Also, do you have any experience with the mid-range molecular determination of parathyroid hormone? Do you think that that has any advantage over the use of the N-terminal or the C-terminal determination?

RESPONSE: Regarding the question on our experience with the hypercalciuria induced by 1,25-dihydroxy vitamin D or with the regular vitamin D, I would like to state that whenever we use 1,25-D for hypophosphatemic rickets patients, we should always use phosphate supplement at the same time. Whenever we stop medications because of hypercalcemia, we should stop both medications. That is, if you encounter hypercalcemia and stop 1,25 dihydroxy vitamin D and continue on the phosphate supplementation, what will happen is, at those very high doses you will promote absorption of phosphate as you hope will happen, but then with hyperphosphatemia--a very, very transient hyperphosphatemia--hypocalcemia, the reciprocal hypocalcemia, will begin stimulating more and more parathyroid hormone secretion. In two of our cases, out of perhaps 15 with hypophosphatemic rickets, we have documented by ultrasound, as well as by kidney biopsy, the presence of nephrocalcinosis. Before we did that, we also had documented at least in one case, a lack of response to calcium infusion which then confirmed our suspicion, our clinical impression of tertiary or autonomous hyperparathyroidism. Ultrasound of the neck documented enlarged parathyroid glands and histologic examination after removal of the parathyroid glands documented the hyperparathyroidism. As I mentioned earlier, the kidney biopsy also documented nephrocalcinosis. Now, we can never be sure in those cases whether the nephrocalcinosis is secondary to the current use of 1,25-D or to the previous use of those super-pharmacological doses of regular vitamin D--as you recall, up to 80,000 units have been used--required to maintain normal phosphatemia and at least some degree of bone healing in those patients. I have information shared with me by our Canadian colleagues who have a lot of experience with renal hypophosphatemic rickets, that every one of those patients studied by ultrasound of the kidney or by kidney biopsy, has been diagnosed as having nephrocalcinosis. So, the treatment of renal hypophosphatemic rickets is frustrating and uncomfortable because the margin between therapeutic benefits and therapeutic toxicity is very narrow. We had hoped that the 1,25-Vitamin D in hypophosphatemic rickets, because of its shorter half-life, might have been an advantage. We are seeing some cases of nephrocalcinosis; future studies in which we will have patients who are only on 1,25-D should be helpful in differentiating between the nephrocalcinosis induced by regular vitamin D_2 and that perhaps compounded by 1,25-D; but, that is into the future. We have several patients who have never been treated with any form of vitamin D except for 1,25-D.

The second point I would like to emphasize regards the hypercalciuria. We have successfully used both hydrochlorothiazide and ameloride to reverse the hypercalciuria and reduce the requirement for a high dose of 1,25-D. As far as the third question (regarding parathyroid hormone determinations), you hear different advocates of measurements of parathyroid hormone fractions and I do not know, at this point, which is the best way to go.

QUESTION: I have a question to the panel, and maybe to the audience concerning the hypercalciuria induced or exacerbated by the use of furosemide in the neonate. Furosemide is used right and left in neonatal units for well-deserved, indicated causes. Would it be justified (or does anybody know if it has already been studied) to use hydrochlorothiazide instead of, or in addition to, furosemide in the neonatal period?

RESPONSE: I have not come across such data. I know of some studies going on, but not completed yet.

RESPONSE: The only study of which I am aware that used thiazide diuretics, is the study from Minnesota on the treatment of respiratory distress syndrome. This study compared furosemide, thiazide or no treatment at all in the outcome or the diuresis that is associated with the improvement of respiratory distress syndrome. But calcium, the hypercalciuric effect was not measured. So, I think that that would have to be studied. Theoretically, if thiazide produced a diuresis, if that were necessary, it would protect and conserve calcium, would have the beneficial effect of reducing calcium excretion. That's speculative because I don't know what forces would be operational in the newborn--whether they would actually reduce hypercalciuria or not.

MODERATOR: What about the hematuria that has been reported to be associated with a certain level of hypercalciuria in older children? Does that happen in the neonate? Does anybody have data on that? What is the mechanism by which hypercalciuria induces or is associated with hematuria?

RESPONSE: I'm not aware of any data.

RESPONSE: I am aware that data are being collected. The work that you refer to reports that 10% of microscopic hematuria is associated with hypercalciuria. We are accumulating data in different age groups concerning microscopic hematuria and the association with hypercalciuria but the data are not ready yet.

RESPONSE: I believe there are some very preliminary data published in a Commentary in which it is stated that some hematuria was noticed in some newborns with nephrocalcinosis who were treated with furosemide. The hematuria and the nephrocalcinosis apparently disappeared within weeks or months, upon discontinuation of the diuretic.

COMMENT: If it is the calcium in the tubules that is the trigger or cause of the damage, then you would expect to see hematuria; but the hypercalciuria induced by the diuretic is very transient and mild. It's relative. You don't see the tremendous effect until you get into heavy furosemide therapy and that usually is on a chronic basis with the infants with Broncho-Pulmonary Dysplasia (BPD). I think the worse case of renal stones I have ever seen was in a nine month old baby, born prematurely, with BPD, who had been on furosemide for nine months. Somebody just happened to notice in a flat plate of the abdomen or maybe in a follow-up chest x-ray that got a little bit low, these tremendous stones. The collecting systems on both sides were filled, like there were moth balls in the renal pelvis. That resolved once the furosemide was stopped and the urine was acidified. They just sort of dissolved, gradually disappeared. They did not have to be surgically removed; I didn't expect that they would disappear, but they did. That was the most dramatic effect I have ever seen.

QUESTION: I would like to ask the panel if they have any knowledge about hypocalcemia in the newborn subjected to phototherapy.

RESPONSE: I'm not aware of any effect that has been reported or any study that has been done, but it is an interesting question. More and more people are doing studies on phototherapy and its deleterious effects. Maybe that would be one to look at, to see if it is bad or not.

COMMENT: I would like to ask questions. I do not have the answers. What has been looked at in these patients with hypocalcemia under phototherapy? Has the parathyroid hormone been measured? Has the magnesium been measured?

COMMENT: You are probably referring to a couple of reviews that appeared in the Yearbook of Pediatrics, 1982-83.

COMMENT: I missed that.

QUESTION: I am told by my Chairman that the vitamin-D requirements in people with vitamin-D resistant rickets decrease as they reach puberty. Is that true or not?

RESPONSE: That has not been my experience. In fact, when we tried to stop 1,25 vitamin D and phosphate supplement after the patients reached adulthood, they would complain that they had muscle weakness and some bone pain. And the parents of children with hypophosphatemic rickets who have rickets themselves and who have lost teeth from spontaneous aveolar changes, all have alluded to improvements in muscular strength and well-being after receiving again 1,25-D and phosphate supplementation. And I have continued some of the patients whose photographs I showed you, on 1,25-D and phosphate at their request, but I am very, very concerned and only if they promise to send me urine for calcium/creatinine determinations would I continue to supply them with the vitamin-D for fear of hypercalcemia. But as far as requirements at the time of adolescence, I don't agree with that observation. I don't see that, in fact, at all.

QUESTION: I have one other question. With your nice and elegant presentation convincing us that indeed PTH seems to induce phosphaturia via cyclic AMP, would you comment on the latest studies that have appeared dissociating cyclic AMP and phosphaturia? If you recall, there was a study published recently in Science where they had two fragments of parathyroid hormone, one that inhibited cyclic AMP--or at least did not stimulate cyclic AMP levels in vitro--and another fragment that stimulated adenyl cyclase activity in vitro and then when those two agents were infused, both of them produced phosphaturia anyway.

RESPONSE: Thank you for the compliments, but you are one up on me. I have not read that article. I will look it up and let you know next week. I am not aware of that study.

COMMENT: The thing that they commented on is that, indeed, PTH increases adenyl cyclase activity and also produces phosphaturia. It seems like those studies that have examined this question have used pharmacological doses of PTH, and that if you use smaller dosages of PTH, you can dissociate the phosphaturia and increase urinary cyclic AMP activity. I was just wondering if you had any ideas on that. The reason I got one up on you is because we sent a paper on adenyl cyclase activity and beta receptors in the kidney and we thought that they need not be related to each other. Therefore, we had to scrounge some articles trying to dissociate certain agents and adenyl cyclase stimulation.

QUESTION: Turning to the target bone disease in those hypophosphatemic patients with low vitamin D, do you know whether or not the bones of those children have been analyzed? Is the predominant lesion indeed osteomalacia as it seems to be on the x-rays, presumably with reduced or absent PTH activity so that you would not expect to have any component of osteosclerosis?

RESPONSE: The studies published in the New England Journal in 1981 reflected your questions. You are just two years behind. But don't give up. So much of your work is so exciting. You just need to be provided with time by your boss to write those papers.

QUESTION-COMMENT: I was very interested in your calcium studies. Do you think the results with the 4.25% dextrose concentration as far as calcium mass transfer relates directly to the ultrafiltration or is there some other effect of glucose that is causing this? Second, what kind of results are seen with changes in albumin loss and glucose concentration?

RESPONSE: Probably, there are several reasons for the negative calcium mass transfer with the high dextrose concentration. One might be, at least in adults, that because the volume of ultrafiltration is higher, momentarily there is a concentration gradient favoring mass transfer into the dialysate. The other explanation might be that we are seeing a patient with an almost constantly normal ionized calcium in serum (due to several mechanisms that we could speculate about), and because of that there is no uptake of calcium into the extracellular fluid but rather calcium loss into the peritoneal fluid because the concentration is higher in the extracellular fluid compartment. Concerning the protein losses, they are higher with the higher dextrose concentration. That has been shown to be so in adults. Since we used only 4.25% in these babies, I couldn't tell you if there would have been any difference with a lower dextrose concentration.

QUESTION: I was involved for a very short period of time with one patient whom I would like to present to the panel members to see what their approach would be. A 17 year old female was admitted a few years ago with encephalopathy secondary to birth trauma manifested by mental retardation, spasticity, and seizure disorder. At that time, the patient was on dilantin and phenobarbital. I don't have the data in my hands and I am not prepared to present the details of the case. She had microscopic hematuria and proteinuria, hypercalcemia, very high alkaline phosphatase, and almost normal serum phosphorus. In a routine chest x-ray there were multiple fractures. The dilantin we know produces calcium problems but she had a seizure disorder and was referred to us as having generalized seizures. All the times I saw her it was more like a twisting or myoclonic seizure though the nurses reported that she had generalized seizures. We placed her on 1,25 vitamin D and she has been getting better. I would like to know what you would have done.

RESPONSE: You have presented the anti-convulsant complicating the conversion by hepatic hydroxylation to 25 D because liver hydroxylase is stimulated by the presence of the anticonvulsants. This is a situation that we see often in institutionalized children with birth trauma (as you described), mental retardation, seizures, etc. We have found that 1,25-D can reverse many of these cases, but we also have some very disappointing results in which, despite fairly high doses of 1,25-D and calcium supplementation, we do not make progress and we get very high urinary calcium excretion partly because these children are not moving around very much. I can only share with you these dismaying results. I think you have done well if this young lady begins to have healing of rickets, and fractures are less and less frequent.

QUESTION: I wonder if the hematuria and proteinuria in this patient have something to do with her problem. The IVP was normal.

RESPONSE: I don't know whether there was any interstitial nephritis or perhaps there already was hypercalciuria and nephrocalcinosis, even preceding your use of 1,25-D because children are less mobile and perhaps consuming too much calcium.

COMMENT-QUESTION: A lot of these anti-convulsants are associated with lupus-induced states. I was wondering if fluorescent anti-nuclear antibodies or serum complement were determined.

RESPONSE: Serum complement was normal, ANA was negative but the anti-DNA was not done.

COMMENT: Then, I would pursue that line of thinking although I am not an expert on SLE. A negative ANA need not indicate absence of some of these vasculitides. You have to measure extractable nuclear antigen as well because of the differences in the sensitivity of the technique. If one is suspecting some sort of a lupus-like syndrome, one should measure not only fluorescent anti-nuclear antibodies but anti-single strand and RNPN extractable nuclear antigen.

COMMENT: I just wanted to add something about the anti-convulsant interference with vitamin D. Not only does the anti-convulsant have a deleterious effect on the hydroxylation rate of vitamin D (to 25-D) in the liver, but it also has extra-hepatic effects on the vitamin's metabolism. There is an interruption of the normal entero-hepatic circulation and since D is a lipid-soluble vitamin, that might be interfered with as well. There are some data to support a possible direct effect on intestinal calcium absorption and even on bone resorption.

QUESTION-COMMENT: Was there a history of repeated urinary tract infections in this patient? Very often mental retardation is associated with some abnormalities in the urinary tract.

RESPONSE: No, and the IVP was normal.

MODERATOR: I would like to ask what is the concept of pregnancy. You were talking about conceptual being the time of the decision. Is that when the parents rent a motel? What is the impact on the baby? Does it carry any physiological importance?

COMMENT: Whether conception occurs in a motel or not, it's only the time that is important. If you didn't understand my editorial comment, you will read articles that will plot functions of maturation in newborn infants for conceptual age. By definition, that is an idea being conceived. Con-cep-tion is actual uniting of the sperm and the egg. That's the one that we think is most important as far as the physiological sequencing is concerned.

MODERATOR: To clarify your point, what you are saying is that we should not use that term.

COMMENT: Conceptual age, by definition, is not grammatically correct.

QUESTION: So, for aliens like me, what would you recommend we should now use, conceptional age rather than conceptual age and make sure we don't get our semantics crossed?

MODERATOR: Our time is up now. I would like to thank everyone for this challenging session. This has been a rewarding Seminar at least for me. The subjects were exciting and the faculty, excellent. We have had a very good group of people in the audience with varying degrees of expertise but, in general, so devoted and interested that the whole effort has been worthwhile. We have had some unfortunate developments but besides that, we can rest satisfied that we have accomplished something not only in sharing of information but also of feelings. We have become acquainted with new people. I would like to thank the faculty, especially the guest faculty, our Pediatric Nephrology group here in Miami, the translators who have done so well with a very tough job which takes a very heavy toll, the staff, Bonnie, Pat, Linda, and Pearl who is going through such a difficult time. To all of you, many, many thanks. Remember, we need to keep improving the Seminar so we need your suggestions and criticisms. We look forward to seeing you next year.

EDITOR'S COMMENTS

This Panel Discussion touched upon some specific and some general subjects pertaining to the neonate; most times the latter were an extension of the former, making it difficult for me even to attempt separating them. Aggressive nutritional approaches in general but mainly as they applied to the neonate with CRF in order to attain growth, mineral metabolism and desirable vs undesirable side effects of therapy, and diuretics, were all discussed. Various basic questions pertaining to bioethical, moral, and medico-legal aspects of work with neonates were asked. "When is the evaluation and treatment of a newborn baby considered research?" was asked, and the implication of this question or the inability to thoroughly answer it, still haunts us. Hopefully, in future Seminars and books we shall dwell on these subjects again and other reference points will be available to us.

V

SPECIAL LECTURES

FUNCTIONAL IMMATURITY OF THE NEWBORN KIDNEY--PARADOX OR PROSTAGLANDIN?

Billy S. Arant, Jr., M.D.

Since learning that glomerular filtration rate (GFR) during the first six months of life could not be factored for body size to be comparable with normal adult values (1), renal function in newborn infants has been considered limited. When 10% sodium chloride was fed to normal subjects, urine flow rate did not increase as much in infants as it did in adults; a conclusion was that sodium excretion in the infants was impaired even though no measurements of sodium had been made (2). When a developmental study of the newborn kidney's capacity to excrete water was performed, newborn infants excreted a greater fraction of an oral water load with each successive postnatal day, but the ability to excrete the water like an adult kidney was not observed during the first two weeks of life (3). The notion followed that the diluting mechanism of the neonatal kidney was limited compared to the adult kidney. When challenged by hydropenia, the inability of the neonatal kidney to concentrate urine to 1200 mOsm/kg like the adult kidney was further evidence of limited renal function in the neonate (4). Renal hydrogen ion secretion or bicarbonate reabsorption seemed reduced in the newborn when urine pH in premature infants remained alkaline during the first week of life while plasma bicarbonate concentrations were below the range of normal adult values (5). Sodium balance has been shown in several studies to be negative in premature infants born prior to 34 weeks gestation. The fractional excretion of sodium (FE_{Na}) in such infants was usually >3.0% (6), and sodium balance remained negative even when sodium was added to parenteral fluids given premature infants (7). Lower maximal tubular transport of PAH, glucose, and phosphate in infants compared to adults provided additional support for the idea that renal function in the neonate was indeed limited. Moreover, lower ratios of maximal tubular glucose reabsorption to GFR and of proximal tubular volume to glomerular surface area provided both physiologic and morphologic evidence favoring the concept of glomerulotubular imbalance with preponderance of glomerular structure and function to explain the differences between the normal kidneys of newborn infants and adults (8).

What is difficult to reconcile with this concept, however, is that regardless of its reported functional limitations the neonatal kidney is adequate to facilitate the abrupt physiologic adaptation of the normal fetus to postnatal life and to support the normal infant during rapid somatic growth. How, then can renal function in the normal neonate be considered limited? When newborn infants were studied at birth and during postnatal life, GFR was not observed to change significantly prior to a conceptional age of 34 weeks gestation (9). Infants born more than 34 weeks after conception exhibited an increase in GFR during the first week of life as described previously in fullterm infants. It can be important in the clinical management of preterm infants to understand that, although an infant may be six weeks old, GFR may not have increased significantly from birth. This observation has been confirmed in subsequent studies (10,11). Like preterm infants, GFR in newborn puppies did not change during the first two weeks of life, but increased only after 14 days of age (12). It is interesting that nephrogenesis in the human kidney is completed at 34 weeks (13) and in the canine kidney at 14 days (14).

One explanation for the failure of GFR to increase during this peculiar period in renal development is that renal blood flow is distributed primarily to the juxtamedullary cortex. Studies in the dog have demonstrated total renal blood flow in the puppy is low at birth, but increases and redistributes to the outer cortex during the second week of postnatal life (15). Micropuncture of superficial nephrons of the dog is not possible before two weeks of age because superficial tubular structures are collapsed and become identifiable only during the third week (16). The developmental increase in renal blood flow depends on a decrease in renal vascular resistance (17), and this occurs paradoxically as systemic vascular resistance is increasing and as blood volume and plasma renin activity are decreasing. Prostaglandin synthesis, measured primarily as prostacyclin, was noted to be increased in puppies at birth and to decrease with postnatal age (18). It is possible that the lower systemic vascular resistance and higher renal vascular resistance at birth can be explained, in part, by increased prostaglandin synthesis in the fetus which not only causes vasodilatation but also stimulates renin release. Studies in newborn infants (19) and puppies (20) have demonstrated a direct relationship between GFR and blood pressure. An increment in GFR following birth, however, is dependent not only on an increase in systemic blood pressure, but also on a decrease in renal vascular resistance.

More recent studies of renal function in human infants contradict some conclusions of earlier studies. For example, urine flow rate in the fetus remains ~10ml/kg/hr between 30 and 40 weeks gestation (21). Moreover, an appropriate response by the newborn kidney to changes in endogenous vasopressin secretion has been observed (22). When preterm and fullterm infants were deprived of fluid for the first 72 hours of life, relative urine volumes were higher on the first day in the least mature infants, but decreased to become similar to that of more mature infants by 72 hours (23); urine flow rate in these infants varied inversely with urinary osmolality. In fact, the highest urinary osmolality exhibited was in the smallest infant. The amount of sodium, potassium, chloride and nitrogen excreted in the urine also was greater in the premature than in fullterm infants. When sodium balance in preterm infants was compared with plasma sodium concentration, FE_{Na} was <1.0% regardless of gestational age in those who were conserving water. However, in infants whose urine flow rates were higher, FE_{Na} remained <1.0% when plasma sodium concentration was <135 mEq/L but varied directly with plasma sodium concentrations >135 mEq/L (24). During osmotic diuresis, FE_{Na} was high regardless of plasma sodium concentration or urine flow rate. When compared with plasma osmolality in the same preterm infants, FE_{Na} was minimal when plasma osmolality was <270 mOsm/kg and increased as plasma osmolality increased; the most pronounced increases in FE_{Na} were observed when the infant was undergoing osmotic diuresis and least when the infant excreted a concentrated urine--these must be considered appropriate, perhaps even "mature" responses by the neonatal kidney. In a recent study, infants <1250 grams were given two fluid regimens during the first week of life so that a daily weight loss of 1.5% or 3% occurred; no difference in morbidity or outcome between groups was observed (25). However, infants given more fluid required supplemental sodium to maintain plasma sodium concentration within the normal range, while infants given less fluid required little or no additional sodium to maintain balance. It would appear that no conclusion regarding renal sodium handling in premature infants can be made unless the variables of fluid intake and urinary osmolarity have been considered.

The inability of the neonatal kidney to excrete a sodium load has been attributed in part to the higher plasma aldosterone concentrations and Na-K-ATPase activity in the distal nephron (26). Puppies in the first and third weeks of life were able to excrete only 10% of an intravenous sodium load within a two-hour period compared with 50% by the adult kidney; however, 2-week-old puppies were able to excrete up to 30% of the sodium chloride administered--more than either 1- or 3-week olds, suggesting that sodium excretion is not a developmental change only, but rather an interplay of additional factors. Moreover, it is unlikely that the higher plasma aldosterone concentrations can account for all factors that determine sodium excretion by the newborn kidney because an inverse relationship between plasma aldosterone concentration and the urinary sodium:potassium ratio in newborn infants has been noted (27). One must conclude, therefore, that aldosterone may not be maximally effective in facilitating sodium reabsorption in the neonatal kidney. When the renal excretion of an intravenous load of sodium chloride in dogs was studied, physiologic saline produced no change in plasma osmolality, but extracellular fluid volume increased (28). Plasma protein concentration was diluted, however, and a fluid shift from the vascular to the interstitial space was measured; plasma volume and mean arterial blood pressure actually decreased after saline loading. It had been assumed previously that administration of isotonic saline would increase plasma volume. Nearly identical findings were reported for fetal lambs (29). When the amount of sodium excreted by the puppy was compared to changes in blood pressure which followed saline loading, it was observed that, regardless of the age of the puppy, sodium was excreted in a mature fashion when blood pressure increased; whereas, when blood pressure decreased, sodium excretion by the kidney at every age was reduced below the expected adult response (28).

In another study of puppies between birth and maturity, glomerulo-tubular balance for glucose was reported to obtain from birth when changes in extracellular fluid volume were avoided (30). When puppies were given 20 ml/kg of normal saline intravenously, glucose reabsorption decreased and glomerulo-tubular imbalance was induced. Measurement of glucose reabsorption following excretion of the saline load saw a return of glomerulo-tubular balance for glucose. Glomerulo-tubular balance for glucose has been reported also for human infants (9,31). Tubular reabsorption of beta-2-microglobulin, another marker advocated for determining maturation of tubular function, decreased as fractional urine flow rate (V/GFR) increased in human neonates (11)--just as observed in adult dogs (32). This observation was independent of the conceptional age of the infant. Glomerulo-tubular imbalance in the neonatal kidney, therefore, can result from factors other than renal development.

The urinary excretion rate of prostaglandins has been found to increase with the maturity of the infant (33). When factored for body weight or urinary creatinine excretion, however, prostaglandin excretion was related inversely to the gestational age of the infant. Speculation as to whether or not the higher prostaglandin excretion rates in newborns have physiologic significance for developmental renal physiology may find support from observations made in children with Bartter's syndrome, a condition in which prostaglandin synthesis is increased. In infants $\leq$30 weeks gestation, urinary PGE_2 and 6keto$PGF_{1}\alpha$ excretion was similar to values measured in an older infant with Bartter's syndrome (24). Similarities in renal function between premature infants and patients with Bartter's syndrome include higher fractional excretions of sodium and potassium, inability to concentrate urine and decreased pressor response to angiotensin II (34). A review of reported observations for the effects of various prostaglandins on renal sodium excretion in mammals found PGE_2 to effect a naturiesis (35). Moreover, furosemide increased urinary prostaglandin excretion in preterm infants and was accompanied by naturiesis, diuresis and increases in PRA, plasma aldosterone concentration and urinary aldosterone excretion (36). In the human adult, furosemide increased the urinary excretion of 6keto$PGF_{1}\alpha$ and sodium, and increased plasma renin activity (37). In addition, prostaglandins can interfere with the renal concentrating mechanism by inhibiting sodium chloride transport in the ascending thick limb of the loop of Henle, by decreasing urea reabsorption in the collecting tubules and by antagonizing adenylcyclase activity to prevent any increases in permeability of epithelial cells--all factors decrease medullary tonicity and the ability of the kidney to concentrate the urine. Moreover, prostaglandins can increase blood flow through the vasa recta and wash out the medullary gradient to decrease medullary tonicity and further impair urinary concentrating ability. Angiotensin II, in increasing doses, can stimulate prostaglandin synthesis by epithelial cells, and when prostaglandin synthesis is inhibited, angiotensin II has a much more potent vasoconstrictor effect on the renal vasculature (35).

We have concluded from these observations that it is possible for the increased biosynthesis of vasodilator prostaglandins in the fetus and neonate compared to the adult to explain some of the paradoxical observations in developmental physiology, i.e., higher cardiac output relative to body weight; lower heart rate when systemic vascular resistance is low; lower blood pressure when plasma renin activity and angiotensin II are increased; attenuated pressor responses to angiotensin II, vasopressin, catecholamines and volume expansion; persistent fetal circulation when systemic vascular resistance is low and pulmonary vascular resistance is high; edema formation at a time after birth when diuresis and weight loss are observed commonly; negative sodium chloride balance when aldosterone is high, higher fractional urine flow rates; lower urinary osmolalities; high renal vascular resistance when systemic vascular resistance is low; and distribution of renal blood flow primarily to juxtamedullary nephrons.

REFERENCES

1. Barnett, H.L.: Kidney function in infants and children. Pediatrics 5: 171, 1950.

2. Dean, R.F.A. and McCance, R.A.: The renal responses of infants and adults to the administration of hypertonic solutions of sodium chloride and urea. J. Physiol. 109: 81, 1949.

3. Ames, R.G.: Urinary water excretion and neurohypophysial function in full term and premature infants shortly after birth. Pediatrics 12: 272, 1953.

4. Polacek, E., Vocel, J., Neugebauerova, L., et al.: The osmotic concentrating ability in healthy infants and children. Arch. Dis. Child. 40: 291, 1965.

5. Edelmann, C.M., Jr.: Maturation of the neonatal kidney. Proc. 3rd Int. Congr. Nephrol., Washington 1966, vol. 3. Basel: Karger, 1967, pp. 1-12.

6. Siegel, S.R. and Oh, W.: Renal function as a marker of human fetal maturation. Acta Paediatr. Scand. 65: 481, 1976.

7. Engelke, S.C., Shah, B.L., Vasan, U. et al.: Sodium balance in very low-birth-weight infants. J. Pediatr. 93: 837, 1978.

8. Edelmann, C.M., Jr. and Spitzer, A.: The maturing kidney. J. Pediatr. 75: 509, 1969.

9. Arant, B.S., Jr.: Developmental patterns of renal functional maturation compared in the neonate. J. Pediatr. 92: 705, 1978.

10. Al-Dahhan, J., Haycock, G.B., Chantler, C. et al.: Sodium homeostasis in term and preterm neonates. I. Renal aspects. Arch. Dis. Child. 58: 335, 1983.

11. Engle, W.D. and Arant, B.S., Jr.: Renal handling of beta-2-microglobulin in the human neonate. Kidney Int. 24: 358, 1983.

12. Arant, B.S., Jr., Edelmann, C.M., Jr. and Nash, M.A.: The renal reabsorption of glucose in the developing canine kidney; a study of glomerulotubular balance. Pediatr. Res. 8: 638, 1974.

13. Potter, E.L. and Thierstein, S.T.: Glomerular development in the kidney as an index of fetal maturity. J. Pediatr. 22: 695, 1943.

14. Horster, M., Kemler, B.J. and Valtin, H.: Intracortical distribution of number and volume of glomeruli during postnatal maturation in the dog. J. Clin. Invest. 50: 796, 1971.

15. Aschinberg, L.C., Goldsmith, D.I., Olbing, H. et al.: Neonatal changes in renal blood flow distribution in puppies. Am. J. Physiol. 228: 1453, 1975.

16. Horster, M. and Valtin, H.: Postnatal development of renal function: micropuncture and clearance studies in the dog. J. Clin. Invest. 50: 779, 1971.

17. Gruskin, A.B., Edelmann, C.M., Jr. and Yuan, S.: Maturational changes in renal blood flow in piglets. Pediatr. Res. 4: 7, 1970.

18. Arant, B.S., Jr., Terragno, N.A. and Terragno, D.A.: Effect of changing plasma volume on blood pressure and prostaglandins in neonatal puppies. Fed. Proc. 38: 359, 1979.

19. Fawer, C-L., Torrado, A. and Guignard, J-P.: Maturation of renal function in full-term and premature neonates. Helv. paediatr. Acta 34: 11, 1979.

20. Kleinman, L.I. and Lubbe, R.J.: Factors affecting the maturation of glomerular filtration rate and renal plasma flow in the new-born dog. J. Physiol. 223: 395, 1972.

21. Wladimiroff, J.W. and Campbell, S.: Fetal urine-production rates in normal and complicated pregnancy. Lancet 1: 151, 1974.

22. Fisher, D.A., Pyle, H.R., Jr., Porter, J.C. et al.: Control of water balance in the newborn. Am. J. Dis. Child. 106: 137, 1963.

23. Hansen, J.D.L. and Smith, C.A.: Effects of withholding fluid in the immediate postnatal period. Pediatrics 12: 99, 1953.

24. Arant, B.S., Jr.: Renal disorders of the newborn infant. In Tune, B.M., Mendoza, S.A., Brenner, B.M. et al. (eds.): Contemporary Issues in Nephrology: Pediatric Nephrology. New York: Churchill-Livingstone, 1984, p. 111.

25. Lorenz, J.M., Kleinman, L.I., Kotagal, U.R. et al.: Water balance in very low-birth-weight infants: relationship to water and sodium intake and effect on outcome. J. Pediatr. 101: 423, 1982.

26. Spitzer, A.: The role of the kidney in sodium homeostasis during maturation. Kidney Int. 21: 539, 1982.

27. Raux-Eurin, M.C., Pham-Huu-Trung, M.T., Marrec, D. et al.: Plasma aldosterone concentrations during the neonatal period. Pediatr. Res. 11: 182, 1977.

28. Arant, B.S., Jr.: Effects of changing plasma volume and osmolarity on sodium excretion by the neonatal kidney. Pediatr. Res. 12: 538, 1978.

29. Brace, R.A.: Fetal blood volume responses to intravenous saline solution and dextran. Am. J. Ob. Gyn. 147: 777, 1983.

30. Arant, B.S., Jr.: Glomerulotubular balance following saline loading in the developing canine kidney. Am. J. Physiol. 4: F417, 1978.

31. Brodehl, J., Franken, A. and Gellissen, K.: Maximal tubular reabsorption of glucose in infants and children. Acta Pediatr. Scand. 61: 413, 1972.

32. Hall, P.W., Chung-Park, M., Vacca, C.V. et al.: The renal handling of beta-2-microglobulin in the dog. Kidney Int. 22: 156, 1982.

33. Arant, B.S., Jr., Stapleton, F.B., Engle, W.D. et al.: Urinary prostaglandin excretion rates and renal function in human infants at birth. Pediatr. Res. 16:317A, 1982.

34. Siegel, S. R.: Decreased vascular and increased adrenal and renal sensitivity to angiotensin II in the newborn lamb. Circ. Res. 48: 34, 1981.

35. Dunn, M.J.: Renal prostaglandins. In Dunn, M.J. (ed.): Renal Endocrinology. Baltimore: Williams and Wilkins, 1983, p 1.

36. Sulyok, E., Varga, F., Nemeth, M. et al.: Furosemide-induced alterations in the electrolyte status, the function of renin-angiotensin-aldosterone system, and the urinary excretion of prostaglandins in newborn infants. Pediatr. Res. 14: 765, 1980.

CONTINUOUS AMBULATORY PERITONEAL DIALYSIS IN INFANTS AND CHILDREN

Edward C. Kohaut, M.D. and Diane Appell, R.N.

In 1923 Putman[1] demonstrated the peritoneum to be a dialyzing membrane and in the same year Ganter[2] first attempted to treat patients with acute renal failure with peritoneal dialysis. Because of numerous complications, use of the procedure was discontinued until 1946, when it was successfully performed on a number of adults with acute renal failure by Seligman and others.[3,4] In 1949 Swan and Gordon[5] reported the use of peritoneal lavage in 5 children with anuria. Stimulated by the work of Grollman[6] and Houck,[7] intermittent peritoneal dialysis (IPD) was used frequently for the treatment of adults with acute renal failure in the 1950s. In the early 1960s reports by Segar et al.[8] and Etteldorf et al.[9] popularized this form of therapy in children.

In 1967 Levin and Winklestein[10] reported the first use of IPD in the treatment of a pediatric patient with chronic renal failure; however, due to lack of a permanent peritoneal access, repeated punctures were required and dialysis was only done monthly in conjunction with vigorous dietary management, which was the main mode of therapy. The development of a chronic peritoneal access device by Palmer, which was refined by Tenckhoff,[11] coupled with the development of automated cycling machines by Boen,[12] provided the capability to treat patients with chronic renal failure with IPD. In 1968 Counts and colleagues[13] initiated an IPD program in children and since then other authors[14-16] have described similar programs.

DEVELOPMENT OF CAPD

In 1976 Popovich et al.[17] first described a new form of peritoneal dialysis. The authors recognized that the peritoneal membrane was inefficient, but demonstrated that if dialysis was done continuously, adequate dialysis could be obtained. They then designed a system that was wearable and portable so that convenient, continuous dialysis could be provided. This form of dialysis reached prominence in 1978 after the publication of the combined experience of doctors Moncrief and Nolph.[18]

Early in the development of CAPD, both Oreopoulos[19] and Popovich[20] predicted that it would be a valuable tool in the treatment of the pediatric patient with chronic renal failure. In 1980 the first preliminary reports of the use of CAPD in children appeared in abstract form.[21,22] In 1981 more extensive experience was reported[23,24] and in the following year Baum et al.[25] presented definitive data demonstrating that CAPD was an attractive alternative to hemodialysis in the pediatric population.

CHRONIC PERITONEAL ACCESS

Many pediatric centers implant chronic (Tenckhoff) catheters for both temporary and chronic peritoneal access. However, rather than utilizing the original Trocar technique, the catheter is usually placed surgically utilizing a procedure similar to that described by Alexander and Tank.[26] This procedure is carried out in the operating room under sterile conditions. The key to this procedure is a purse-string suture that is placed around the peritoneal cuff securing the catheter to the peritoneum. This assures an adequate peritoneal seal. Originally these authors utilized a two-cuffed catheter; however, due to a high incidence of erosion of the subcutaneous cuff the procedure was modified to use only the peritoneal cuff. Whether a subcutaneous cuff is needed remains controversial. Vugneaux et al.[27] also support the use of a single peritoneal cuff in children. Some fear that elimination of the subcutaneous cuff may lead to an increase in tunnel infections. Originally, the catheter was placed in the mid-line. However, many centers now place the catheter through the lateral edge of the rectus muscle. This seems to have further reduced the incidence of dialysate leakage.

Catheter outflow obstruction due to omental wrap is a significant cause of catheter failure.[28] Although data are not available, it seems to be more common in the pediatric population. Alexander and Tank[26] have reduced this complication by excising a window in the omentum and directing the catheter through the window so that the catheter is well below the omentum. Others have performed omentectomies at the time of catheter insertion. Various modifications to Tenckhoff catheter have been made in an attempt to eliminate omental wrap as a complication. These include: the coiled Tenckhoff, the Toronto western catheter, and finally the Ash column-disc catheter. Further experience with these catheters is required to assess their efficacy in children. Another common cause of catheter failure is obstruction with fibrin. This may occur when a patient develops peritonitis, and it can be avoided if heparin is added to the dialysate when peritonitis is present.

DIALYSIS SOLUTIONS

During the development of CAPD in children a number of innovative procedures were required to adapt this method to smaller patients. At first dialysate was only available in 2 liter bottles, even those individuals treating adults were required to transfer solutions into bags. The small volumes required for the pediatric patient were transferred from the larger bottles to small bags by either the hospital pharmacy[29] or at home by the parents.[30] This increased the cost of the procedure[29] as well as the chance of dialysate contamination. In July of 1980 dialysate became available in 500 cc. and 1000 cc. bags as well as the standard two liter bag. This stimulated more widespread use of this procedure in the pediatric patient. Dialysate has since become available in 250 cc., 750 cc., and 1500 cc. bags. Most patients can now be treated with commercially available standard solutions. In August of 1982 a service was introduced (Baxter-Travenol) that provides patient specific volumes on a prescription basis, making it possible to dialyze any size patient with safely prepared solutions.

Standard solutions have always been used in the young patient on CAPD. In 1982 it was found that many patients on CAPD, both adults and children, had low or low normal serum bicarbonate and mildly elevated serum magnesium.[31] A new solution was, therefore, formulated which had a lower magnesium content and higher lactate concentration.

There is considerable interest in formulating a dialysate with an osmotic agent other than glucose. Amino-acid solutions have been utilized.[32] This may have advantages especially in the pediatric patient where maintainance of nitrogen balance is critical. However, the cost of such a dialysate may be prohibitive for general use.

ULTRAFILTRATION

It has been reported that the ultrafiltration rate in small infants is less than that of adults and older children during long-dwell dialysis.[33] Ultrafiltration in peritoneal dialysis is directly related to the magnitude of the osmotic gradient across the peritoneal membrane and the length of time the gradient exists. Due to glucose absorption from the dialysate, the osmotic gradient falls with increasing dwell time. Increased ultrafiltration can be produced with shorter dwell times. Therefore, with IPD this problem was not noted in small infants.[34] However, it was a problem with the longer dwell times used in CAPD in infants.[33]

When CAPD was initiated in children, the dialysate volume used was extrapolated from adult experience. Therefore, if a 70 kg adult required a 2000 cc. dialysate volume, a child would require about 28 cc./kg. Thus, initially a dialysate volume of 20 to 35 cc./kg was recommended. However, the peritoneal surface area does not have a linear correlation with weight. Putiloff[35] in 1884, and more recently Esperanca and Collins,[36] performed direct measurements of the peritoneal surface area. Both authors found that infants had more than twice the peritoneal surface area per unit weight than adults. Increased surface area led to an increased peritoneal efficiency as demonstrated by increased urea clearances.[36] Presumably this increased efficiency gives rise to increased glucose reabsorption, decreased osmotic gradient, and reduced ultrafiltration. If the dialysate volume for an infant is extrapolated by surface area (2000 cc./1/73m2) or (1200 cc./m2) rather than weight, then the fall in osmotic gradient related to time approximates that seen in the adult patient[37] Studies comparing peritoneal clearance of puppies and adult dogs suggest that the increase in efficiency is due not only to the increased surface area, but also to other factors unique to the peritoneal membrane of the young animal.[38] However, further studies in young children suggest that the area permeability product may be less than an adult when scaled for body weight.[39] One possible explanation for this discrepancy is that the children studied in the latter study were older than the patients previously studied.[37] The difference between dialysate volumes calculated by weight or surface area becomes less significant as the patient increases in size.

RESULTS OF CAPD IN CHILDREN

Determining actuarial patient or procedure survival for CAPD in children is difficult since most pediatric dialysis units treat patients a relatively short time prior to transplantation. Baum et al.[25] noted that short term actuarial survival of CAPD patients was no different than a similar group treated with hemodialysis. In a survey of four pediatric centers, Alexander[40] found survival rates on CAPD to be higher than a population of children on hemodialysis reported by the EDTA.

The complications associated with CAPD are significant: peritonitis is seen at a rate of 1.7 episodes per patient year[41]. The organisms most often associated with peritonitis are similar to those encountered in adults, namely Staph epidermitis, Staph aureus and Alpha strep.[24] Occasionally peritonitis is associated with gram negative organisms and rarely Candida. The diagnosis of peritonitis is most commonly made by the caretaker who notes the dialysate drainage is cloudy. Rarely, patients have presented with abdominal pain and/or fever prior to noting cloudy dialysate. Therapy is immediately instituted by adding Cefazolin (200 mg./L) and Gentamycin (8 mg./L) to the dialysate. Patients rarely require hospitalization as many have minimal or no symptoms. We do admit most of the patients with peritonitis who are less than 1 year of age, as we have found that many will have reduced intakes and require gavage feedings to prevent rapid protein depletion. Antibiotics are adjusted dependent on the culture results and treatment is continued for seven days. If the dialysate does not clear in three days despite appropriate antibiotic therapy, the catheter may have to be removed. If the patient has rebound peritonitis (cloudy fluid developing soon after antibiotics are discontinued) with the same organism, the catheter is probably infested and replacement indicated.

Exit site infection is less common in our experience, since we have used single cuff catheters. The diagnosis is apparent when an exudate is found at an inflammed catheter exit site. Cultures are taken and usually an anti-staphlococcal penecillin is started pending culture results. This complication, as an isolated event, is usually not significant, however, it may lead to catheter tunnel infections and/or peritonitis with possible loss of the catheter.

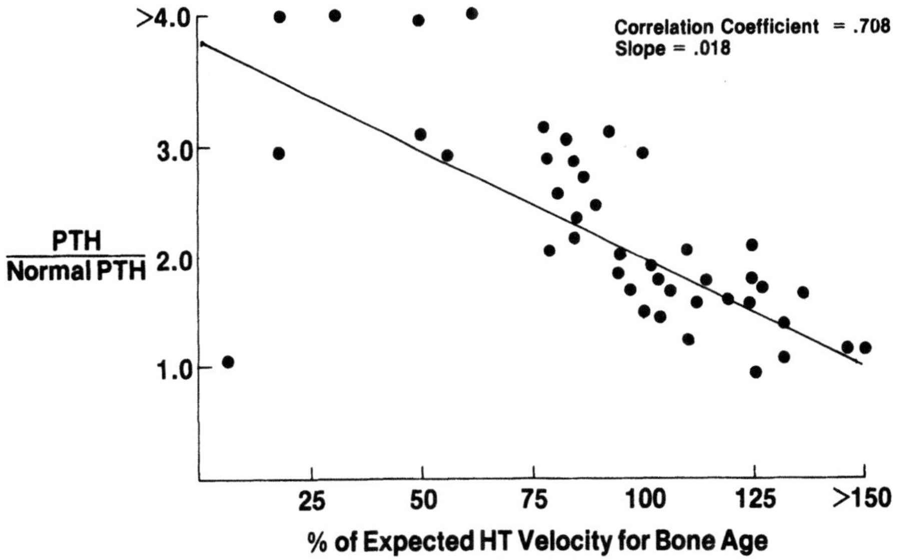

FIGURE 1. Parathormone (PTH) assays were done monthly. Each data point represents an average of three monthly measurements. Since the type of PTH assay changed during the study period, PTH is expressed as a ratio of actual/normal. A correlation coefficient of .708 demonstrates a significant correlation between growth and control of secondary hyperparathyroidism.

Hyponatremia has been noted in our population due both to inadequate ultrafiltration and net sodium loss. Many of our infants have required sodium supplements to maintain normal serum sodiums. Since caloric intake is essential, we do not want to limit oral fluids. Therefore, we must have relatively high rates of ultrafiltration. The loss of sodium in the dialysate cannot be equaled by the relatively small amount of sodium in the formula. Many of the infants have reached end stage renal failure secondary to lesions commonly associated with renal sodium wastage. This group of patients has a higher incidence of hyponatremia. Hyponatremia associated with weight gain is more often seen in our older patients and is reversed by increased ultrafiltration.

Hypokalemia is a frequent complication of CAPD. This is also seen in adults on this mode of therapy and is poorly understood.[18] The patients with the most significant hypokalemia are usually those with the poorest protein intakes.

Hypovolemia can be a lethal complication of CAPD. This is a particularly difficult problem in infants. If the infant becomes anorexic, developes diarrhea, or vomiting, we would advise either gavage feeding at home or hospitalization. An alteration of the dialysis schedule may be indicated. Even if the patient does not progress to shock, during a period of

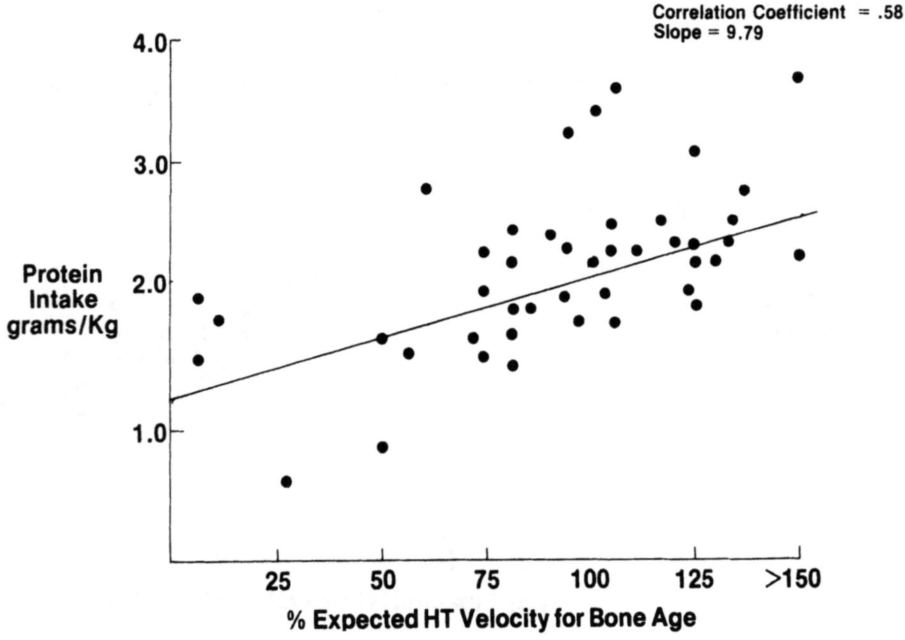

FIGURE 2. Protein intake was assessed in a similar manner as caloric intake. Protein intake in grams/Kg is plotted against growth. A statistically significant correlation coefficient of .58 is reached.

anorexia or gastroenteritis, he may start a downhill course which resulting in protein depletion and a prolonged period of poor growth.

Other complications of CAPD include hernias, both incisional and inguinal, persistant dialysate leak and "parent burnout"[41]. The demands placed on the parents of children, and especially infants, on CAPD are numerous. They not only have to do the bag changes, but perform all the usual tasks a parent needs to provide. The pressure placed on these parents to assure adequate intake to a child that may not be hungry are frustrating. Many of our parents are also taught to pass N-G tubes for feeding. To help avoid "burnout", we have always attempted to train both parents, as well as an alternate caretaker when possible, however, at the end of a year our parents are very anxious for the child to receive a transplant.

Patients on CAPD appear to have better control of azotemia, hypertension and anemia than their peers on hemodialysis[24]. This may not be true of renal bone disease. The CAPD procedure itself does not appear to have any beneficial effect on

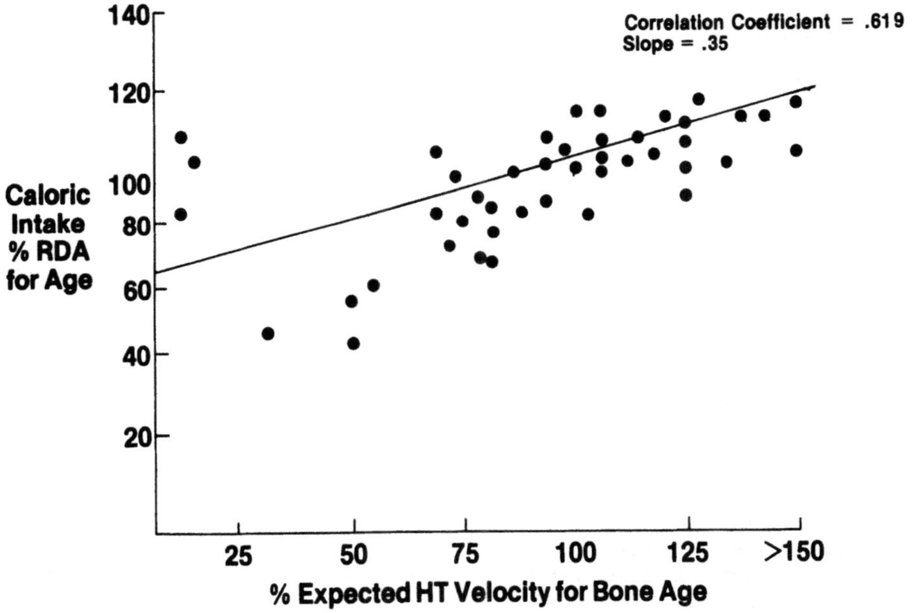

FIGURE 3. Caloric intake expressed as a percent of RDA for age is plotted against growth. Each data point represents an average of three monthly evaluations. Three day diet diaries were used for this study. A significant relationship between these factors is demonstrated by a correlation coefficient of .619.

secondary hyperparathyroidism[41], which is one measure of renal bone disease. In fact, because of the demand for increased protein intake, which increases phosphate intake, hyperphosphatemia may be more difficult to control. Also, long dwell dialysis results in increased loss of certain metabolites of vitamin D[42] resulting in increased supplementation. However, with aggressive therapy with phosphate binders and 1,25 dihydroxycholecalciferol parathormone levels may approach normal[43].

GROWTH AND NUTRITION

Growth failure in patients with renal insufficiency and end stage renal failure has been well documented. Patients treated with hemodialysis rarely will have normal growth[44,45]. The initial reports from centers who have evaluated growth in their CAPD populations are encouraging. Growth rates from four centers are summarized in the following table.

Author	PATIENTS	HEIGHT VELOCITY 100% or greater	% OF EXPECTED 70-100%	<70%
Stefanidis[46]	17	6	6	5
Kohaut[43]	11	4	5	2
Baum[25]	6	average growth 83% of expected		
Salusky[47]	21	average growth near normal		

In an attempt to discover why some of our patients grew well and others did not, we broke the time our patients were on therapy down into three month patient periods. We then measured various biochemical and nutritional parameters and correlated these to height velocity. Height velocity correlated best with control of secondary hyperparathyroidism (Figure 1). There was a positive correlation with protein and energy intake (Figure 2, 3). There was also a weak correlation with control of acidosis. We concluded that patients with end stage renal failure on CAPD could grow normally if parathormone levels were controlled to at least twice normal, that protein intake exceed 2 grams/Kg, and energy intake exceed 100% of RDA for age[42].

The effect CAPD might have on other factors which may effect growth, such as vitamins and trace elements in unknown. One infant in our program developed clinical zinc deficiency. Since that time we have supplemented diets of infants with a trace element packet similar to those provided patients on total parenteral nutrition.

INFANTS TREATED WITH CAPD

The aggressive treatment of young infants with renal failure bring to the surface as many social and moral questions as it does questions pertinent to their therapy. Betts and

McGath[48] gathered data which demonstrated that those patients born with renal insufficiency have very poor growth in the first year or two of life, and then grow at a near normal rate through childhood. If "catch-up" growth is not possible, it follows that children left untreated early will remain small despite later therapy. Rotundo et al.[49] followed twenty-three patients with renal insufficiency in the first year of life and found that twenty had serious and permanent neurological dysfunction in follow-up. These data suggest that if normal growth and neurological function is to be maintained, then therapy for renal insufficiency should be early and aggressive. However, enthusiasm for early therapy must be weighed against the social, emotional and financial cost incurred. This is especially true at this point, since we cannot be sure early therapy will prevent the above complications. Our approach to this problem has been to first provide the patient with aggressive nutritional support coupled with routine medical management. If the patient does not thrive with this approach the parents are educated in CAPD and given the option to place their child on this form of therapy.

Therapy for the infant on CAPD is basically similar to that of the older child and adult with some notable exceptions. Since the infant cannot reach a fluid source unaided, his thirst mechanism is not operational, and fluid intake must be controlled. We have had more problems with low intake rather than excessive intake. Therefore, we have a minimum amount of fluids our patients must take each day. If they do not take this, the rest is given by gavage feeding. This minimum is calculated by adding insensible losses, residual urine output and dialysis ultrafiltration. In those patients where residual output is small, we would rather increase ultrafiltration and, thus, preserve caloric intake rather than limiting fluids. As discussed previously, ultrafiltration is often dependent on providing a dialysate volume of 1200 cc./m^2. Often our ability to do this is limited by the patient's respiratory capacity. Infants may require more frequent, shorter dialysis dwell times to effect ultrafiltration. Our older patients with intakes of 2 grams/Kg protein may grow normally, however, many of our infants on CAPD are taking four to six grams/Kg of protein/day. The following is an example of our infant formula prescribed for a 4 Kg baby.

Similac-20 450 cc./day
Three tablespoons of Propac/day
One tablespoon of MCT Oil/day
Four tablespoons of Polycose/day (powder)

	Formula	Propac	MCT Oil	Polycose	Total
Energy, kcal	302	54	116	128	600
Protein, grams	7	16			19

Utilizing this type of formula, we have been successful in meeting the nutritional demands of our infants. What the ideal energy and protein intake of infants on CAPD is not known. Urea nitrogen appearance rates of our patients are consistently lower than one would predict from protein intake[50]. Whether this is because we are not getting reliable dietary intake data, or whether the excess nitrogen is consumed in anabolism is not known. As our patients get older, the caretaker often starts substituting solids for formula. We discourage this as predictably they substitute with a food that has reduced caloric density and lower protein content.

Conley et al.[51] have treated three infants under six months of age with peritoneal dialysis. They have not utilized traditional CAPD, but rather have designed a system using a Y-tubing which allows them to do multiple (7-10) exchanges a day while only entering the system once. This allows the use of lower dialysate volumes and should reduce the incidence of peritonitis. They have provided aggressive nutritional support with constant N-G feedings. Two of these three patients have been successfully transplanted after reaching appropriate size. The third expired. Alexander[52] initiated CAPD in two children at less than six months of age. One is alive on CAPD, the other died. He also advocates constant gavage feedings to maintain adequate intake. The following table combines the above data with our own:

Patients Started on Dialysis <6 months of age	Alive on CAPD	Alive func Graft	Dead
14	4	6	4

This mortality rate of 29% is considerable higher than seen in any other series of older patients treated with chronic peritoneal dialysis. Unfortunately no control data is available. One would assume the mortality rate in a similar group of patients left untreated would be much higher.

The experience of all three centers emphasizes the importance of nutritional management inthe care of the young infant with renal failure. Gavage feedings either constant or intermittent was universal, as was the use of caloric supplements. The patients treated by Conley received 3.5-4.5 grams/Kg of protein, currently our infants are being fed diets with 4-6 grams/Kg of protein.

When our infant CAPD program started, our goal was to have our patients reach 10 Kg prior to transplant. However, two of the four infants transplanted weighed only 8 Kg. They were transplanted early because of "parent burnout". Children who have been on CAPD do as well after renal transplantation as those who have been on hemodialysis[53].

SPECULATIONS

The available data would indicate that it is possible to treat young infants with CAPD. Although the mortality rate is higher than is reported in older children and adults, many patients have done well. Most of the above patients were started on dialysis as a last resort. There are not enough data as yet to state that early dialysis will avoid the complications unique to the infant with renal failure or insufficiency.

Jones et al.[54] assessed growth, body composition and nutritional status in 21 children who had advanced renal failure presenting in the first year of life. Striking similarities were noted when this group was compared to a group of patients with protein-calorie malnutrition. The authors suggested that protein depletion early in life may lead to certain adaptive mechanisms which enable the patient to grow at a near normal rate but limit the possibility of "catch up" growth. If adequate dietary intakes of protein were provided to these infants, possibly early growth failure could be avoided. Mehls et al.[55] demonstrated that the rat with renal failure requires a greater nitrogen and calorie intake to grow than a normal rat. Theoretically we could then avoid early growth failure by providing normal or above normal intakes of protein and calories. However, this may be difficult to do while still maintaining acid-base balance, normal calcium-phosphate metabolism and controlling azotemia. Therefore, dialysis may be required.

Progressive and permanent encephalopathy is another serious complication seen in children who develop renal failure early in life[49]. Although it appears that it is more serious than the encephalopathy noted in children who developed protein-calorie malnutrition in early life, some similarities exist[56]. These data re-emphasize the special nutritional needs of the infant with renal failure or insufficiency. If these needs cannot be met while still controlling fluid and electrolyte status, or if the patient develops uncontrolled uremia, dialysis may be required.

There have been and will continue to be rapid advances in the mechanics of peritoneal dialysis. These advances will further reduce the incidence of infection and make the procedure more convenient. Hopefully, we will also learn more about the unique requirements of the infant with renal failure.

REFERENCES

1. Putnam, J.T.: The living peritoneum as a dialyzing membrane. Am. J. Physiol. 63: 548, 1923.

2. Ganter, G.: Dialysis of blood in living subjects. MMW. 70: 1478, 1923.

3. Seligman, A.M., Frank, H.A., Fine, J.: Treatment of experimental uremia by means of peritoneal irrigation. J. Clin. Invest. 25: 211, 1946.

4. Frank, H.A., Seligman, A.M., Fine, J.: Treatment of uremia after acute renal failure by peritoneal irrigation. JAMA. 130: 703, 1946.

5. Swan, H., Gordon, H.: Peritoneal lavage in the treatment of anuria in children. Pediatrics. 4: 586, 1949.

6. Grollman, A., Turner, L.B., McLean, J.A.: Intermittent peritoneal dialysis in nephrectomized dogs and its application to the human being. Arch. Int. Med. 87: 379, 1951.

7. Houck, C.R.: Problems in maintenance of chronic bilaterally nephrectomized dogs. Am. J. Physiol. 176: 175, 1954.

8. Segar, W.E., Gibson, R.K., Rhomy, R.: Peritoneal dialysis in infants and small children. Pediatrics. 27: 603, 1961.

9. Etteldorf, J.N., Dobbin, W.T., Swenney, M.J., Smith, J.D., Whittington, G.L., Sheffield, J.A., Meadowsn, R.W.: Intermittent peritoneal dialysis in the management of acute renal failure in children. J. Pediatr. 60: 327, 1962.

10. Levin, S., Winklestein, J.A.: Diet and infrequent peritoneal dialysis in chronic anuric uremia. N. Engl. J. Med. 277: 619, 1961.

11. Tenckhoff, H., Schechter, H.: A bacteriologically safe peritoneal access device. Trans. Am. Soc. Artif. Intern. Organs. 14: 181, 1968.

12. Boen, S.T., Moon, C., Curtis, P.K. et al.: Periodic peritoneal dialysis using the repeated puncture technique and an automated cycling machine. Trans. Am. Soc. Artif. Intern. Organs. 10: 409, 1964.

13. Counts, S., Hickman, R., Barbaccio, A. et al.: Chronic home peritoneal dialysis in children. Trans. Am. Soc. Artif. Intern. Organs. 19: 157, 1973.

14. Feldman, W., Balisk, T., Drummond, K.: Intermittent peritoneal dialysis in the management of chronic renal failure in children. Am. J. Dis. Child. 116: 30, 1968.

15. Brouhand, B.H., Berger, M., Cunningham, R.J. et al.: Home peritoneal dialysis in children. Trans. Am. Soc. Artif. Intern. Organs. 25: 90, 1979.

16. Day, R.E., White, R.H.R.: Peritoneal dialysis in children. Arch. Dis. Child. 62: 56, 1977.

17. Popovich, R.P., Moncrief, J.W., Decherd, J.F., Bomar, J.B., Pyle, W.K.: The definition of a novel portable, wearable equilibrium peritoneal dialysis technique. Abstr. Am. Soc. Artif. Intern. Organs. 5: 64, 1976.

18. Popovich, R.P., Moncrief, J.W., Nolph, K.D., Ghods, A. J., Twardowski, Z.J., Pyle, W.K.: Continuous ambulatory peritoneal dialysis. Ann. Intern. Med. 88: 449, 1978.

19. Oreopoulos, D.G.: The coming of age of continuous ambulatory peritoneal dialysis (CAPD). Dial & Trans. 8: 460, 1979.

20. Popovich, R.P., Pyle, W.K., Rosenthal, D.A. et al.: Kinetics of peritoneal dialysis in children. In Moncrief, J.W., and Popovich, R.P. (eds.): CAPD Update. New York: Masson Publishing, USA, 1981, p. 227.

21. Alexander, S.R., Tseng, C.H., Maksym, K.A. et al.: Early clinical experience with continuous ambulatory peritoneal dialysis (CAPD) in infants and children. Clin. Res. 28: 131A, 1980.

22. Oreopoulos, D.G., Katirtzoglou, A., Arbus, G. et al.: Dialysis and Transplantation in young children. Br. Med. J. 1: 1628, 1979.

23. Balfe, J.W., Vigneus, A., Willumsen, J., Hardy, B.E.: The use of CAPD in the treatment of children with end stage renal disease. Perit. Dialy. Bull. 1: 35, 1981.

24. Kohaut, E.C.: Continuous ambulatory peritoneal dialysis: A preliminary pediatric experience. Am. J. Dis. Child. 135: 270, 1981.

25. Baum, M., Powell, D., Calvin, S.: Continuous ambulatory peritoneal dialysis in Children. N.E.J.M. 307: 1537, 1982.

26. Alexander, S.R., Tank, E.S.: Surgical aspects of continuous ambulatory peritoneal dialysis in infants, children, and adolescents. J. Urol. 127: 501, 1982.

27. Vigneaux, A., Hardy, B.E., Balfe, J.W.: Chronic peritoneal catheter in children--one or two cuffs. Perit. Dial. Bull. 1: 151, 1981.

28. Potter, D.E., McDaid, T.K., Ramirez, J.A.: Peritoneal dialysis in children. In Atking, R.C., Thomason, N.M., Farrel, P.C. (eds.): Peritoneal Dialysis. New York: Churchill Livingstone, 1981, p. 356.

29. Shmerling, J., Kohaut, E.C.: Costs and social benefits of CAPD in a pediatric population. In Moncrief, J.W., Popovich, R.P. (eds.): CAPD Update. New York: Masson Publishing, 1981, p. 189.

30. Alexander, S.R., Tseng, C.H., Maksym, K.A., Campbell, R.A., Talwalkar, Y.B., Kohaut, E.C.: Clinical parameters in continuous ambulatory peritoneal dialysis for infants and children. In Moncrief, J.W., Popovich, R.P. (eds.): CAPD Update. New York: Masson Publishing, 1981, p. 211.

31. Kohaut, E.C., Balfe, J.W., Potter, D.E. et al.: Hypermagnesemia and hypocarbia in pediatric patients on CAPD. Perit. Dial. Bull. 3: 41, 1983.

32. Williams, P.F., Marliss, F.B., Anderson, G.H., et al.: Amino acid absorption following intraperitoneal administration in CAPD patients. Perit. Dial. Bull. 3: 124, 1982.

33. Kohaut, E.C., Alexander, S.R.: Ultrafiltration in the young patient on CAPD. In Moncrief, J.W., Popovich, R. P. (eds.): CAPD Update. New York: Masson Publishing, 1981, p. 221.

34. Lorentz, W.B., Hamilton, R.W., Disher, B. et al.: Home peritoneal dialysis during infancy. Clin. Nephrol. 15: 194, 1981.

35. Putiloff, P.: Materials for the study of laws of growth of the human body in relation to the surface areas of different systems: The trial on Russian subjects of plaingraphic anatomy as a means of exact anthropometry--One of the problems of anthropology. Sib. Br. Russian. Geog. Soc. October 29, 1884, Omsk, 1886.

36. Esperanca, M.J., Collins, D.L.: Peritoneal dialysis efficiency in relation to body weight. J. Pediatr. Surg. 1: 162, 1966.

37. Kohaut, E.C.: Effect of dialysate volume on ultrafiltration in small children. Eur. J. Pediatr. 140: 174, 1983.

38. Elzouki, A.Y., Gruskin, A.B., Baluarte, J.H., Polinsky, M.S., Prebis, J.W.: Developmental aspects of peritoneal dialysis kinetics in dogs. Pediatr. Res. 15: 853, 1981.

39. Morgenstern, B., Pyle, W.K., Gruskin, A. et al.: Transport characteristics of the pediatric peritoneal membrane. Proceedings of the A.S.N., 122A, 1983.

40. Alexander, S.R.: Personal communication, 1983.

41. Alexander, S.R.: Pediatric CAPD Update--1983. Perit. Dial. Bull. 3: S15, 1983.

42. Guillot, M., Garabedian, M., Lavocat, C. et al.: Evaluation of 25-hydroxyvitamin D and Vitamin D binding protein losses in thirteen children on continuous ambulatory peritoneal dialysis. Int. J. Pediatr. Nephrol. 4: 99, 1983.

43. Kohaut, E.C.: Growth in children treated with continuous ambulatory peritoneal dialysis. Int. J. Pediatr. Nephrol. 4: 93, 1983.

44. Kleinknecht, C., Broyer, M., Gagnadoux, M. et al.: Growth in children treated with long term dialysis. Ad. in Nephrol. 9: 133, 1980.

45. Chantler, C., Carter, J.E., Bewick, M. et al.: Ten years experience with hemodialysis and renal transplant. Arch. dis. Child. 55: 435, 1980.

46. Stefanidis, C.J., Hewitt, I.K., Balfe, J.W.: Growth in Children receiving continuous ambulatory peritoneal dialysis. J. of Ped. 102: 683, 1983.

47. Salusky, I.B., Fine, R.N., Nelson, P. et al.: Nutritional status of pediatric patients undergoing CAPD. Kid. Int. 21: 177, 1982.

48. Betts, P.R., McGrath, G.: Growth pattern and dietary intake of children with chronic renal insufficiency. Br. Med. J. 2: 189, 1974.

49. Rotundo, A., Nevins, T.E., Lipton, M., Lockman, L.A., Mauer, S.M., Michael, A.F.: Progressive encephalopathy in children with chronic renal insufficiency in infancy. Kid. Int. 21: 486, 1982.

50. Blumenkranzt, M.J., Kopple, J.D., Moran, J.K. et al.: Nitrogen and urea metabolism during continuous ambulatory peritoneal dialysis. Kid. Int. 20: 78, 1981.

51. Conley, S.B., Brewer, E.D., Gandy, S. et al.: Normal growth in very small infants on peritoneal dialysis: 18 months experience. Program and Abstracts, National Kidney Foundation Twelfth Annual Clinical Dialysis and Transplant Forum, Chicago, Ill., p. 8, 1982.

52. Alexander, S.R.: Personal communication, 1984.

53. Balfe, J.W.: Use of CAPD in children prior to transplantation. Proceedings, Second Annual National Conference on CAPD, Kansas City, February 15-17, 1982.

54. Jones, R.W.R., Rigden, S.P., Barratt, T.M. et al.: Growth failure in children with ESRD. Pediatr. Res. 16: 784, 1982.

55. Mehls, O., Ritz, E., Gilli, G. et al.: Nitrogen metabolism and growth in experimental uremia. Int. J. Pediatr. Nephrol. 1: 34, 1980.

56. Dodge, P.R.: Influence of protein-calorie malnutrition on the human nervous system. In Dodge, P.R., Prensky, A.L., Feigin, R.D. (eds.): Nutrition and the developing nervous system. St. Louis: C.V. Mosby, 1975, p. 305.

VI

WORKSHOP

WORKSHOP: CASE PRESENTATIONS AND DISCUSSION

Jose Strauss, M.D., Moderator

MODERATOR: Four cases are going to be presented. I don't know how many of you have been in workshops like this. They are rather unique in that we spend half an hour discussing a case which is intended to bring out some special point. Open and active participation is welcomed. Try to bring out some of the points made in the formal presentations or any other points that you may want to bring in. The first case is to be presented by Dr. Carolyn Abitbol.

DR. ABITBOL: The patient was a 2.3 kg infant born at 34 weeks gestation to a 32 year old gravida 3, para 2, aborta 0, female who had had a 65 pound weight gain during pregnancy. There was also mild gestational hypertension during the pregnancy. Early onset of labor followed spontaneous rupture of membranes. The delivery was uncomplicated and Apgars were 8 at 1 minute and 9 at 5 minutes. He was fed Similac formula and was discharged home at nine days of age with a weight 30 gms less than his birth weight. He was tolerating formula well and gaining weight until 6 weeks of age when he developed a seborrheic type rash over his face and neck and began to lose weight. At nine weeks of age he was admitted to the hospital for evaluation of failure to thrive.

At the time of his admission, BUN was 85 mg/dl, creatinine 1.8 mg/dl, albumin 4.6 g%, sodium 128 mEq/L, potassium 1.8 mEq/L, chloride 100 mEq/L, CO_2 40 mEq/L, hematocrit 28%, hemoglobin 9.5 g%. Stool fat was positive on one occasion. An IVP was normal.

He was treated with ampicillin for suspected sepsis but later was changed to Keflin because he developed a scalp abscess. He was begun on parenteral alimentation after two weeks of hospitalization and persistence of his electrolyte abnormalities. Subsequently, he developed Klebsiella sepsis which required treatment with gentamicin and ampicillin. Blood pressures were reported as normal or low at all times.

At the time of consultation (Fig. 1), physical examination revealed an extremely cachectic, irritable, hypertonic black male infant; weight was 2.0 kg, length 51 cm, BP 70/40 mm Hg, pulse 120 b/min, temperature 96°F. The fontanelle was open and flat. There was a scaling erythematous rash over the calvarium with erythema and periorbital edema; the pharynx was clear; the chest was clear to auscultation. Cardiac examination revealed a grade II/VI systolic ejection murmur at the left lower sternal border; no gallops were audible. The abdomen was soft; the liver was palpable, three cm below the right costal margin; the spleen was not palpable; no masses were palpable. GU Exam: the phallus was circumcised; the scrotum was poorly developed, but rugated; there was one testicle palpated in the right inguinal canal; the left testicle was not palpated. The hips would not abduct due to the patient's hypertonicity; the hands were held clasped closed and when forced open, demonstrated a fungal rash. Neurologically, the patient was opisthotonic but no localizing signs could be demonstrated.

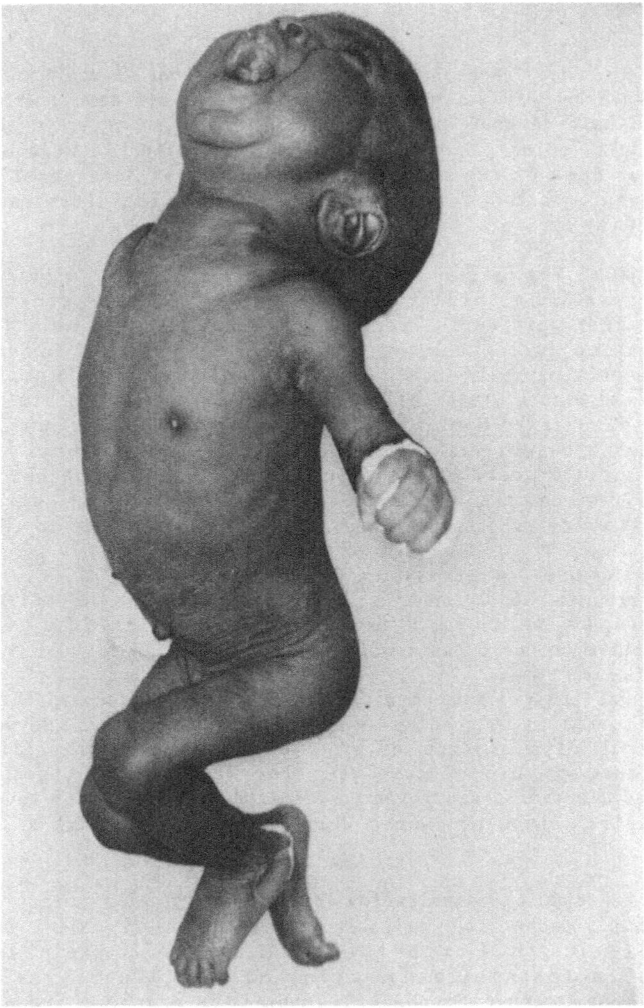

Figure 1

Laboratory data: BUN 44 mg/dl, creatinine 1.5 mg/dl, sodium 128 mEq/L, potassium 2.5 mEq/L, chloride 70 mEq/L, CO_2 38 mEq/L. Urinary sodium > 120 mEq/L, urinary potassium 44 mEq/L, FE_{Na} 17%; plasma renin activity 25 ng/ml/hr, urinary aldosterone 17 ng/day, both of which were elevated above normal values. Urine volume ranged from 480 to 600 ml/day and free water clearance ranged from 2 to 5 ml/min/hr.

The clinical diagnosis of Bartter's Syndrome was made. Renal biopsy was performed at one year of age; a histological section is shown in Figure 2.

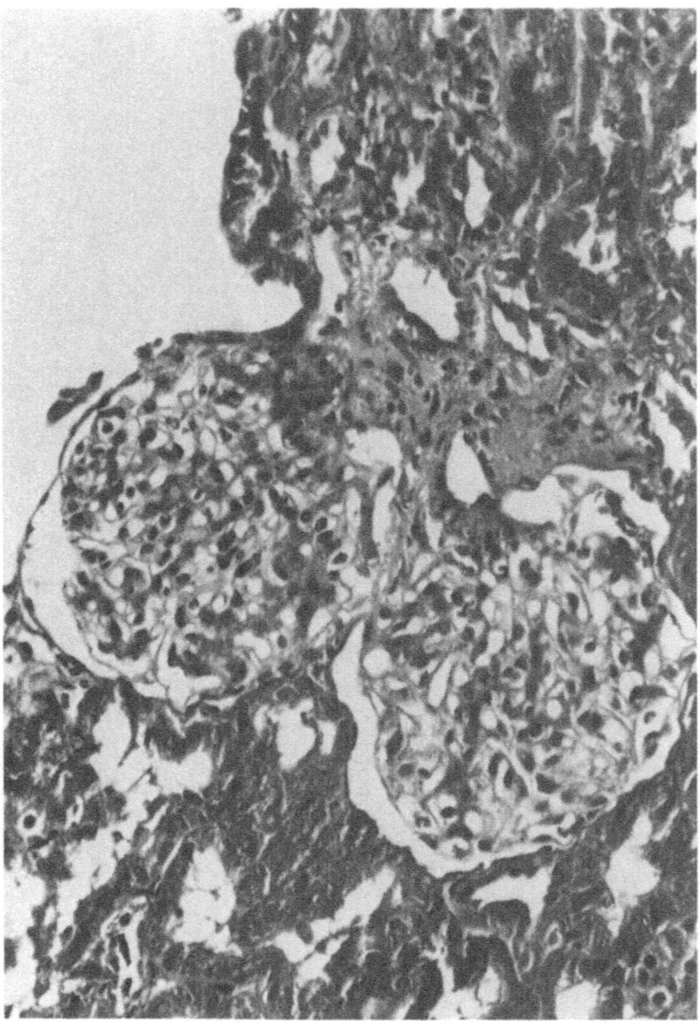

Figure 2

Treatment consisted of potassium chloride in 10% solution by gradual increases in the dose to 15 mEq/kg/day and sodium chloride supplement at 2 mEq/kg/day. Free water and dietary calorie supplements were also provided; free water was forced to one liter per day and calorie intake was increased to 150 - 180 calories/kg/day by adding Polycose and corn oil to the formula. After six months (Fig. 3), the patient had shown excellent catch-up growth with his weight increasing to the 25th percentile and his length to the 10th percentile. With maintenance of all electrolyte supplements and of high free water intake, renal function returned to normal with serum creatinine of 0.5 mg/dl and electrolytes as follows: sodium 144 mEq/L, potassium 3.5 mEq/L, chloride 97 mEq/L, CO_2 30 mEq/L.

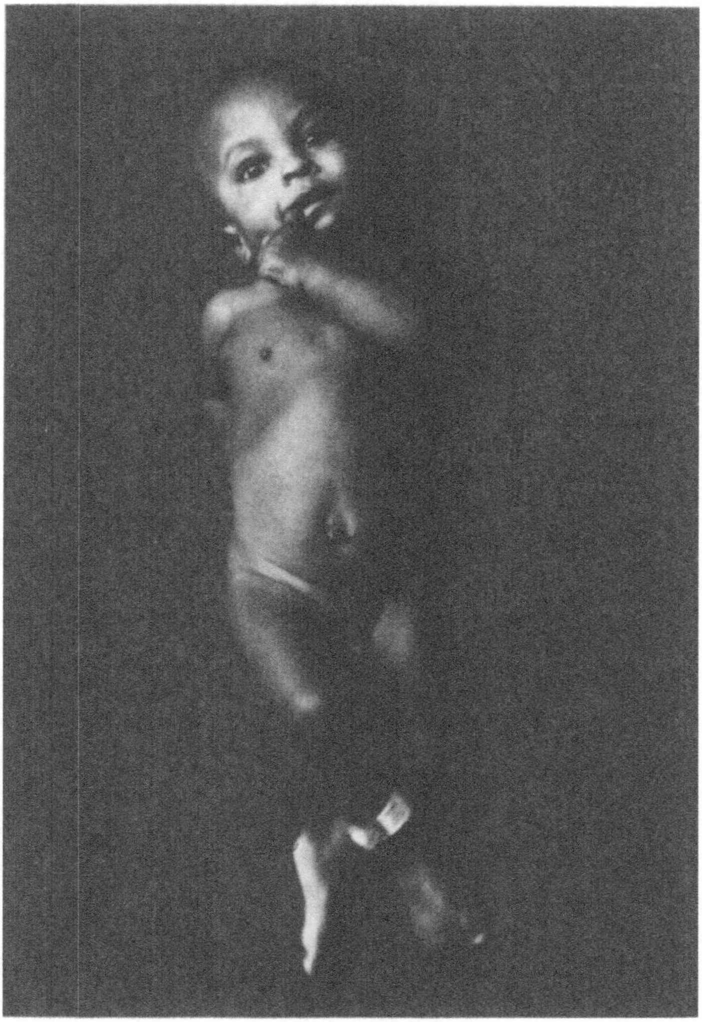

Figure 3

MODERATOR: Thank you Dr. Abitbol. Would the Panelists please join us here for the discussion?

QUESTION: Somewhere along the line was urinary chloride measured?

RESPONSE: Yes.

COMMENT: The things that are of interest are the hypokalemia and hyponatremia at the time of first presentation with a normal serum chloride.

DR. ABITBOL: The chloride was measured on multiple occasions and always exceeded 115 mEq/L. At some point, on one occasion, it was over 200 mEq/L. I did not tell you that in the report; I should have. I don't believe that initial chloride. That is what was reported by the laboratory but it seemed uncanny.

QUESTION: Out of proportion?

RESPONSE: Yes.

QUESTION: When he was begun on Motrin, how rapidly did you see improvement or better control?

RESPONSE: I didn't include that part of his history (which was included in the Case Summary you were given) mainly because he had already shown considerable improvement from his initial supplementary therapy. I became concerned that perhaps he needed some sort of therapy like Motrin. At that point, I decided to use it and I really didn't know what to follow. So, what I did follow were his free water clearances and distal delivery of chloride, if you wish. Those seemed to get better but the follow-up was somewhat sporadic and they were all done on fractional urines or timed urines in the office for one or two hours. I'm not really sure that they really demonstrated response to the therapy.

QUESTION: What were your thoughts on his neurological examination, his hypertonicity in the face of hypokalemia? How do you put that together? Was there something else?

RESPONSE: No. Legitimately, I took a picture of this, or maybe illegitimately. I took this picture before I ever saw his electrolytes. I thought that this was just an extremely malnourished infant. I was asked initially to consult because of his malnutrition and their inability to manage this problem. They had no idea that this was a primary electrolyte problem. So, I thought that this was malnutrition.

QUESTION: In the nine day stay in the hospital, was that just staying with mother or was there a problem at birth, following birth?

RESPONSE: I don't remember. This was at a community hospital. I don't remember the initial circumstances.

COMMENT-QUESTION: I am fascinated by your presentation. There are certain atypical features in your patient. As you may know, another group has reported a series of patients in the American Journal of Diseases of Children, perhaps three years ago, in which they try to differentiate in infants, early onset Bartter Syndrome and late onset Bartter Syndrome. The prognosis for infants with early onset Bartter Syndrome is generally very poor; they just do not do well; they are malnourished. They do not, however, present with the features that you presented: hypertonicity, and susceptibility to infections. So, it could be coincidental; the child could just happen to be more susceptible because of malnutrition. I think you have done extremely well for the patient. As you may know, too, the long term use of prostaglandin inhibitors, in Dr. Bartter's own experience, had not been very good in that, when a patient was treated only with prostaglandin inhibitors, there were escapes from treatment and the hypokalemia returned and few of his patients on a long term basis did well with prostaglandin inhibitors alone. In fact, the treatment of his choice was usually only with potassium supplementation and perhaps spironolactone. He did not, while he was still alive, seem to favor prostaglandin inhibitors nor aspirin because his experience with his fairly large series did not seem to bear out the initial enthusiasm. I am currently following four patients with Bartter's Syndrome, some who were originally of Dr. Bartter's own series. Perhaps not all of you know what happened to the two index cases of Bartter's Syndrome. He went to Georgetown, do you remember? Dr. Bartter reported his two index cases in 1962. I remember those years because that was the time I graduated from medical school. I began reading about his cases in 1964. Little did I know that I would be working with Dr. Bartter towards the end of his tenure at the NIH. One case never returned for follow-up and presumably died of chronic renal insufficiency, probably from interstitial nephritis. Another one, I believe, also died, had a histological examination of the kidney and also showed interstitial nephritis. Of course, the characteristics of the juxtaglomerular apparatus with the hypoplasia have been widely documented. And yours were some of the most beautiful JG apparatus I have seen in a long, long time. Why did the two glomeruli stick together so closely? You must have a nice needle that put them together.

COMMENT-QUESTION: As my colleague has mentioned, some of the clinical features of this patient are somewhat atypical: the seborrheic rash, one or two episodes of septicemia, and the interesting neurological findings, which one does not ordinarily see with hypokalemia, the severe opistotonus. Can we definitely make a diagnosis of Bartter's Syndrome simply based on the fact that they are potassium wasting and that they have hypertrophied J-G apparatus on renal biopsy?

COMMENT: It is always an ongoing debate between those of us who believe in the Bartter's Syndrome and those who think that it is a conglomerate of everything. According to the latest work of Dr. Bartter and his associates, you would need to have a chloride reabsorption defect in the thick ascending loop of Henle in order to establish the syndrome. But not all of us are willing to catheterize a patient and give the standard water loading dose to study the chloride transport. I'm sure you are aware that in the American Society of Nephrology meeting several months ago, there were reports from San Francisco that perhaps water loading and saline loading provide quite divergent results and perhaps call into question some of the initial studies on the syndrome. As I am sure you also are aware, some of us have published data concerning a sodium reabsorption defect also. Some have documented a distal sodium reabsorption defect. I, along with others, have documented a proximal sodium reabsorption defect that overwhelmed the distal tubule; so, if one only studies the distal tubule sodium reabsorption, one could delineate a defect but it could have been due to flooding of the sodium that is not reabsorbed in the proximal tubule. Of course, the study done by Dr. Bartter and his associates was not done with sodium chloride loading, if I remember correctly, and therefore casts doubt on the questions that the San Francisco group is asking about the original series of patients with Bartter's Syndrome. I would accept this as Bartter's Syndrome because you have no other cause for the hypokalemia. For this age it is hard to imagine a fictitious hypokalemia from the use of diuretics which can happen even in very masculine football players; stars on the football field, for some reason, want to take furosemide and induce hypokalemia. It is very difficult to differentiate in those cases. However, in a child of this age, unless one were to invoke that the parents were giving the child furosemide or some other diuretic, it would be hard to imagine why there is potassium wasting, as Dr. Abitbol so nicely documented. But, of course, if there is persistent hypokalemia one can have a concentration defect, one can have the J-G apparatus hyperplasia secondary to persistent hypokalemia. So, it is a process of exclusion which, on the long term follow-up described, I would accept as a case of Bartter's.

COMMENT: He is now six years old and of normal weight and height. He continues to need at least 15 mEq, sometimes 20 mEq/kg/day of potassium. He has required increasing doses of potassium.

COMMENT: The other condition we have to consider is surreptitious vomiting which would give rise to hypochloremia, but that can be easily differentiated if you check the urinary chloride which would then be very, very low. But, again, it is hard to imagine a child this early in life who has surreptitious vomiting.

QUESTION: I had a question on the catch-up growth. If I recall it right, somebody studied the long term effect on growth patterns of children with Bartter's Syndrome. What I gather from the follow-up studies is that it seems that before they reach puberty, no matter what treatment they were on, they were below the fifth percentile. Right after puberty, no matter what treatment they were on, they started to have catch-up growth.

COMMENT: You are correct. That study, which was published in Nephron in 1979, I believe, summarized the experience working with children with Bartter's. However, one must be aware of the study from Toronto where the early onset Bartter's Syndrome really do not do well. I don't believe that the Nephron study separated Bartter's Syndrome into late onset and early onset ones. That study was primarily on the late onset Bartter's Syndrome which are really the cases we saw at the NIH, not early onset ones. It is up to us pediatricians in the community to pick up the early onset Bartter's Syndrome.

MODERATOR: Where do we stand in terms of that proposal that there was an actual linkage between the proximal and distal tubules? At one point in one EM study of a Bartter's patient we thought we saw such a structure. I believe we called Dr. Bartter and discussed that with him. Would you like to comment on that?

COMMENT: There were three pieces of work incomplete at the time of Dr. Bartter's death in May 1983. One was what you mentioned and another was electronmicroscopic findings of the basement membrane which they were working on. The third was the defect in sodium entry into cells; some early data on this were published in the JCI. I hope that they are still working on the syndrome and those of us outside the NIH who are working on the syndrome would cast some light on it. I think that is about the best way in which I can put it.

MODERATOR: Thank you very much. We go now to the next patient, Case #2, which is an interesting comparison--a reverse in some ways--of the first case. That is the case being presented by one of our distinguished Guest Faculty.

CASE PRESENTATION: This is a 24 month old white male infant who was diagnosed as having hyperkalemia at seven weeks of age.

The patient was in his usual state of health until approximately seven weeks of age when he developed persistent vomiting for two days and refusal to feed. He was also noted to have lost weight on the day of admission. Except for a right inguinal hernia, the admission physical examination was grossly normal. On routine blood tests, he was noted to be hyperkalemic. This was confirmed by numerous determinations from non-hemolyzed samples obtained by venopuncture. Except for one CO_2 of 17.6 mEq/L, all serum CO_2 determinations were greater than 21 mEq/L. The BUN and serum creatinine remained within normal limits. A creatinine clearance was performed which was 52 ml/min/1.73m^2 (normal value at seven weeks: < 42-90 ml/min/1.73m^2). The fractional potassium excretion was abnormally low and ranged between 2.4 and 11%, FeNa% was < 1.0%. A renal sonogram was normal. Initial urine and serum aldosterone and plasma renin were normal at this time. Serum aldosterone 130 ng/dl (normal range 30-130 ng/dl); urine aldosterone 5 mcg/24 hours (normal 2-26); and peripheral renin 7.86 ng/ml/hour (normal: mean 6.3 $\pm$ .97 SEM at three months).

The patient was placed on PM 60/40 formula feedings and he was started on furosemide (FEK^+ increased to 22%). He was discharged from the hospital and was followed as an outpatient.

He was readmitted approximately 2 1/2 weeks after discharge for a chlamydia pneumonia and hyperkalemia. He was treated with erythromycin and his furosemide dose was increased. After one week, he was discharged.

Since discharge about two years ago, he has been followed as an outpatient by Pediatric Nephrology. Fractional K^+ excretion has ranged between 14 and 21% and serum K^+ has been 4.3 to 6.0 mEq/L. About 18 months ago, he was admitted for further evaluation. At the time of admission, physical examination was unremarkable. Inulin clearance was 67 ml/min/1.73^2 and creatinine clearance, 66 ml/min/1.73^2 (normal value at eight months: 58 to 160 ml/min/1.73m^2). A 12 hour trial period off furosemide demonstrated a fall in fractional K^+ excretion to 5.9%; after furosemide (2 mg/kg) was given, FEK^+ increased to 29.6%.

He continued to receive furosemide on a daily basis since discharge until about nine months ago, at which time (15 months of age), he was admitted to the hospital to re-evaluate his need for daily furosemide. Two 24 hour urine collections were obtained: during the first collection, the patient was receiving furosemide and during the second collection, he was off furosemide. Since there was no difference in the FEK%, he was maintained off furosemide. Serum aldosterone had decreased to 62 ng/dl; at no time was the patient hyperchloremic.

Since then, his serum potassium has remained between 4.4 and 5.0 mEq/L. He has been doing quite well and has been developing appropriately.

MODERATOR: Any questions?

QUESTION: At seven months of age, the serum aldosterone was 162 whereas the upper limit of normal for your laboratory for serum aldosterone is 130? Does that indicate a hyperaldo at that point? How would you interpret that finding?

RESPONSE: Unfortunately, that was taken at the time that he was on furosemide.

QUESTION: So, he might have had a contracted extracellular volume?

RESPONSE: That's how we interpreted it. Anyway, the reason I am presenting this patient is to try to see if the panel agrees if: 1) this is a pseudo-hyperaldosteronism type two, similar to that described in San Francisco. I don't think so because he is not acidotic; 2) this is a potassium secretory defect per se.

COMMENT-QUESTION: To interpret aldosterone respone to volume contraction, do you have normals to assess how much aldosterone or renin to expect in a normal state after volume contraction? We need that in order to see if we can make some sense of those aldosterone levels. Are they really high? It would be also interesting to relate the aldosterone excretion in 24 hours to the prevailing serum potassium. It has been suggested that we should interpret aldosterone based on the prevailing serum potassium concentration rather than as an isolated figure. But that might be a second point. Do you have some feeling about how much aldosterone you expect in that laboratory--with volume contraction? Two times base line? Three times base line? How much do you expect? I don't have an answer locally and that is one of the questions we have been confronted with. How much renin or aldosterone is expected?

COMMENT: I think that the patient seems to be responsive to changes in volume in the sense that his renin and aldosterone are going parallel on several occasions. The levels you mentioned as normal for serum aldosterone for your laboratory, is that normal for a potassium of 6-7 mEq/L? If plasma potassium concentration is the more potent stimulus to aldosterone secretion, the predominant one, it looks like there is no response to rises in potassium in this particular patient. There seems to be no difficulty in his reabsorbing sodium before, during, or after furosemide. It seems appropriate that somehow sodium is being reabsorbed all along the nephron, but potassium is not being secreted and aldosterones are not appropriately high for the serum potassium concentrations.

COMMENT-QUESTION: That relates to the question I asked this morning about the tubular sensitivity or insensitivity to selected functions. It is interesting that, if we postulate that this patient might have a combination of lack of aldosterone response and mild insensitivity of the tubule to respond to aldosterone specifically (because obviously it does respond to furosemide since fractional excretion of potassium goes up and serum potassium goes down), why does he not lose sodium? Is it only a selective aspect of potassium handling?

RESPONSE: One of the things we could have done would have been to infuse super-normal levels of mineralo-corticoids which we were unwilling to do. I thought at one time that under most circumstances, one of the evidences of aldosterone effect is the ratio of sodium/potassium in the urine. That is, if the sodium/potassium ratio is less than one, usually that will indicate an aldosterone effect. There are certain exceptions: for example, in mineralo-corticoid escape, that does not hold true. So, if you look at the urine sodium/potassium ratio in this patient, except on one occasion, they were all less than one which would be prima facie evidence of aldosterone effect. Therefore, I think that there is enough evidence here that this tubule was responding to aldosterone--may not be as complete as you would like but it was responding.

COMMENT-QUESTION: Could the tubule be in fact responsive to aldosterone but the adrenals not be responsive to hyperkalemia? So that every time this patient got volume depleted for whatever cause, then you would see an aldosterone response but not the aldosterone response that should have been stimulated by his hyperkalemia?

COMMENT-QUESTION: Looking at those urine sodium/potassium ratios, would this degree of avid sodium reabsorption, which may be the result of volume depletion, make it hard to interpret aldosterone effects? If there is very little sodium being delivered, the potassium is not being secreted. You've got low fractional excretion of potassium and you've got high serum potassium levels with normal aldosterone.

REPONSE: That is the point. What happened which is not listed in the report is that the patient got a sodium load but the sodium/potassium ratio was still low. Well, the problem is, is this level high, low, or appropriate for this patient? One thing, though, is that if you go through the definition of hyperaldosteronism, the classic one, you certainly wouldn't call this patient hyperaldosteronemic. He just didn't have high serum levels of aldosterone. So, the questions are: 1) is the amount of aldosterone being secreted appropriate for this serum level of potassium?; and 2) is there adequate response? Since I didn't know aldosterone secretory rates and I don't know how much should be secreted at a particular point in time, I think that the only conclusion you could make from this is that: 1) the aldosterone levels are not low, and 2) the tubule is responding to the aldosterone effect. Because of this, I don't think that you would tend to blame aldosterone secretion or effect but, rather, that the reason that it has very little effect is because the defect in the tubule is primarily a potassium secretory defect. If you want to call that pseudo-hyperaldosteronism, that is ok with me.

COMMENT: But, then, you've got the specific isolated potassium situation and most pseudo-hyperaldosteronisms will have a deviation in the plasma sodium concentration.

RESPONSE: That is exactly the point for this presentation. In the usual pseudo-hyperaldosteronism (Type I) you do have a defect in sodium reabsorption; then, in the pseudo-hyperaldosteronism Type II it is a chloride shunt that is involved but these patients have hyperchloremic acidosis. So, based on these different findings in concert, I don't think that you could blame aldosterone in this patient.

COMMENT: I would agree. We'll just call this "His complex".

RESPONSE: I'm not trying to call this "my syndrome". I know that my boss has his own syndrome of renal alkalosis; he thinks it's different from Bartter's.

MODERATOR: Have we exhausted this case? Let us then go to Case #3 which will be presented by Dr. Michael Freundlich.

DR. FREUNDLICH: This baby is a 33 weeks AGA girl born on November 21, 1983; Apgar's 7 and 8, and birth weight 1520 g. Shortly after delivery, she developed the clinical picture of Hyaline Membrane Disease; an umbilical arterial catheter was placed and antibiotics (ampicillin 200 mg/kg/day and gentamicin 5 mg/kg/day) for suspected sepsis were begun, all of which were dicontinued after 48 hours. Initial blood pressure was 52/29 (mean 42) mmHg by transducer.

By day six of life, she was in room air and blood pressure was 60/54 by Dinamap. Electrolytes were normal, Ca 9.4 mg/dl. That same day the patient developed bradychardia and required assisted ventilation. An umbilical arterial catheter was placed again; BUN was 21 mg/dl and creatinine 1.4 mg/dl. The next day, a loud heart murmur was heard, BP was 100/50 mmHg, and a Patent Ductus Arteriosus (PDA) was diagnosed. The left femoral pulse was diminished; the urine was positive for proteinuria and hematuria. Electrolytes remained stable (serum potassium 4.3 mEq/L, CO_2 24 mEq/L).

On day 10 of life, the PDA was surgically ligated; during the immediate postoperative course, shock was corrected with blood and parenteral fluids. On December 2, 1983 (12 days old) she was stable; however, arterial blood pressures were around 100/80 mmHg with the means ranging from 65 to 82. BUN was 16 mg/dl and creatinine 0.8 mg/dl. A plasma renin was obtained that subsequently was revealed to be 207 ng/ml/hr. Apresoline, initially 1 mg IV every four hours, required progressive increase up to a total cumulative daily dose of 9 mg/kg. Blood pressures remained around 100/80 mmHg. The urinary sodium concentration was 46 mEq/L and slight hematuria and proteinuria were still present. Aldomet, 10 mg/kg/day in four divided doses over 30-60 minutes IV infusion, was added on December 6, 1983, as well as Lasix 3 mg/kg/day. The next day blood pressure was 112/80, and the Aldomet was doubled. Pulse remained stable around 170/minute. Urine output throughout all this period was adequate; slight hyponatremia (126 mEq/L) was corrected and Lasix was discontinued.

On December 9, 1983, captopril was initiated at 0.25 mg/kg/dose/ 12 hours. After one dose, the blood pressure fell to 70/50 mmHg. Aldomet was discontinued that day and Apresoline weaned off over the next 24 hours. The renal scan revealed decreased flow to the right kidney. The dose of captopril was eventually stabilized at 0.5 mg /6 hours. The patient is also on hydrochlorothiazide 2 mg/kg/day. Arterial blood pressures are around 80-70/50-40, mean 40-42 mmHg. Most recent serum creatinine is 0.6 mg/dl and the urine is negative for blood and protein.

MODERATOR: Thank you for this presentation. Now, we will open the discussion.

QUESTION: How is it that the mean blood pressures you are reporting are 40 to 42 with diastolics around 40? Am I reading that right?

DR. FREUNDLICH: You are right in your observation. Those numbers really do not represent actual measurements, but rather the most representative values over a period of several weeks. What I tried to do, was to take the most representative measurements throughout the observation period.

QUESTION: Was the scan done before or after captopril?

DR. FREUNDLICH: Before the captopril.

COMMENT-QUESTION: Some time ago we did a study on puppies that I never published where we gave saralasin intravenously. We noticed that GFR decreased in spite of the fact that the blood pressure remained normal. As you know, captopril can decrease renal function. I did notice that the serum creatinine was around 0.6 mg/dl. Did you notice any change in renal function or serum creatinine throughout the observation period?

DR. FREUNDLICH: This serum creatinine of 0.6 mg/dl is the most recent one and is the lowest. Serum creatinine has been higher during the clinical course, and has been coming down progressively; I hope it stays down. I do not have recent measurements of GFR, but we will obtain it since the baby is still in the hospital.

QUESTION: Could you kindly tell us a little bit more about the shock picture which occurred right after surgery? The reason why I am asking this is because, as we all know, one cause for early onset renal artery stenosis may be a thrombosed ductus and the baby could have gone into shock as a consequence of the thromboembolic episode rather than from blood loss. Was there a simple explanation for the shock?

DR. FREUNDLICH: I really couldn't answer specifically the question. I should say that immediately following surgery the baby presented with hypertension, poor peripheral circulation and shock; blood and fluids were administered, and within 6 to 12 hours the baby was hemodynamically stable again. So, clearly it was associated with the surgery.

COMMENT: This is a textbook example of hypertension induced by renal artery thrombosis. This is a premature who had an indwelling arterial catheter and showed a rise in arterial blood pressure from a base line of 52/29 to 100/50 mmHg and who had a patent ductus. In our series, about 50% of the children had a ductus. The diminished left femoral pulse is compatible with thrombotic occlusion of that vessel. The presence of proteinuria and hematuria are also quite characteristic. I would echo what was just said in that some patients, including infants, develop renal artery thrombosis following ligation of a patent ductus arteriosus. But this child clearly had hypertension before the ductus was ligated. It has been postulated that transient hypertension may occur following ligation of the ductus due to shifting of volume from the pulmonary into the systemic circulation. However, persistent hypertension would suggest a thrombotic phenomenon since, after several days of diuresis, the hypertension secondary to volume expansion should have subsided. I am also concerned about the potential deleterious effect of captopril on GFR in those infants; however, I am not aware of any reported case so far. One might expect that problems may occur, particularly since captopril alters the balance between efferent and afferent arterole resistance. This might lead one to suspect that functional problems may have developed in the affected kidney particularly, as noted, on the GFR. It has been proposed that this may be a useful clinical test in making the diagnosis of renal artery stenosis. I have never done that, but I suppose somebody will come up with a study with positive results. The exquisite sensitivity of this infant to captopril, I think, is also not uncommon and the use of low doses of the drug, as you have done, is very appropriate because one can overshoot and make these patients very hypotensive. So, it is appropriate to start on a low dose and increase progressively, per dose, until you start to see an effect. I believe in Minnesota it was found that dosages as low as .05 mg/kg can affect blood pressure. The renal scan picture is again quite characteristic, not only the diminished uptake by the affected kidney, but also a delay in the peak on the renogram and a pseudo obstructed picture with retention of the isotope in the kidney.

MODERATOR: Could you continue on the subject you were addressing earlier in the Seminar about the management of hypertension in infants as compared to older ages with one drug as opposed to several anti-hypertensive agents?

COMMENT: This is an example, obviously, of the fact that what I proposed to do, is not always feasible.

MODERATOR: Are not other people doing differently than what you are proposing?

COMMENT: That is quite likely. We treat hypertension when the measurements are above what we consider the 95th percentile for age and weight, and that oftentimes is a guesstimate since much of the data are not available in low birth weight infants. In infants who are asymptomatic and borderline, we will often follow without treatment, especially if they are older prematures or full term infants. We usually are quite successful in using single therapy, either a diuretic or a vasodilator like hydralazine in combination with sodium restriction. But, occasionally we have had to use multiple drugs. Usually what we do is start out with a diuretic and add hydralazine as you did. Our next drug of choice would probably be propranolol and if that is not successful, we would go as a last resort to captopril. I follow that sequence basically because I am more familiar with diuretics, hydralazine and propranolol in terms of their use and side effects, than I am with captopril and we have a more cumulative long term experience with those drugs than we have with captopril. However, there are occasional cases like this one where we have to use multiple drugs and still do not have a good control of blood pressure. In our experience, in all the cases except one, we have been able to wean patients off medications over a period of time. Usually, when the blood pressure remains stable over a one to two month period, we start tapering one drug at a time. There is one child with whom I have been peripherally involved who had a left renal artery thrombosis, was not responsive to accepted doses of anti-hypertensive medications, and was found at four to six months of age to have decreased femoral pulses. This child had an aortogram done early in life and was found to have a normal aorta; then, he was restudied at six months of age and was found to have an acquired coarctation of the abdominal aorta at the level of the renal artery thrombosis. That child is currently being treated by another physician with medications since the family has rejected any surgical intervention. It has been quite difficult to control the hypertension. This is the first case I am aware of with acquired coarctation of the aorta secondary to renal artery thrombosis.

COMMENT-QUESTION: It is not infrequent for a neonate who has renovascular hypertension to have also pulmonary pathology like bronchopulmonary dysplasia, wheezing or something else. Would that change your approach in terms of the drugs to use in controlling hypertension?

RESPONSE: Theoretically, it would; initially, we were quite hesitant to use beta blockers in children with chronic lung disease or in those who presented with congestive heart failure as a consequence of hypertension. We really have not encountered problems in that area. I would indeed avoid using a beta blocker if faced with a child who had a bronchospastic component.

QUESTION: How often do you encounter mild tachycardia with the use of hydralazine, enough to warrant discontinuation of the medication?

RESPONSE: Actually we see it quite frequently. We had one child who developed paroxismal atrial tachycardia; however, most neonates tolerate it satisfactorily. What we have seen is a resistance to the action of hydralazine; one should suspect that resistance is present if tachycardia does not develop after the drug is administered. We always insist on getting recordings on pulse rate following administration of hydralazine to see if we have had a substantial response.

MODERATOR: That is a very good question and I wonder if we could spend a little more time on that one. We have been told by our Clinical Pharmacology colleagues that you can actually induce myocardial infarction especially in the presence of hypoxia. But even without hypoxia, they say that the workload on the heart is so extreme with the administration of hydralazine that you have to be very careful not to damage the myocardium. We have never seen it, but we always ask about tachycardia and if there is prominent tachycardia even as a baseline, we are cautious, may completely avoid the use of peripheral vaso-dilators and use an alternative drug like a beta blocker. How do you react to this question?

RESPONSE: It is indeed a difficult situation since the beta blocker also has a deleterious effect on the myocardium. I have not seen ischemia developing in the infants on whom we have used hydralazine; although I must say I have not looked very closely except for EKGs. I think the bulk of the experience with myocardial infarction has been tachycardia superimposed on an arteriosclerotic adult heart. A similar situation might occur with the administration of theophylline in the newborn period as opposed to the adult. It seems that in the presence of a permeable intact coronary arterial system, we really don't run into problems, but we could conceivably run into those problems in the future. Another problem that we have not encountered but has been described in adults is the aspect of withdrawal from the beta blocker with fatal tachycardia. We do tend to taper our patients quite carefully off the beta blockers as has been recommended in adults. But, until now we have not seen that problem or poor myocardial performance induced by chronic beta blockade.

COMMENT: I have always been puzzled by the question of why we use Aldomet in the neonate, because I am sure we are all aware that Aldomet does not act, at least effectively, without the patient being in the erect position. I see it in all chapters and monographs as recommended in the treatment of hypertension in the neonate. I should say that I also use it; however, intellectually, I would like to question the experts why indeed do we use it with the obvious lack of an upright position in a newborn. I would also like to share some experiences with the rest of the group here. Surprisingly, we have seen quite a lot of hypertension in neonates with our superb cardiovascular surgeon. We have continued to see a lot of aneurysm of the aorta interrupting blood supply to the kidneys and I had several good experiences utilizing Turnamine, a specific beta blocker, which requires only one daily administration. Instead of using Inderal after starting with diuretics and Apresoline, instead of going to Aldomet, I would go to either Inderal or very quickly switch to the specific beta blocker Turnamine with fairly good results. I am also very pleased to see that you no longer see proteinuria or hematuria in this patient which is reassuring since captopril can cause membranous nephropathy and one sign would be heavy proteinuria.

COMMENT: I must confess that although I also recommend Aldomet, I have not used it in years. However, I think that its effect can be seen without postural changes and probably there are several levels of action for the drug. One of those levels is on the central nervous system, and as such sometimes it can obscure neurological signs because of its central effect in patients with hypertension and neurological symptoms. I suppose that you should comment on that since it is in your area of expertise.

COMMENT: As everybody knows in this panel, the benefit of Aldomet is due to its alpha II agonist effect. It is stimulant in the central nervous system and it will decrease peripheral sympathetic outflow. If one believes that there are a lot of circulating cathecolamines in the newborn, one can assume then that it can work without assuming the upright position. It was believed that Aldomet was converted into a pseudo neuro-transmitter called alpha-methyl-norepinephrine; yet, it is a very powerful vaso-constrictor, it is an alpha II agonist. The other point I wanted to make, with your permission, is that Turnamine is the trade name and the generic name is atenolol. I would like to add one more point and that is to raise a word of caution to the use of those drugs in the neonatal period, particularly in patients with broncho-pulmonary dysplasia who, according to our neonatologists, could easily have bronchial spasm.

MODERATOR: What about the different beta blockers? There are some data that suggest that some beta blockers like propranolol reduce GFR while there are other drugs that do not, or in fact might increase GFR. What is the opinion of the panel concerning that point?

COMMENT: I am, indeed, familiar with those studies; when we gave propranolol to our puppies for a period of six months doses of 6 to 18 mg/kg/day, we noticed no change in plasma creatinine over that period of time. However, we didn't look at the inulin or creatinine clearance.

COMMENT: As you know, most of those studies were concerned with people who had already low GFRs to begin with and when they were given propranolol, the GFR decreased further. We had a patient whose GFR decreased with propranolol and once we stopped it, her GFR increased again. Whether propranolol should or should not be given when the GFR is decreased is one thing that people talk about indeed but this remains a question. One of the agents that was reviewed recently in the New England Journal of Medicine is nedulol. It is also one dose medicine and it was suggested that the drug did not decrease renal blood flow and maybe if you are worried about it, nedulol might even have intrinsic dopaminergic activity and thus have a vasodilator effect.

COMMENT: I just want to go back to Aldomet. I also have wondered why pediatricians state as a second line drug the use of Aldomet. I stopped using it about 10 years ago because mainly I was dealing with adolescent hypertension, that was before umbilical artery catheters, and in addition to having compliance problems with teenagers, we saw their school performance deteriorate markedly. "A" students went into failing grades after one month of having therapy, and never achieved really good control of blood pressure anyway. All this was reversible once Aldomet was stopped. Teenagers had undesirable side effects without really good control of blood pressure; so, we stopped using it and I went to guanethidine about whose side effects I did not worry much because I could monitor them; they were not a problem psychologically. That was obviously before beta blockers. You did not have much to choose from. I have not found an occasion to use Aldomet since then.

MODERATOR: We also have found side effects from the use of Aldomet like breast engorgement. Yet, guanethidine was not less frustrating.

COMMENT: I am surprised that your teenager was in good shape after Aldomet because there is a high incidence of impotence with the drug.

COMMENT: I have been impressed with the discussion of the panel and I was also wondering why I have touted the use of Aldomet, particularly when I listen to the panel. I guess I never have been that impressed with the drug; but I saw that a whole lot of people recommended it and I thought it was me and not the drug. Certainly, hypertension can cause heart failure in the newborn and it is obviously much too late to do anything about hypertension. One statement that would occur to me is that we spent the last 30 minutes talking about the terrible side effects of all the medications that are used for hypertension. I wonder if the panel could address the issue of indications for treatment. When are we really treating a potentially dangerous disease and when are we treating some numbers?

RESPONSE: That is an excellent question. I don't know and I don't think anybody knows what the morbid consequences are of non-treatment of mild to moderate hypertension in newborns. I think that we know that hypertension can cause significant sequelae like congestive heart failure and neurological problems. I have been impressed by the poor correlation between the absolute number I get for blood pressure and the absence or presence of symptoms. I have seen babies asymptomatic with marked elevation of blood pressure, but I have seen others with what I would consider mildly elevated blood pressures who developed neurologic problems and congestive heart failure. But in the totally asymptomatic infant, who's got no evidence of end-organ effect and an elevated blood pressure, I really don't think we know; it is a very good question.

COMMENT: I would like to add a question in that same respect. Yes, indeed, you take a newborn and you put him on therapy; but, how do you monitor blood pressure? It is difficult enough under ideal circumstances to have a quiet, undisturbed blood pressure, treated or untreated. And there comes a time when this baby is ready to be discharged to go home; do you teach the mother to take blood pressures? Do you send the baby home with a monitor? How do you handle that?

RESPONSE: I have developed a rather sneaky technique to measure blood pressure in my clinic. If the baby is breast feeding I put the child in a room with the mother and ask her to start breast feeding, leave the room dark, and I sneak in while the child is at the breast. If the baby is bottle feeding, I do the same thing or else I'll ask the mother when the child usually sleeps. You have to be very careful that you get the cuff around the arm and get the blood pressure before the baby wakes up.

COMMENT: What we have done is sent visiting nurses to the home of the baby for blood pressure recordings and the mother brings the numbers to us.

COMMENT: I would like to mention that whenever you send nurses home or see the patient in the office, make sure that the blood pressure is documented vis-a-vis the time the antihypertensive medication was given. We have seen that children have their blood pressures measured one hour after the drug is given and not measured prior to the next dose; we often get a most optimistic reading. It is important that we record what time that blood pressure was taken and its relation to the drug administration.

COMMENT: One drug that I guess you did not mention the other day is the use of Minoxidil in the newborn. I am sure some people are using it.

COMMENT: I have never used it, and I am not sure I would feel comfortable using it. I would prefer using another drug. I am sure the parents will not appreciate the physical changes noted with the use of it. As you know, hirsutism is a major side effect.

COMMENT: Going back to the pre-captopril era, I had the opportunity to use Minoxidil in an infant who was in severe congestive heart failure. He was severely hypertensive and everything else failed. Diazoxide would work for about two hours before there was a need for further treatment and we tried everything else, so we used Minoxidil. The effect was as dramatic as Dr. Freundlich reported with this particular case and gave us a few weeks in which we were able to regroup, trying to figure out what was going on and then decide what to do prior to the development of any of those undesirable physical attributes of Minoxidil.

COMMENT: I have not used Minoxidil in infants, but in adults you would need a beta-blocker and a loop diuretic to minimize the reflex tachycardia and salt retention. After a short period, though, adults are better controlled with more conventional drugs.

QUESTION: What were the clotting studies like? What is the role of anticoagulants in the treatment of renal thrombosis?

RESPONSE: In the first dozen patients we studied, two had clotting studies suggesting disseminated intravascular coagulation; the rest were normal. We have not used anticoagulants, either heparin or streptokinase. Recanalization occurs in most instances; in fact, 70% of our infants have shown some restoration of function of the thrombosed renal vessel and about 10% have failed to show functional restoration. A large collaborative study will be required to assess whether anticoagulants would be of use.

MODERATOR: Thank you for your participation. We have to move on to the next case.

MODERATOR: Another distinguished Guest Faculty will present our last case (#4).

CASE PRESENTATION: A four and a half year old white male was brought to the hospital for evaluation of short stature and bowed legs. He was 52 cm tall and weighed 3.4 kg. Delivered normally after his mother's uncomplicated pregnancy, the child had exhibited normal early development: he walked at 11 months, talked at nine months and achieved toilet training at three years of age. Teeth erupted at eight months. Linear growth declined shortly after 18 months of age and progressive bowing of the lower extremities was noted from approximately two years of age. Although the patient's diet was described as grossly normal without evidence of any food intolerance, dairy products were consumed in limited quantities because of associated "leg cramps".

The medical history was remarkable for repeated gum infections necessitating the removal of eight teeth, and a large occipital prominence noted since one year of age, resulting in some deformity of the skull. The family history was positive for "bowed legs" in both maternal grandfather and a great-grandmother. In addition, the patient's mother had "vitamin-D resistant" rickets.

On physical examination the patient was a well-nourished, intelligent male, with obvious bowing of the femurs. The arms were normal, and an occipital bulge were appreciated. Examination of the head, eyes, ears, nose and throat was within normal limits; the thyroid was not palpable. The chest excursion was normal; bony prominences were appreciated on the fifth and sixth ribs near the mid-clavicular line bilaterally. Cardiac and abdominal examinations were also within normal limits. There were normal male genitalia. The deformities of the extremities were as noted above. Motor strength and coordination were considered normal. Neurological examination was interpreted as normal; although the gait was awkward secondary to the bowing, the station was normal and fine motor coordination was good.

Laboratory data upon initial presentation included a hematocrit of 40 vol% (hemoglobin of 14.5 gm%) and a WBC of 6600/mm^3 with a normal differential. The specific gravity of the urine was 1.026, the pH 7.1. Microscopic examination of the urine revealed 0 RBC, 1 to 5 WBC/HPF, and no casts or bacteria. The serum electrolytes included a sodium of 135 mEq/L, potassium of 4.3 mEq/L, chloride 104 mEq/L and CO_2 of 24 mEq/L. The BUN was 7 mg/dl, the serum creatinine 0.5 mg/dl, and the total serum protein 6.7 g/dl (albumin 4.3 g/dl). Uric acid was 3.9 mg/dl, magnesium 1.5 mEq/L, and protein electrophoresis demonstrated a slight decrease in gamma globulins, quantitatively 0.7 g/dl. Serum calcium was 9.5 mg/dl, phosphorus 2.0 mg/dl and alkaline phosphatase was 453 IU (elevated for age). Tubular reabsorption of phosphate was 89% and phosphate clearance 4.2 ml per minute. Radiographic studies revealed marked rachitic changes in all long bones, with a bone age of only two and a half years. Chest x-ray demonstrated splaying of the anterior end of the ribs bilaterally, and fragmentation of the humeral epiphysis. The epiphyseal line was noted to be jagged and widened. Pelvic films revealed irregularity and slight fragmentation of the femoral head, with flattening and irregularity of the metaphyses bilaterally. The femoral necks were short. The lower legs showed lateral bowing of the distal femoral metaphyses. Similar changes were also noted in tibia and fibula bilaterally. There was slight scaphocephaly on the skull film; the coronal and saggital sutures were closed and fused.

The possibility of renal tubular acidosis was excluded on the basis of a normal ammonium chloride test. The absence of diarrhea, steatorrhea or other evidence of malabsorption, and the absence of glycosuria and a normal 24-hour amino acid excretion, argued against the diagnosis of malabsorption and Fanconi's syndrome, respectively. Calcium absorption was demonstrated to be decreased.

The diagnosis at the conclusion of the patient's initial evaluation was "vitamin-D resistant" rickets. In accordance with the then accepted hypothesis that the disease was secondary to the inability to convert vitamin D_3 to active metabolite 25-hydroxycholecalciferol, the patient was begun on 25-hydroxycholecalciferol.

The patient received 25-hydroxycholecalciferol for approximately eight months, and although he subjectively improved in strength and stamina, there was no significant bone maturation. His therapy was thus changed to phosphate supplementation. Over subsequent months, 25-hydroxycholecalciferol was intermittently reinstituted without noticeable improvement. The orthophosphate was increased to the limits of gastrointestinal tolerance. Growth, however, responded only minimally.

At nine years of age, the patient was noted to have a serum calcium of 9.5, phosphate of 2.0-3.0 mg/dl, alkaline phosphatase of 420 IU, BUN 11 and creatinine of 0.5 mg/dl. A 24-hour urine collection was remarkable for a calcium of 18 mg, phosphate of 2000 mg and a creatinine of 440 mg. Serial muscle enzymes (including aldolase, CPK and SGOT) were all within normal limits. A neuromuscular examination and an electromyogram were normal. Therapy with dihydrotachysterol and supplemental orthophosphate was initiated. The response was disappointing, with less than 2 cm of growth over two years.

By age 11, the bone age was nine and the rachitic changes persisted. Although the serum calcium remained within normal limits, the phosphorus continued to be depressed. A lower extremity fracture required 14 weeks to heal.

But, at age 14, he was begun on 1,25-dihydroxycholecalciferol, while continuing phosphate supplementation, and a dramatic improvement was achieved. Within months his growth accelerated so markedly that by age 15, his height velocity was 14.1 cm/year, which is 235% of that expected for his chronologic age. His most recent admission was at age 15 for calcium balance studies, and at that time his serum calcium was 9.8 mg/dl, phosphate was 4.9 mg/dl, and rachitic changes were no longer appreciated radiologically.

MODERATOR: That is a very nice case. Since time is limited, perhaps you would like to make some comments as to what you think the messages are with that patient.

COMMENT: I would be delighted to do that. The radiographs on this patient show the wrist before 1,25 dihydroxyvitamin D substituted the other forms of vitamin D. You can see that there is loss of provisory zone of calcification in the distal radius and ulna and irregularity and widening of the epiphyseal plate. Within six months of 1,25 vitamin D, are the beginnings of healing and 12 months after initiation of therapy with 1,25 D, there is marked healing, continued healing. There is a lesson here. That is, short of 1,25 dihydroxyvitamin D, even when this child was being taken care of by outstanding people, with the conventional treatment of either vitamin D_2 at fairly high doses of up to 60,000 units or higher, or with 25 hydroxy D alluded to in the history presentation, bone healing did not occur. We were puzzled. We did not understand, because previously hypophosphatemic rickets was not thought to be related to a vitamin D metabolic disorder; it was thought to be a genetically determined phosphate leak of the renal tubule. However, there are two lines of evidence to show that there has to be some effect from abnormal vitamin D metabolism to permit us to use high doses requiring--forcing us--to use doses sometimes as high as 4 micrograms of 1,25 dihydroxyvitamin D a day in children. That is, huge amounts without causing hypercalcemia, surely causing hypercalciuria. I would like to bring out certain points about pathogenesis. That is, it has been shown that in the untreated patients with renal hypophosphatemic rickets, 1,25 vitamin D concentrations in the blood are low. Low in terms of the hypophosphatemia and low compared to normal control subjects. So, there seem to be problems with D metabolism. Then, data published from Montreal in the hypophosphatemic mouse, the genetically determined hypophosphatemic mouse which is the only animal model for this condition, showed that if one produces hypocalcemia by a calcium deficient diet in this hypophosphatemic rickets mouse compared to normal controls, the hypocalcemia progressively being produced should result in more and more 1,25 dihydroxyvitamin D production. I was also shown that normal rats will have production of 1,25 vitamin D in relationship with hypocalcemia but in the hypophosphatemic mouse there is a depression of the set point for the production of 1,25 vitamin D. So, this gives us the possibility that we can transfer results of animal studies to human; this may or may not be permissible but it is the best evidence we have so far of a defect in 1-hydroxylase in the mitochondria of the kidney that usually produce 1,25 dihydroxy vitamin D. The second line of support, of course, are the data from Wisconsin in children with hypophosphatemic rickets as well as that from Duke University in the untreated adults with hypophosphatemic rickets in which 1,25 vitamin D concentrations in blood were in fact very low. So, this gives us the rationale of why we have to use increasing doses of 1,25 vitamin D in order to achieve correction of the rickets, and why with the other forms of vitamin D, we are unable, because of these defects in 1-hydroxylase, to achieve correction. This explains many paradoxes that we as clinicians just trying to treat patients with what seems to be the best therapy, have not been able to explain until the data were published five months ago (September 1983).

MODERATOR: The statement has been made that 25-hydroxy vitamin D may have a stronger bone effect, at least in renal patients, than the 1,25 vitamin D. In the Multicenter Study, we are studying 1,25 vitamin D. Would you like to elaborate on that?

COMMENT: I would be pleased to say what I understand the situation to be. There are very nice data which would imply that 25-hydroxy D has better healing and fewer complications in certain cases of renal osteodystrophy. However, in renal hypophosphatemic rickets, if we are to accept the evidence that I just presented of a lowering of the set point for 1,25 vitamin D production because of the defect in the mitochondria of 1-hydroxylase, and if we are to accept the data of low 1,25 D production in the serum in the untreated cases, then using 25 D, as this patient had in the hands of noted figures at the NIH, there is no way of overcoming the defect of conversion to the active metabolite unless one uses super pharmacological doses of vitamin D derivatives. By mass action, one can push the remaining 1-alpha-hydroxylase to produce enough 1,25 to achieve healing of the rickets. That is a possibility.

QUESTION: Let me ask you a question now that you have convinced us that, indeed, there is a defect of 1,25 conversion in hypophosphatemic rickets. How do you distinguish this condition from vitamin-dependent rickets described some time ago?

RESPONSE: Good point. We do not know why vitamin D-dependent rickets, which are reported primarily from Canada, are different. Since there is in vitamin D-dependent rickets clearly a defect in conversion from 25 to 1,25 D, why in these cases of renal hypophosphatemic rickets, now that we are showing a difference in set point, it is not a complete defect in conversion. It is a difference in set point for production of 1,25 D; we do not see all the other consequences of D deficiency, as you would expect to see in vitamin D dependent rickets who are not treated. I cannot explain it all. Hopefully, after tomorrow's presentation when you actually will see the data, perhaps at that point you will be more convinced; but, we still could not explain these differences which is probably one reason we still continue to study this fascinating problem.

COMMENT-QUESTION: Could we get back to the question that you raised, expanding this to children with chronic renal insufficiency and bone disease? I wonder what are the panel's feelings about the proposal of some individuals that one form of vitamin D might be more effective than another form in treating bone disease.

COMMENT: We have certainly seen an improvement and a reduction in progression of bone disease since we have started using 1,25 D versus dihydrotachysterol (DHT). We have had no access to the newer metabolites.

COMMENT: I don't really know how to answer that question effectively. I think that there are also studies in adults that suggest that 25 might have an advantage over 1,25 although this certainly is not my line of expertise. The thing that bothers me is that, supposedly, 1,25 works in concert with parathormone and that you can produce even more osteoclastic activity to raise serum calcium, which is the desired end effect, is that not true?

COMMENT: Very good points. There are receptors, binding sites in the parathyroid gland for 1,25 dihydroxy-vitamin D. Accumulating evidence in the last few years has shown that 1,25 vitamin D probably has direct inhibitory effect on parathyroid hormone secretion itself. However, I would submit that 1,25 vitmain D alone is not the answer; it probably would require in many cases, a certain balance between 1,25 D, 24-25 D, and perhaps 25 D or 25 that becomes 24-25 D. A certain balance, a certain ratio that would be optimum for bone healing that otherwise could not be achieved. That is what the future will hold: a certain balance between these metabolites in specific cases.

COMMENT: I agree with the last comment. I don't think we have the answer but the only observations we know, more from adults than from children, is that 25 is more effective in the osteomalasia component of bone disease, and 1,25 might be more effective in the hyperparathyroid component. Since the majority of children reported in the literature have mixed disease (osteomalasia and hyperparathyroid components), already it has been suggested that maybe a combination of 25 and 1,25 might be the most healthy one.

MODERATOR: Since you are the one who asked the question, would you like to state your position?

COMMENT: I have no position. I would like to underline the fact that those studies, at least those that were presented in Germany, really involve a very small number of patients--just a handful in each category, so I think that larger studies are indicated. The other wrench in the works is the whole question of aluminum. Especially in a small group of patients, one might have problems within that group. One or two or more patients had problems with aluminum toxicity.

COMMENT: That is a lot of food for thought, a lot of food at the table for those of us who work in the vitamin D and parathyroid hormone field.

COMMENT-QUESTION: Correct me if I'm wrong, but there are now studies to indicate that there are really patients with true vitamin D-resistant rickets; that is, they are given 1,25 vitamin D and they don't respond. I thought I read that in the JCI sometime last year.

COMMENT-RESPONSE: I missed that article. Concerning true vitamin D resistance, there are cases in my experience in which we had to use such high doses of 1,25 D that we were worried. We used doses as high as 4 mcg/day for some of these cases of renal hypophosphatemic rickets all the time. We are now trying to modify our treatment in response to our observations of hypercalciuria at high vitamin D dosages. By lowering the dose when we use hydrochlorothiazide in conjunction with amiloride, we have found that we can reduce the hypercalciuria and induce a sustained elevation of the hypophosphatemia in these hypophosphatemic rickets patients. This particular patient that I have presented here was referred to me a couple of years ago. He was being treated with 4 mcg/day. This data will be shown tomorrow. We are now able to use the diuretic, hydrochlorothiazide, in conjunction with amiloride to fairly good ends without the complications to be expected of diuretics.

MODERATOR: Thank you very much.

PARTICIPANTS

AND

INDEXES

PARTICIPANTS

Program Chairman

Jose Strauss, M.D., Professor of Pediatrics; Director, Division of Pediatric Nephrology, University of Miami School of Medicine, Miami, Florida.

Guest Faculty

Raymond D. Adelman, M.D., Associate Professor of Pediatrics; Director, Division of Pediatric Nephrology, University of California at Davis, California.

Diane Appell, R.N., Head Nurse, Dialysis Unit, Children's Hospital of Alabama, Birmingham, Alabama.

Billy Arant, Jr. M.D., Professor of Pediatrics, Division of Pediatric Nephrology, University of Texas Southwestern Medical School, Dallas, Texas.

James C. M. Chan M.D., Professor and Vice Chairman, Department of Pediatrics, Medical College of Virginia; Director of Pediatric Nephrology, Children's Medical Center, Virginia Commonwealth University, Richmond, Virginia.

Pedro Jose, M.D., Professor of Pediatrics; Chief, Pediatric Nephrology, Georgetown University Medical Center, Washington, D. C.

Edward C. Kohaut, M.D., Professor of Pediatrics, University of Alabama, Birmingham, Alabama.

Local Faculty

Carolyn Abitbol, M.D., Assistant Professor of Pediatrics, Division of Pediatric Nephrology, University of Miami School of Medicine, Miami, Florida.

Paul Benke, M.D., Ph.D., Associate Professor of Pediatrics, Division of Genetics, University of Miami School of Medicine, Miami, Florida.

Cherry Charlton, R.N., Head Nurse, Pediatric Dialysis Unit, Jackson Memorial Hospital, Miami, Florida.

Rosa Diaz, R.N., CAPD Charge Nurse, Pediatric Dialysis Unit, Jackson Memorial Hospital, Miami, Florida.

Michael Freundlich, M.D., Assistant Professor of Pediatrics, Division of Pediatric Nephrology, University of Miami School of Medicine, Miami, Florida.

Marcela Garcia, R.N., Neonatal Intensive Care Unit, Jackson Memorial Hospital, Miami, Florida.

Tilo Gerhardt, M.D., Associate Professor of Pediatrics, Division of Neonatology, University of Miami School of Medicine, Miami, Florida.
Jorge Lockhart, M.D., Associate Professor of Urology, University of Miami School of Medicine, Miami, Florida.

Emmalee Setzer, M.D., Assistant Professor of Pediatrics, Division of Neonatology, University of Miami School of Medicine, Miami, Florida.

George Sfakianakis, M.D., Associate Professor of Radiology, Division of Nuclear Medicine, University of Miami School of Medicine, Miami, Florida.

Jose Strauss, M.D., Professor of Pediatrics; Director, Division of Pediatric Nephrology, University of Miami School of Medicine, Miami, Florida.

Paul Tocci, Ph.D., Associate Professor of Pediatrics, Mailman Center for Child Development, University of Miami School of Medicine, Miami, Florida.

Carlos Vaamonde, M.D., Professor of Medicine, University of Miami School of Medicine; Chief, Renal Section, Miami Veterans Administration Medical Center, Miami, Florida.

Gaston Zilleruelo, M.D., Associate Professor of Pediatrics, Division of Pediatric Nephrology, University of Miami School of Medicine, Miami, Florida.

*Other Contributors

Uri Alon, M.D., Nephrology Section, Children's Medical Center, Department of Pediatrics, Medical College of Virginia, Health Sciences Division of Virginia Commonwealth University, Richmond, Virginia.

Philip L. Calcagno, M.D., Professor and Chairman, Department of Pediatrics, Georgetown University Medical Center, Washington, D. C.

Mary E. Carlin, M.D., Adjunct Assistant Professor, Division of Genetics, Mailman Center for Child Development, University of Miami School of Medicine, Miami, Florida.

Nuria Dominguez, M.D., Department of Pediatrics, University of Miami School of Medicine, Miami, Florida.

Gilbert M. Eisner, M.D., Professorial Lecturer, Department of Physiology and Biophysics, Georgetown University Medical Center, Washington, D. C.

Robin A. Felder, Ph.D., Instructor in Pediatrics; Director, Pediatric Renal Research, Division of Pediatric Nephrology, Georgetown University Medical Center, Washington, D. C.

Anne Feuer, M.S., Research Associate, Departments of Pediatrics and Pathology, Mailman Center for Child Development, University of Miami School of Medicine, Miami, Florida.

Robert D. Fildes, M.D., Assistant Professor of Pediatrics, Division of Pediatric Nephrology, Georgetown University Medical Center, Washington, D. C.

Rita M. Fojaco, M.D., Departments of Pediatrics and Pathology, University of Miami School of Medicine, Miami, Florida.

Robert J. Geller, M.D., Division of Clinical Pharmacology, Departments of Internal Medicine and Pediatrics, University of Virginia, Charlottesville, Virginia.

Joseph A. Misiewicz, M.D., University of Miami School of Medicine, Miami, Florida.

Brenda Montane, M.D., Department of Pediatrics, University of Miami School of Medicine, Miami, Florida.

Charles L. Stewart, M.D., Fellow, Division of Pediatric Nephrology, Georgetown University Medical Center, Washington, D. C.

James F. Winchester, M.D., Associate Professor of Medicine; Director, Hemodialysis, Hemoperfusion, and Transplantation Services, Georgetown University Medical Center, Washington, D. C.

*Co-authors

AUTHOR INDEX

Abitbol, C., 107, 147, 189, 235
Adelman, R., 23, 87
Alon, U., 157, 223, 241
Appell, D., 279
Arant, B., 11, 183, 271

Benke, P., 135

Calcagno, P., 17
Carlin, M., 135
Chan, J., 157, 199, 223, 241

Dominguez, N. 147

Eisner, G., 17

Felder, R., 3, 17
Feuer, A., 135
Fildes, R., 17
Fojaco, R., 135
Freundlich, M., 107, 147, 189, 235

Geller, R., 199

Jose, P., 3, 17, 97

Kohaut, E., 279

Misiewicz, J., 135
Montane, B., 147

Sfakianakis, G., 165
Stewart, C., 97
Strauss, J., 107, 147, 189, 235

Vaamonde, C., 49

Winchester, J., 97

Zilleruelo, G., 107, 147, 189, 235

SUBJECT INDEX

Absent kidney, 136
Acid base
  disturbance, 193
  status, 39
Acidosis, 157, 176, 286
Acro-Renal Syndrome, 142
Acro-Renal-Mandibular Syndrome, 142
Acro-Renal-Ocular Syndrome, 142
Acute dialysis, 107
Acute renal failure, 53, 97, 279
  diagnosis of, 122
Adenocarcinomas, 200
Adolescents, 236
Adrenergic receptors
  development of, 3
Adrenoceptor, 3
Advanced age, 53
Advanced renal failure, 235, 289
Albumin, 110, 124, 126, 186
Aldomet, 311
Aldosterone, 158, 305
  secretion, 3
Alkali therapy, 161
Alkaline phosphate, 230
Allopurinol, 58
Alpha adrenoceptors, 3
Aluminum toxicity, 319
Ambulatory peritoneal dialysis, 279
Amikacin, 93
Amiloride, 230
Aminoaciduria, 162
Aminoglycoside
  administration, 131
  drug interactions, 62
  nephrotoxicity, 58, 87, 127
  therapy, 128
  toxicity, 126
Ammonia, 158
Amphotericin, 100
Anasarca, 107
Anemia, 285
Angiocath, 116
Angiography, 33
Angiotensin, 11
Anomalies, 147
Anorexia, 285
Antibiotics, 87
Anti-convulsants, 267
Anti-hypertensive agents, 27
Anti-hypertensives, 42
Antinatriuresis, 4
Antineoplastic drugs
  nephrotoxicity, 65
Anuria, 279
Anuric infants, 98
Argyle, 109
  catheters, 115
Arteriograms, 35
Artificial spincters, 176
Aspirin, 56
Autoimmune disorder, 247
Automated cycling, 279
Azotemia, 98, 107. 285

Balance, 17
Bartter's Syndrome, 302
Beckwith-Wiedemann, 138
Beta
  adrenoceptors, 3
  blocker, 310
Beta 2
  microglobulin, 130
  bicarbonate, 157, 186
  dialysis, 120
  solutions, 213
Bicitra, 161
Bilateral
  hydronephrosis, 154
  versus unilateral, 154
Binding sites, 241
Biopsies, 118
Bladder
  capacity, 169
  infection, 177
  needle aspiration, 154
Bleeding, 108

Blood, 38
  buffers, 157
  effect of volume change, 35
  pressure regulation, 11
  pressure measurement, 23, 313
  volume, 11
Body composition, 289
Bone, 242
  collagen, 242
  deformities, 224
  disease, 285, 318
  resorption, 242
  structure, 237
B.O.R. Syndrome, 139
Branchio-oto-renal, 139
Breast tumors, 200
Buffers, 157

Calcitonin, 207
Calcium, 189
  carbonate, 161
  concentrations, 183
  excretion, 172
  intake, 223
  losses, 237
Caloric intake, 285
Calyceal blunting, 138
cAMP, 3
CAPD, 151, 235, 279
Captopril, 27, 44, 308, 309
Cardiac
  failure, 107
  output, 11
"Catch-up" growth, 289
Catecholamines, 3
Catheter
  chest tube, 109
  failure, 280
  outflow obstruction, 280
  tunnel infections, 283
Cephalotin
  and aminoglycosides, 62
Cerebral
  edema, 108
  hemorrhages, 37
Cerebrohepatorenal Syndrome, 140
Chest tube catheter, 109
Chlorothiazide, 27
Cholangiocarcinomas, 200
Cholestyramine resins, 162
Chromosome
  syndromes, 139
  studies, 144
Chromosomes
  added, 139
  deleted, 139
Chronic
  peritoneal access, 280
  renal failure, 147, 280
Chrostek, 199
Circulating
  parathyroid hormone, 242
  volume, 235
Cisplatin nephrotoxicity, 67
Citrate-containing products, 204
Citrate excretion, 172
Coarse skin, 245
Collagen synthesis, 242
Comparative nephrotoxicity, 60
Congenital
  anomalies, 147
  hypoparathyroidism, 247
Congestive heart failure, 55, 110
Continuous
  ambulatory peritoneal
  dialysis, 235, 279
  intravenous ultrafiltration, 116
CRF, 149
Cryptophthalmus Syndrome, 142
Cyclers, 279
Cyclic AMP, 241, 265
Cyclic dialysis, 279
Cystic diseases, 149
Cytoxic agents, 207

DADS, 165
Daily activities, 236
DB-CAMP, 212
Dehydration, 54, 202, 223
Developmental sodium handling, 17
Dextrose, 110
D. George Syndrome, 247
Diabetes mellitus, 54
Diabetic ketoacidosis, 162
Diafiltration, 119
Diagnostic imaging, 165
Dialysate, 110
  extravasation of, 108
  volumes, 282
Dialysis, 107, 118, 151, 209, 235, 279
  solutions, 281
  ultrafiltration, 287
Diarrhea acidosis, 162
Diazoxide, 27
Digital subtraction angiography, 165
Diffuse mesangial sclerosis, 42
Diffusion, 235
Dilutional acidosis, 39, 162
Diphosphonates, 209
Disequilibrium, 108, 235
Distal RTA, 169
Distal solute delivery, 19

Distressed physicians, 121
Diuretics, 27, 71, 207, 310, 319
Dopamine, 4, 37, 123
  receptor development, 3
Dopaminergic control, 6
Dose and toxicity, 61
Down's Syndrome, 139
DSA, 165
Drug
  interactions, 52
  related disorders, 204
Drugs
  combinations of, 63
  non-steroidal anti-inflammatory, 68
Duplicated collecting system, 138
Duration of therapy, 61
Dysmenorrhea, 71
Dysmorphic Syndromes, 135, 202

Ear
  anomalies, 139
  pits, 139
Early hypocalcemia 183, 189
Edema, 108
EDTA, 209
Encephalopathy, 266, 289
End-stage
  failure, 284
  renal disease, 178
Energy intake, 286
ESRD, 150, 235, 284
Estrogen, 3
Ethics Committee, 260
Ethical considerations, 238
Evaluation, 174
Excessive intake, 287
Excretory urography, 165
Exit site infection, 283
Experimental dialysis, 261
Extracellular
  blood volume, 235
  fluid, 235
Extracorporeal system, 111

Family unity, 236
Fanconi Syndrome, 93, 224
Fetal
  Alcohol Syndrome, 137
  calcium, 183
  hydantoin syndrome, 137
  intervention, 153, 154
Fetus, 153
Fibrin, 110
Filtered phosphate, 223

Fluid
  and electrolyte balance, 125
  intake, 287
  therapy, 185
Flux studies, 237
Fractional sodium excretion, 17, 172
Fraser Syndrome, 142
Functional immaturity, 271
Furosemide 27, 88, 121, 122, 185, 263

Gastroenteritis, 285
Gastroschisis, 119
Gavage feeding, 287
Gentamicin, 88
  and cyclosporin A, 62
  ototoxicity, 130
GFR formula, 50
Glomerular filtration rate, 50
Glomerulosclerosis, 152
Glomerulotubular balance, 274
Glycols, 100
Glycosuria, 162, 224
Glucocorticoids, 204
Glucocorticosteroids, 208
Glucose, 29, 274
  absorption, 237
Growth, 44, 236, 283
  failure, 34, 224, 286
  retardation, 158
  velocity, 230

Heart rate, 11
Heavy metals, 100
Height
  for age, 230
  velocity, 229
Hematuria, 264
Hemihypertrophy, 138
Hemodialysis, 235
  priming the system, 119
Hemodynamic determinants, 11
Hemoperfusion, 97
Heparin, 110
Hernias, 285
High dextrose concentration, 266
High pressure bladders, 176
Home, 236
Homeostatic functions, 97
Hormonal losses, 237
Horseshoe kidney, 138
Hyaline membrane disease, 107
Hydralazine, 27, 310, 311
Hydrochlorothiazide, 230
Hydrogen ion
  metabolism, 157
  retention, 173

Hydronephrosis, 148
Hypercalcemia, 200, 201, 206, 241, 250,
  medication-related, 202
Hypercalcemic states, 199
Hypercalcitoninemia, 189, 191
Hypercalciuria, 189, 230, 250, 262
Hyperchloremic metabolic acidosis, 158
Hyperkalemia, 158
Hypernatremia, 40
Hyperparathyroidism, 43, 189, 200
  secondary, 283
Hyperphosphatemia, 189, 190
Hyper-reninemic states, 71
Hypertension 23, 34, 42, 56, 285, 309, 313
  causes of, 24
  systemic, 26
Hypertonic glucose, 235
Hyperglycemic, 110
Hyperuricemic, 56
Hyperuricosuria, 56
Hypocalcemia, 183, 189, 203, 245
Hypocalcemic states, 199
Hypokalemia, 284, 301
Hypokalemic muscle weakness, 158
Hypomagnesemia, 189, 190, 213, 245
Hyponatremia, 284, 301
Hypoparathyroidism, 193, 213
  sporadic, 247
Hypophosphatemia, 286
Hypophastemic rickets, 223, 317
Hypoplasia dysplasia, 149
Hypoplastic kidneys, 138
Hypoproteinemic, 110
Hypothyroidism, 213
Hypovitaminosis D, 216
Hypovolemia, 36, 284
Hypoxic
  acute renal failure, 129
  neonate, 110

Idiopathic hypoparathyroidism, 213
Imaging, 165
Immobilization, 202
Independence, 236
Indium, 41
Innervation, 4
Insensible losses, 287
Insufficient PTH, 241
Insulin response, 110
Intermittent peritoneal dialysis, 279
Interstitial fluid, 108, 113
Intoxication, 108
Intracellular messengers, 3
Intractable acidosis, 107
Intraperitoneal catheter, 235
Intrauterine life, 153
Intravascular volume, 113, 205
Intravenous angiography, 166
In utero
  false diagnosis, 173
  intervention, 175
Ionized calcium, 184, 241
IPDS, 279
Isoproterenol, 4
IVP, 34, 165, 173, 174

Jugular vein, 111

Kallikrein, 19
Klippel-Feil Syndrome, 138
Kidneys
  sodium chloride vs sodium bicarbonate, 39

Lactic acidosis, 107, 120, 162
Late neonatal hypocalcemia, 189
Leukemia, 200
Limb of Henle, 19
Liver
  disease, 55
  hydroxylase, 266
Long-dwell dialysis, 281
Low phosphate milk, 213
Low-set ears, 139
Lymphidemia Hyperparathyroidism Nephropathy Syndrome, 142
Lysosomal phospholipidosis, 129
Lysozyme, 130

Magnesium, 241
  depletion, 60
Malformations, 135, 147
Malignancies, 200
Mannitol, 58, 110
Maternal hyperparathyroidism, 247
Mean arterial pressure, 11
Meckel Syndrome, 140
Medication-related hypercalcemia, 202
Mental retardation, 245
Metabolic acidosis, 35
Metabolite balance, 319
Methoxychlorane, 100
Methyldopa, 27
Mezlocillin, 93
Middle molecules, 235
Mineral metabolism, 236

Mineralization, 242
Minoxidil, 314
Mithramycin, 207
Mitochondrial
  abnormalities, 129
  changes, 129
Moon-face, 245
Mortality rate, 288
MT, 237
Mucocutaneous candidiasis, 247
Mullerian Aplasia, 140
Multiple myeloma, 55, 200
Muscle spasm, 199
Myelomeningoceles, 178
Myocardium, 311

Natriuretic factors, 19
NFDR Syndrome, 142
N-G tubes, 285
Neonatal
  hypercalcemia, 138
  hypertension, 23
  hypocalcemia, 183, 189
  tetany, 190, 209
Nephrocalcinosis, 158, 171, 250
Nephrotic Syndrome, 56, 110
Nephrotoxic agents, 97
Nephrotoxicity, 49, 87, 126
  criteria for, 49
  drug-related factors, 52
  patient-related factors, 52
  prevention of, 58
Net acid excretion, 157
Netilmicin, 89
Neurofaciodigitorenal Syndrome, 142
Neurogenic bladder, 149, 177
Neurological dysfunction, 287
Neurotransmitters, 3, 19
Neutra-Phos, 230
Newborn
  kidney, 271
  nephrotoxicity, 51
Nitrogen balance, 281
Nitroprusside, 27
NMR, 166
Nomogram, 244
Noonan Syndrome, 138
Norepinephrine, 4
"Normal", 37
NSAIDS nephrotoxicity, 68
Nuclear magnetic resonance, 166
Nutrition, 259, 262, 286
Nutritional
  intake, 236
  management, 288
  support, 287

Obesity, 245
Obstructive failure, 98
Old age, 53
Oliguric states, 98
1,25-dihydroxy-vitamin D, 184, 224, 241
1,25 vitamin D, 317, 318
Omental wrap, 280
Oncotic pressure
  intracapillary, 113
Ontogeny, 5
Oral phosphate, 208
Organic
  acids, 162
  solvents, 100
Osmotic
  agents, 281
  gradient, 235
  water permeability, 18
Osteoclasts, 242
Osteocytes, 242
Ototoxicity, 129
Overgrowth Syndromes, 138
Oxytocin, 19

PAH, 165
Parathormone, 283
Parathyroid extract, 212
Parathyroid hormone, 184, 241, 265, 283
  excretion, 41
  losses, 238
  resistance, 245
  secretion, 318
Parathyroidectomy, 209, 223
"Parent burnout", 285
Passive diffusion, 235
Patient work-up, 175
Pelvic kidneys, 138
Perforation, 108
Peripheral vasodilators, 113
Peritoneal
  catheter, 115
  dialysis, 107, 115, 235, 279
  efficiency, 282
  losses, 237, 238
  mass transfer, 237
  surface area, 282
Peritonitis, 108, 280
Permeability product, 282
Persistent dialysate leak, 285
pH, 157
Phagocytes, 242
Phentolamine, 4
Phosphate
  concentrations, 184
  intake, 286

Phosphate
  tubular reabsorption, 223
  wasting, 224
Phosphates, 208
Phosphorus removal, 237
Phosphaturia, 265
Phototherapy, 99, 264
Plasma water, 111
Polycitra-K, 161
Polycystic dysplastic kidney, 136
Polypharmacy, 129
Posterior urethral valves, 147, 149
Postsynaptic receptors, 3
Potassium depletion, 60
Potter's Syndrome, 135
Prematurity, 203
Prenatal
  nephrology, 174
  sonography, 153
Prerenal failure, 98
Primary V-U reflux, 149
Procainamide, 57
Propranolol, 27, 312
Prostaglandin, 271
  -angiotensin interactions, 11
  inhibitors, 302
  synthetase inhibitors, 56, 209
Protein, 43
  intake, 284
Proteinuria, 56, 152, 311
Protons, 157
Proximal tubule, 18
Prune Belly Syndrome, 140, 149
Pseudohyperaldosteronism, 305
Pseudohypoparathyroidism, 245
PTE, 212
PTH, 184, 241, 265, 283
  excretion, 41
  losses, 238
  resistance, 245
  secretion, 241, 318
Pulmonary
  edema, 107
  renal hypoplasia, 154

"Quality of life", 259

Rachitic bone diseases, 224
Radial Ray Aplasia, 142
Radiant warmers, 99
Radiocontrast nephrotoxicity, 53
Radiographic studies, 165
Radioisotope
  scintigraphy, 165
  tomography, 165
Reflux, 177
Rehydration, 205
Relative permeabilities, 18
Renal
  anomalies, 177
  aplasia, 136
  artery, 25
  blood flow, 4
  failure, 97, 98, 235
  hemodynamics, 3
  hypoplasia, 138
  injury, 49
  malformations, 135, 143, 150
  osteodystrophy, 236
  pelviectasis, 138
  replacement therapy, 235
  scan, 33, 34, 174
  sodium handling, 17
  transplantation, 202
  threshold, 244
  toxicity
  tumors, 200
Renal artery
  stenosis, 138
  thrombosis, 33, 309, 310
Renal failure
  definition, 122
  indices, 123
Renal function deterioration, 150
Renal hypophosphatemic rickets
  metabolic aspects, 223
Renal insufficiency
  pre-existing, 53
Renal neurotransmitter receptors, 5
Renal Tubular Acidosis, 157, 169
  classification, 171
Renal tubular ecstasia, 138
Residual urine output, 287
Resistance to PTH, 241
Results disagreements, 173
Rheumatoid diseases, 71
Rickets, 223
Risk factors, 49
Robert's Syndrome, 140
Rokitansky Syndrome, 140
RTA, 157, 169
  classification, 171
Rubenstein-Taybi Syndrome, 140

Salicylates, 100, 162
Salt load, 18, 39
Salt-poor albumin, 110
"Salt-wasting", 41
Saphenous vein, 111
Schinzel-Giedion Syndrome, 142

School attendance, 236
Secondary congenital anomalies, 176
Septic shock, 113
Serum phosphorus, 183
Shock, 113
Shohl's solution, 161, 175
Short stature, 224
Shorter dialysis dwell, 287
Single
  cuff catheters, 283
  hypoplastic kidney, 138
  umbilical artery, 139
Slow bleed, 38
Sodium, 38
  fractional increase of, 124
  load, 41, 273
  modelling, 125
  reabsorption, 18, 38, 307
  renal handling of, 40
Sodium bicarbonate, 161
Sodium chloride vs sodium
  bicarbonate, 39
Sodium handling
  developmental, 17
Sodium nitroprusside, 27
Sodium sulfate, 209
Soft catheter, 109
Solute
  shifts, 235
  transport, 235
Sonographic assessment, 153
Sorbent hemoperfusion, 97, 101
SPECT, 165
Sporadic hypoparathyroidism, 247
Stroke volume, 11
Subcutaneous space, 109
Subperiosteal mineralization, 226,
Substance P, 19
Surgical
  intervention, 178
  reconstruction, 151
Sympathetic nervous system, 6
Symptomatic patent ductus, 36
Syndrome identification, 144
Systemic hypertension, 26

Tachycardia, 310
Tc-99m, 165
Tenckhoff catheter, 109, 115, 116
  237, 279
TES, 166
Tetany, 190, 199
Thiazides, 216
Third ureter, 138
Thirst mechanism, 287
Thyroid cancer, 200
Thrombectomy, 42
Thrombosis, 41
Thrombus, 25
Thyroxine, 3
Titratable acid, 158
TmP/GFR, 244
Tomograms, 166
Tomographic imaging, 166
Total
  parenteral nutrition, 162
  peripheral resistance, 11
Toxicity, 49
Trace elements, 286
Transcellular volume, 235
Transmembrane pressure, 111
Transmission, 37
Transplantation, 151, 202
Trisomy, 18, 139
Trocar technique, 108, 280
Trocath, 109
Trousseau, 199
TRP, 244
Tubular
  memory, 131
  reabsorption, 223
  sensitivity, 306
Turner's Syndrome, 139
Type IV RTA, 170
25-hydroxyvitamin D, 184, 224, 245

Ultrafiltration, 107, 117, 120, 121,
  281
Ultrasonography, 165
Ultrasound, 33
Umbilical
  artery catheter, 25
  vessels, 111
Undetermined anion gap, 162
Unilateral
  reflux, 177
  vs bilateral, 154
UP junction obstruction, 14
Upper limb/renal malformations
  syndrome, 142
Uretero-pelvic junction, 149
Uretero-vesico junction, 149
Urethral valves, 147
Urinary
  diversion, 150
  Kallikreins, 20
  osmolality, 273
  tract, 147
Urine flow, 99, 123
UV junction obstruction, 149

V.A.C.T.E.R.L. Syndrome, 140
Valves, 147
Vascular
  access, 235
  disease, 55
  resistance, 113
  volume expansion, 122
Vasoconstrictor effect, 4
Vasodilators, 113
Vasodilator prostaglandins, 275
Vasodilatory effects, 4
Vasopressin, 272
Vesico-ureteral reflux, 149
Vessel size, 235
Vitamin D, 189, 203
  deficiency, 191
  metabolites, 237
  preparations, 214
  requirements, 265
Vitamin D-dependent rickets, 203, 318
Vitamin D-resistant rickets, 316
Vitamins, 286
Volume
  expansion, 40
  osmolality, 39

Water load, 39
Williams Syndrome, 138
Wilm's tumor, 138

X-linked dominant, 229

Zellweger Syndrome, 140

GPSR Compliance

The European Union's (EU) General Product Safety Regulation (GPSR) is a set of rules that requires consumer products to be safe and our obligations to ensure this.

If you have any concerns about our products, you can contact us on ProductSafety@springernature.com

In case Publisher is established outside the EU, the EU authorized representative is:

Springer Nature Customer Service Center GmbH
Europaplatz 3
69115 Heidelberg, Germany

Batch number: 10682323

Printed by Printforce, the Netherlands